The Edgar Cayce Handbook for Health Through Drugless Therapy

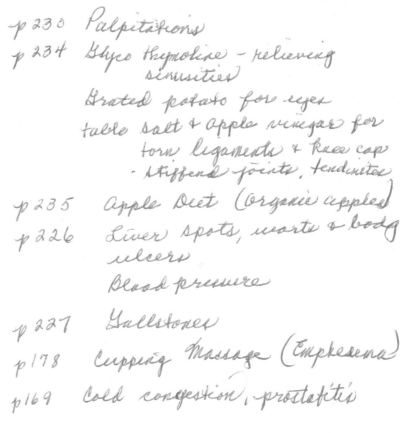

p102 - Asthma, Emph, Cupping massage to break chest & back congestion

p224 Colonic (distention, fullness) shortness of breath etc

p284 Superfluous Hair

p286 Hair loss - balding
p289 Eye Strain
p296 Normalcy of the salivary glands

p297 Varicose veins

p298 Moles, Warts, Cysts

p311 Gervital 3 (Anti Depressent) Aging & liscensed

p230 Palpitations

p234 Glyco thymoline - relieving sinusities
Grated potato for eyes
table salt & apple vinegar for torn ligaments & knee cap - stiffened joints, tendinites

p235 Apple Diet (Organic apples)

p226 Liver spots, warts & body ulcers
Blood pressure

p227 Gallstones

p178 Cupping Massage (Emphesema)

p169 Cold congestion, prostatitis

The Edgar Cayce Handbook for Health Through Drugless Therapy

Harold J. Reilly, D.Ph.T., D.S.,
and Ruth Hagy Brod

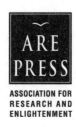

ARE
PRESS

ASSOCIATION FOR
RESEARCH AND
ENLIGHTENMENT

A.R.E. Press • Virginia Beach • Virginia

Note to Readers: It is essential that you consult a physician before trying any of the remedies and exercises contained in this book, and in no case should you try any of them without the full concurrence of your physician. It is also important that you do not discontinue the treatment and diet prescribed by your doctor.

Copyright © 1975 by Harold J. Reilly

Revised Edition
ISBN 0–87604–482–8

1st Printing, February 2004

A.R.E. Press
215 67th Street
Virginia Beach, VA 23451–2061

Library of Congress Cataloging in Publication Data

Reilly, Harold J.
    The Edgar Cayce handbook for health through drugless therapy.
Bibliography: p.
    Includes index.
    ISBN 0–02–601960–4
    1. Hygiene. 2. Cayce, Edgar, 1877–1945. I. Brod, Ruth Hagy, joint
author. II. Title. [DNLM: Parapsychology. 2. Therapeutic cults. WB960 R362]
RA776.5.R43   613   74–30015

Illustrations by Ray Cullis

Cover design by Richard Boyle

Printed in the United States of America

To Betty

Who I feel was sent to me by Edgar Cayce to help me carry on the work which has made this book possible.

H. J. R.

To Albert

Beloved husband, friend, and partner who makes all things possible.

R. H. B.

"This, then—that the *spirit*, the soul, the *elements* of the *active* forces, use those por-tions *of* the physical body as their temple during an earth's experience." (311-4)

"For, all healing comes from the One Source. And whether there is the application of foods, exercise, medicine, or even the knife—it is to bring [to] the consciousness of the forces within the body that aid in reproducing themselves—[which is] the awareness of Creative or God Forces." (2696-1)

" . . . at least one week out of each month should be spent in beautifying, preserv-ing, rectifying the body—if the body would keep young, in mind, in body, in pur-pose. This doesn't mean that the entity should spend a whole week at nothing else." (3420-1)

Editorial Notes for This Edition

Care has been taken in the preparation of this edition to preserve the content and intent of the authors, while reformatting the layout to make the book easier to use.

Wherever possible, ancillary concepts, quotations, and anecdotes have been shifted into boxes or margin spaces for handy reference. Footnotes have been gathered as endnotes at the end of the book, while titles of books, which the authors either referred to or quoted from, have been consolidated in a bibliography at the back. Updated lists of reference books on Cayce's life, diet, health, and remedies have been inserted in appropriate chapters. Some of the statistical charts have been updated along with the Sources of Supply.

NOTE: Quotations from the Edgar Cayce readings are identified by two numbers, e.g., 262–15. The first set of numbers refers to the individual or group who received the reading, while the second refers to the sequential number of the series of that particular reading. In the example cited, "262–15," this was the fifteenth reading given to Study Group #1 assigned the number "262."

—The Editors

Contents

Acknowledgments

Completing this book has been a three-year project that would have been impossible without the dedicated help of many people who believe in and were inspired by the spiritual, mental, emotional, and physical wisdom in the Cayce readings.

The authors wish to use this opportunity to thank those who shared their personal experiences with us and the many friends and colleagues who have assisted us in our work.

We wish to acknowledge and thank the following for their very special help:

Hugh Lynn Cayce for his perceptive Foreword and reminiscences;

Gladys Davis Turner, Lucille Kahn, Hugh Lynn, Dr. Pat Reilly, and Dorothy Reilly for helping us reconstruct the history of Edgar Cayce and our family;

J. Everett Irion, Violet Shelley, and the editorial, library, and administrative staffs of the A.R.E. in Virginia Beach, Virginia;

Volunteers Rhoda Boyko, who assisted Mrs. Brod for two years in researching and typing the excerpts from the Cayce Medical Circulating Files; Rudolph Boyko, who helped his wife; Albert T. Brod, who did endless copying, checking, correcting, and reading; Andrew Grossman, who assisted with many chores;

Artist Jacqueline Mott, who added last-minute illustrations to those commissioned and executed by Ray Cullis;

And Doctors William A. McGarey, John Joseph Lalli, and Edith Wallace for reviewing the manuscript and for their helpful criticism and suggestions.

A special tribute to the significant leadership and courage in fighting for the consumer's right to health and pollution-free air, water, and food of the following congressional committee and subcommittee chairmen and appreciation for the transcripts of their hearings:

Senators Richard S. Schweiker (R.-Pa.), Gaylord Nelson (D.-Wis.), William Proxmire (D.-Wis.), Philip A. Hart (D.-Mich.), and Congressman James J. Delaney (D.-N.Y.).

To Dr. Roger J. Williams, director of the Clayton Foundation Biochemical Institute of The University of Texas, our profound appreciation and respect for his great book, *Nutrition Against Disease* (New York, Pitman Publishing Co., 1971), from which we have quoted extensively.

We also wish to extend our thanks to the following:

E. M. Abrahamson and A. W. Pezet, *Body, Mind and Sugar*, New York, Pyramid Books, 1951;

Ted Burke, "Recipes for Rejuvenation," *Harper's Bazaar*, March 1973;

Cathryn Elwood, *Feel Like a Million*, New York, Pocket Books, 1965;

Frank Glenn and Arthur J. Okenaka, "Study of a 167-Year-Old-Man," *Journal of the American Geriatrics Society*, July 1964;

Mrs. Edward Henderson, director of the American Geriatrics Society and editor of the *Journal*;

Josef P. Hrachovec, *Keeping Young and Living Longer*, Los Angeles, Calif., Sherbourne Press, 1972;

William A. McGarey, *Edgar Cayce and the Palma Christi*, Edgar Cayce Foundation and Medical Research Bulletins of the Edgar Cayce Foundation;

The Metropolitan Life Insurance Co., for its weight and longevity charts;

Proceedings of the Conference on Aging, sponsored by the Huxley Institute, New York, March 6, 1972;

Corinne H. Robinson, *Normal and Therapeutic Nutrition*, New York, Macmillan Publishing Co., Inc., 1972;

Neil Solomon, *The Truth About Weight Control*, New York, Stein & Day, 1972;

Jess Stearn, *Edgar Cayce—The Sleeping Prophet*, Garden City, N.Y., Doubleday & Co.; New York, Bantam Books, 1968;

C. M. Taylor and O. F. Pye, *Foundations of Nutrition*, New York, Macmillan Publishing Co., Inc., 1966;
Renee Taylor, *Hunza Health Secrets*, New York, Award Books, 1969;
Carlson Wade, *Magic Minerals: A Key to Better Health*, New York, Parker Publishing Co., 1967;
Maurice Zolotow, *Marilyn Monroe: A Biography*, New York, Harcourt, Brace & Co., 1960.

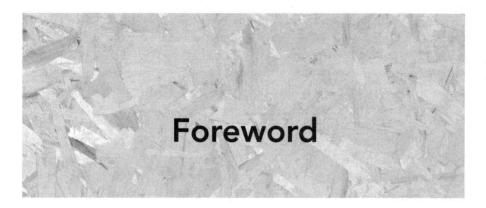

Foreword

This, then—that the spirit, the soul, the elements of the active forces, use those portions of the physical body as their temple during an earth's experience.

(311-4)

Harold Reilly, one of America's outstanding physiotherapists, has helped more people make practical use of data in the Edgar Cayce physical readings than any man I know. One reason for this is the man himself, for Dr. Reilly is one of the most positive, energetic, and practical persons I have ever known. He inspires confidence; he obviously practices what he preaches. He is friendly, enthusiastic, and possesses a wonderful sense of humor. A conversation with Dr. Reilly persuades you, a treatment from him convinces you, that your body can do more than you ever expect from it. He inspires self-respect.

Another reason Dr. Reilly has been so successful in helping others use the Edgar Cayce readings is because his philosophy of health was already in alignment with the philosophy of health expressed in the readings when his name was first mentioned in these readings. Surprisingly, his name was mentioned several years before the two men met in person. This bond at the level of the mind, and yet at the level of the spirit, too, led hundreds of people to seek out Harold Reilly at both his institute in Rockefeller Center and his farm in New Jersey. They met him also in his books, *The Secret of Better Health* and *Easy Does It*, and later in the books of many others who wrote about him and his work with the Edgar Cayce readings—two of which were Thomas Sugrue's *There Is a River* and Jess Stearn's *Edgar Cayce—The Sleeping Prophet.*

Both Edgar Cayce and Harold Reilly were more concerned with keeping people well and finding causes of illness than in curing symptoms. In the readings the many suggestions dealing with exercise, diet, packs, and hydrotherapy are frequently treatments for which the individual him- or herself, rather than another person, must take the responsibility. Even the treatments that needed to be administered by another person—such as manipulation, colonics, packs, etc.—were therapies designed to help the body help itself. Here in *The Edgar Cayce Handbook for Health Through Drugless Therapy*, you will find encouragement and, more important, specific ways in which to help yourself regain physical, mental, and emotional stability and a new attitude toward living.

For, all healing comes from the One Source. And whether there is the application of foods, exercise, medicine, or even the knife—it is to bring [to] the consciousness of the forces within the body that aid in reproducing themselves—[which is] the awareness of Creative or God Forces. (2696-1)

Edgar Cayce talked about the importance of the apple diet, castor oil packs, fume baths with special oils for special ailments, specific types of massage, and a variety of valuable diets. But it was Harold Reilly who first began to help people put the treatments together. It was he who encouraged and, indeed, inspired them to follow through until they began to discover that they could get fantastic results at times.

This is a "how to" book. Here are details on treatments with supportive material from the world of science, which by now has confirmed many of the basic concepts in the Edgar Cayce readings. Harold J. Reilly began working with these concepts more than forty-five years ago.

Probably you will not read this book by starting at the beginning and going right through it. Perhaps you will look first for your own particular need. If so, you will discover that Dr. Reilly and Mrs. Brod have organized the material under precise chapter headings, and their cross-references will be invaluable guides both to your problems and to the Cayce-Reilly treatments.

When you have started your own body working on your specific need, you'll want to go back and read the whole book. You'll find a variety of material which can help you and which you'll want to share with your friends. You'll discover that the three people who put this book together obviously enjoyed it—Dr. Harold Reilly, Betty Billings, who assists him in his work, and Ruth Hagy Brod, who researched the material and helped Dr. Reilly write this book. It becomes very clear that these people believed very sincerely in the material they wrote about and that their personal experiences and experiences with hundreds of others confirm their conclusions.

The famous phrase with which Edgar Cayce from a trance state opened thousands of psychic readings, "Yes, we have the body," begins to make real sense in this book. We must begin where we are. If we cannot heal ourselves, how can we be channels of healing for our fellow human beings? Here, completely blended, are the ingredients for the physical, mental, emotional, and spiritual balance that everyone seeks.

—Hugh Lynn Cayce

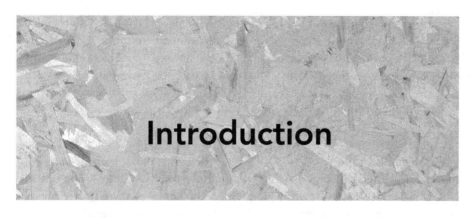
Introduction

I. About Edgar Cayce

Although hundreds of books have been written about Edgar Cayce, for some of you this may be the first introduction to the man who has been called the "sleeping prophet of Virginia Beach," "America's most mysterious man," "religious seer," and medical telepathist or clairvoyant.

Many of his contemporaries knew the "waking" Edgar Cayce as a gifted professional photographer. Others (predominantly children) admired him as a warm and friendly Sunday school teacher. His family knew him as a wonderful husband and father. However, the "sleeping" Edgar Cayce was an entirely different figure—a psychic known to thousands of people from all walks of life who had cause to be grateful for his help. Indeed, many of them believed that he alone had either saved or changed their lives when all seemed lost. The "sleeping" Edgar Cayce was a medical diagnostician, a prophet, and a devoted proponent of the Bible.

Even as a child on a farm near Hopkinsville, Kentucky, where he was born on March 18, 1877, Edgar Cayce displayed powers of perception which seemed to extend beyond the normal range of the five senses. At the age of six or seven he told his parents that he was able to see and talk to "visions," sometimes of relatives who had recently died. His parents attributed this to the overactive imagination of a lonely child who had been influenced by the dramatic language of the revival meetings that were popular in that section of the country. Later, by sleeping with his head on his schoolbooks, he developed some form of photographic memory that helped him advance rapidly in the country school. This gift faded, however, and Edgar was only able to complete the seventh grade before he had to go to work.

By the age of twenty-one he had become the salesman for a wholesale stationery company. At this time he developed a gradual paralysis of the throat muscles, which threatened to cause the loss of his voice. When doctors were unable to find a physical cause for this condition, hypnosis was tried but failed to have any permanent effect. As a last resort Edgar asked a friend to help him reenter the same kind of hypnotic sleep that had enabled him to memorize his schoolbooks as a child. His friend gave him the necessary suggestion and, once he was in a self-induced trance, Edgar came to grips with his own problem. Speaking from an unconscious state, he recommended medication and manipulative therapy, which successfully restored his voice and repaired his system.

A group of physicians from Hopkinsville and Bowling Green, Kentucky, took advantage of his unique talent to diagnose their own patients. They soon discovered that Cayce needed to be given only the name and address of a patient, wherever he was, to be able to tune in telepathically to that individual's mind and body as easily as if they were both in the same room. He needed no other information regarding any patient.

One of the young M.D.s, Dr. Wesley Ketchum, submitted a report on this unorthodox procedure to a clinical research society in Boston. On October 9, 1910, The *New York Times* carried two pages of headlines and pictures. From that day on troubled people from all over the country sought help from the "wonder man."

When Edgar Cayce died on January 3, 1945, in Virginia Beach, Virginia, he left documented stenographic records of the telepathic clairvoyant statements he had given for more than 6,000 different people over a period of forty-three years. The Association for Research and Enlightenment, Inc. (the A.R.E.), a psychical research society, was formed by Cayce in 1931 to preserve and research this data. Its library in Virginia Beach contains copies of 14,145 of Edgar Cayce's psychic readings, stenographically recorded. Of this number 9,541, or about 67 percent, describe the physical disabilities of several thousand persons and suggest treatment for their ailments.

For a great many physicians, medical studies of treatment patterns for a number of major physical diseases seemed to suggest the advisability of testing Edgar Cayce's theories. With this in mind, the physical readings have been made available to a clinic in Phoenix, Arizona. Through written reports and conferences, information on results of treatments have been made available to M.D.s and osteopaths.

The Edgar Cayce readings constitute one of the largest and most impressive records of psychic perception ever to emanate from a single individual. Together with their relevant records, correspondence, and reports, they have been cross-indexed under thousands of subject headings and placed at the disposal of psychologists, physicians, students, writers, and investigators who still come, in increasing numbers, to examine them.

The A.R.E. continues to make the information available in its library, through distribution of *The Complete Edgar Cayce Readings on CD-ROM,* on its Web site (www.edgarcayce.org), and through its many publications. The organization also initiates investigation and experiments into the readings and promotes conferences, seminars, and lectures.

Dr. Harold J. Reilly's forty-five years of clinical experience with the readings constitute an invaluable addition to the record.

II. About Harold J. Reilly

Dr. Harold J. Reilly was one of the leading exponents of drugless, natural physical therapy. He was recognized as one of the most outstanding physiotherapists in the world, and doctors came from all over the globe to study with him.

Dr. Reilly was born on the Lower East Side of New York City in 1895 and grew up in the Van Ness section of the Bronx, the eldest of seven brothers and sisters—all of whom became physiotherapists with the exception of one sister. At twelve he organized an exercise and athletic club in the family home basement. In 1916, after graduating from the National Eclectic Institute, he immediately entered the United States Army and served on the Mexican border with the 102nd Engineers, teaching jujitsu and wrestling. It was when he left the army that he took his degrees from Ithaca College and Eastern Reserve University. He also was graduated from the American School of Naturopathy and the American School of Chiropractise, and completed two years of study in osteopathy.

For several years Dr. Reilly studied at Battle Creek, Michigan, with Dr. John Harvey Kellogg, inventor of breakfast cereals and the electric cabinet, and pioneer in preventive medicine. Also during his varied career Dr. Reilly ran a health farm for the rehabilitation of alcoholic and drug addicts in Sullivan County, New York. In 1924 he established in New York City the Physicians Physiotherapy Service at 1908 Broadway, and in 1935 opened the famous Reilly Health Institute in Rockefeller Center.

Dr. Reilly's impressive educational and professional background encompassed eight degrees, including doctor of science from Eastern Reserve University, master in physiotherapy from Ithaca College, and doctor of physiotherapy from Van Norman University of California. In addition, he was a fellow of the College of Sports Medicine, fellow of the Emerson University Research Council, diplomate of the National Board of Physical Therapy, and director of physiotherapy and rehabilitation of the Edgar Cayce Foundation.

He served fourteen terms as president of the New York State Society of Physiotherapists, was chairman of the Council of Licensed Physiotherapists of New York State, and legislative chairman of the Physiotherapy Grievance Committee appointed by the Board of Regents of the University of the State of New York. He was licensed in four states and Canada.

For more than thirty years, the Reilly Health Institute in Rockefeller Center was a health mecca for prominent people: government leaders such as the late Secretary of State Edward Stettinius, former Attorney General Herbert Brownell, Congressman James Delaney, and ex–Governor Nelson A. Rockefeller; business tycoons such as the late David Sarnoff, Capt. Eddie Rickenbacker, L. Victor Weil, and Jack Kriendler, owner of the 21 Club; and labor leaders such as George Meany, David Dubinsky, Alex Rose, and John L. Lewis. These represent just a few of the many notables who repaired the ravages of responsibility and stress under the direction and healing hands of Dr. Harold J. Reilly, the institute's founder and director.

Dr. Harold J. Reilly was one of the leading exponents of drugless, natural physical therapy. He was recognized as one of the most outstanding physiotherapists in the world, and doctors came from all over the globe to study with him.
—**Introduction**

For several years Dr. Reilly studied at Battle Creek, Michigan, with Dr. John Harvey Kellogg, inventor of breakfast cereals and the electric cabinet, and pioneer in preventive medicine.
—**Introduction**

After the fine conditioning of Harold J. for eighteen years, I feel that everyone should live the life of Reilly. —**Bob Hope**

The inscription on Bob Hope's photograph, which hung among many others in Reilly's office, read, "After the fine conditioning of Harold J. for eighteen years, I feel that everyone should live the life of Reilly."

"Oh, there's nothing so bad, but Reilly can fix it," said Burgess Meredith on his photograph.

From Eddie Albert: "Dr. Reilly had a lot to do with my enjoying life as far back as 1935. He still has."

Many writers and poets—Robert Frost, John Erskine, Bob and Millie Considine, Morey Bernstein, and Fannie Hurst—eloquently expressed their admiration and appreciation in photo inscriptions or in their books. For example, Maurice Zolotow, author of *Marilyn Monroe: A Biography*, wrote: "To Harold J. Reilly, who would have made me as voluptuous as Marilyn Monroe if I had been a woman."

Jess Stearn, in the first edition of his book *Edgar Cayce—The Sleeping Prophet*, wrote: "For my Dear Friend and Mentor, Harold J. Reilly, without whom this book would have been far less." Stearn's book was inspired by Dr. Reilly and largely written at Reilly's farm.

Thomas Sugrue autographed his *There Is a River* with these words: "To Harold J. Reilly, the best doctor on the face of the earth—even some of the arthritic angels must yearn for his ministrations. But above all, I am proud that he was Edgar Cayce's friend and that he is mine."

"Builder of happiness and more effective people" is how the Reverend Norman Vincent Peale described Dr. Reilly, while Hugh Lynn Cayce, in his book *Venture Inward*, wrote as follows: "To Harold—who has helped many people start this Venture Inward as Edgar Cayce conceived it."

Nor were all his clients celebrities. Many were simply suffering human beings referred to him by one or more of the 3,000 practicing physicians, osteopaths, and dentists who sent their patients to him.

Despite his own impressive credentials and record, Dr. Reilly is best known for his unusual and close association with Edgar Cayce, the "sleeping prophet" of Virginia Beach, who began sending cases to Dr. Reilly in 1930—almost two years before the two men met. At the time, Reilly had never heard of Edgar Cayce and did not suspect that the referrals were coming from a psychic.

By the time Cayce died in 1945, he had referred more than a thousand patients to Dr. Reilly and had mentioned him hundreds of times by name in the trance readings in which he diagnosed and prescribed treatment for a wide variety of medical complaints.

In *Edgar Cayce—The Sleeping Prophet*, Jess Stearn describes Dr. Reilly as a "portable repository of practical Cayce therapy." Certainly he was the unquestioned living authority on the health secrets in the Cayce "readings." Most of the dozens of books on Cayce, totaling millions of dollars in sales, celebrate Dr. Reilly's rare skills and understanding of the Cayce treatments and his success in applying them. Dr. Reilly was not only a "master" of the Cayce theories, *but had clinically tested and sifted them in over forty-five years of active practice*. The ultimate fusion of Cayce's psychic powers tapping some source of "universal knowledge" and Reilly's empirical and scientific experience produced an invaluable treasury of health guides that seemed to work when properly administered. They now can be made available to thousands of readers seeking some sensible way out of the polluted maze of modern living.

Despite the overtones of mystery that are present when a clairvoyant of Cayce's reputation is involved, there is no great mystery in the affinity between the two men—one a psychic and one a physical scientist. They shared an identical philosophy of health: in Dr. Reilly's words, "Medicine and most doctors aim at curing a specific ailment. The Cayce 'readings' and the Reilly therapy aim at producing a healthy body which will heal itself of the ailment. We try to understand Nature and work with Nature. Then the body cures itself."

When Dr. Reilly closed the Reilly Health Institute in 1965 and "retired" to his farm in New Jersey, he donated his physiotherapy equipment to the A.R.E. and established a physiotherapy clinic there, trained its therapists, and agreed to serve as its supervisor, a post he held until his death in 1987. He also set up the Physiotherapy Department of the A.R.E. Clinic in Phoenix, Arizona, and trained its personnel. However, it was not easy for Dr. Reilly to stay in retirement. When some of the patients he had been caring for—for example, David Dubinsky, who had been a "Reilly regular" for over forty years—insisted on their weekly treatment, Dr. Reilly agreed to come to New York one day a week and made arrangements to share an office with another doctor in the Capitol Theatre Building. But the time spent in the New York office expanded into two and then three days a week, and soon Dr. Reilly was working almost as hard as he had been when he was running the institute.

When the Capitol Theatre Building was demolished, Dr. Reilly embarked on what he hoped was his second retirement. It didn't last any longer than the first because, with the publication of *Edgar Cayce—The Sleeping Prophet* and other books, a steady stream of men and women from all over the country began making pilgrimages to his New Jersey farm.

Helping him at the farm was his hard-working associate, Miss Betty Billings. She was a graduate of the University of North Carolina, where she received her B.S. in nutrition. She served her residency at Dayton Miami Valley Hospital in Ohio and worked as a clinic dietician at Duke University Hospital and New York Hospital–Cornell Medical Center. She also held a degree in physiotherapy.

Miss Billings first became acquainted with Dr. Reilly in the late 1950s, when she came to him seeking help for her paralyzed mother, after all the orthodox medical avenues of help had been exhausted. She was so impressed by his treatment of her mother that she left the New York Hospital–Cornell Medical Center, where she had been working as a nutritionist–dietician, and joined the Reilly staff at Rockefeller Center. She worked with Dr. Reilly—later marrying him—until his death at 92, and both she and the doctor were in great demand as speakers and health consultants.

Dr. Reilly said of her: "I always had a feeling that Betty Billings was sent to me by Edgar Cayce . . . Nutrition is so important in the Cayce therapy, but I was pretty weak in the technicalities of counting grams of everything, figuring recommended daily allowances, and keeping up with all the new research in this complicated field. I guess Cayce wanted us to work together."

To Harold J. Reilly, who would have made me as voluptuous as Marilyn Monroe if I had been a woman. —**Maurice Zolotow**

In Edgar Cayce—The Sleeping Prophet, *Jess Stearn describes Dr. Reilly as a "portable repository of practical Cayce therapy."*

The basic philosophy of all my work is that I consider myself a teacher and interpreter of the Cayce readings; for the Cayce readings were given for individuals, and I have had to draw on my own background and knowledge and experience to interpret what he wanted, and then teach people what to do. **—H.J.R.**

He is a great professional and a wonderful human being.
—Nelson A. Rockefeller

Dr. Reilly, like Edgar Cayce, specialized in "medical rejects"—those who had abandoned all hope of obtaining help from conventional drug–oriented therapies. His success in treating "hopeless" patients further spread his fame, until the patient pressure at the farm grew far beyond his capacities and those of Miss Billings to handle. As a consequence, he announced that he would have to limit his practice to members of the A.R.E.

"I wanted to discourage patients—especially those who might not take the therapy seriously," he explained. "And besides, if they do not understand the Cayce philosophy of the unity of body, mind, and spirit, and their consciousness is not attuned to the necessary level, it takes too long to get results; sometimes it never happens."

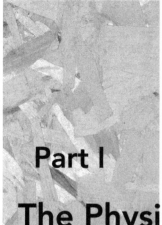

Part I

The Physical Body Is the Temple

1

Prevention:
The Key to Lifelong Health

A forty-two-year-old man asked Edgar Cayce, "How long should I live in this incarnation?" (866–1)

"To a hundred and fifty!" the sleeping prophet of Virginia Beach replied.

To other questioners, Cayce replied that if a person lived properly, ate wisely, didn't worry too much, and kept an optimistic outlook on life, he could live to be 120 or 121 years of age.

To someone who asked, "Then also it is true [that] one may preserve youth?" Cayce answered, "One may preserve youth even as [it] is desired, will they pay the price as is necessary."

"That is, one must consider the diet, as well as application of knowledge obtained from within?" the man continued, pressing for more details.

"To be sure," Cayce replied. (900–465)

Cayce's view of our potential longevity and youth is consistent with the natural laws of the universe as we find them in the animal kingdom. According to biologists, the life span of a species is from eight to ten times the age at which it is first capable of reproduction. Theoretically, then, humans should live to at least 120 to 150 years of age.

Scientists working on geriatrics and longevity in countries all over the world are saying that the average life span of a human being should be about 140 years. Cellular researchers believe that, since it is possible to keep certain cells alive indefinitely in an optimum nutritional environment, theoretically it could be possible for humans to live forever.

Dr. Augustus B. Kinzel, former president of the Salk Institute for Biological Sciences, predicts that "man's dream of never aging will become a fact and notable progress will be evident as early as 1980."

Even a past president of the conservative American Medical Association, the late Dr. Edward L. Bortz, of Philadelphia's Lankenau Hospital, speculated that there is no reason why, by the year 2000, we should not all be living to at least 100 years of age.

In fact, there are places in the world where men and women are presently alive, healthy, and capable of reproducing well past the century mark—notably Abkhazia, in the region of the Caucasus Mountains, in the Soviet Union; Vilcabamba, in Ecuador; and the land of the Hunzas, an independent state of Pakistan.

Later, in Chapter 15, we shall discuss the lifestyles of these remarkable people in some detail, as well as many facets of research into this fascinating subject and some of the Cayce-Reilly guides for your own personal use at home. For the moment, it suffices to point out that their lifestyle is consistent with the Cayce recipe for longevity and prolonged youthfulness.

Paradoxically, while science is working hard to present us with the gift of added years, people are suffering increasingly from chronic and degenerative diseases. Dr. Max Bircher-Benner, one of the great medical pioneers and champions of preventive medicine, said many years ago, "The realm of the incurables has expanded alarmingly. So also has the ability of the medical profession to prolong life artificially. But it was not the Creator's intention that Man should live by the aid of crutches or turn the planet into one vast hospital for the sick."[1]

I corresponded with Dr. Bircher-Benner until his death in 1939 and we shared a common philosophy of health—particularly the importance of prevention in medicine. After all, few of us would choose to stay alive a few more years as invalids, a burden to ourselves and to our families. It is not enough to add more years to life. It is how much life you have left in those years that counts.

In this regard, modern medical science, despite its many impressive achievements in curtailing infections and treating disease, is not doing as well in preventing illness and keeping us well. It is health that we all want—not just better health care. Since we have renewed our friendship with the Chinese, we might emulate one of their old customs and pay doctors when we are well, instead of when we are sick.

Today, modern man and woman (and their children) are an endangered species. The health of the American people is undergoing a gradual deterioration. The need is for more and larger hospitals, more medical schools turning out more doctors, new drugs, and vast sums for research. In 1971, then–President Richard M. Nixon asked federal officials to draft a program that would make Americans the healthiest people in the world. The report revealed that although Americans spend more money for health care than any other nation, their aggregate health is worse than that of most other industrialized countries. We have more cancer, heart disease, diabetes, mental illness, arthritis, and birth defects than any other industrialized nation in the world. We rank fiftieth in total life expectancy. Americans are less healthy than they were twenty years ago and our life expectancy is going down. The president charged his then–Secretary of Health, Education and Welfare, Elliot L. Richardson (and former attorney general), with "finding out what is necessary to make this country healthier than any other country in the world."

He had just to look around the country at the everyday life of its citizens.

We are surrounded on all sides by stealthy enemies, all the more malignantly deceitful and dangerous because they tiptoe about in such attractive disguises and are so quiet. The eight deadliest of these in our modern lifestyle are hidden in the air we breathe; the water we drink; the methods of food production, shipping, processing, and marketing; the family kitchen, where the great American diet is planned and executed (no pun intended); the dependence on the family automobile, which has immobilized us into heart disease and other killing ailments when it doesn't kill or maim us outright on the road, and its companion in crime, the TV set; the friendly neighborhood corner drugstore, which has turned us into a nation of pill-poppers and assisted our children into drug addiction; and the "job," with its killing stresses of insecurity, competition, ruinous "coffee breaks," and business lunches.

We do not have to succumb to these enemies. If we are willing to exert the effort and discipline to use them, protective measures are available to us. "An ounce of prevention is worth a pound of cure" in health as in all other aspects of life.

But now a medical man, Dr. Bircher-Benner, tells us, "My brothers, your life is on wrong lines. Try to recognize the dangers threatening your health and learn how to avoid them, before it is too late. Prevention is possible, provided you take it seriously; it will be effective if you are strong and determined."[2]

After fifty-five years of treating the sick and recycling and building health, fitness, and vitality in thousands of individuals, I have learned that people take better care of their cars and their lawn mowers than they do of their bodies and their health. Over and over I have heard the lame excuse, "But I haven't the time to exercise, to watch my diet, to do all the things you say I should do."

I invariably reply, "You don't have time to keep well, but you will find the time to be sick, won't you?"

Less wax on the car and more peanut oil on the body should be the rule in households for a stronger, healthier population.

Although I am a physiotherapist, my specialization for over fifty-five years has been in treating and recycling the complete person: the one who reflects in his or her body and mind the impact of the external world upon him/her. I have said many times that the same blood that flows through the intestines flows through the brain; but I can reverse that and say that the blood that flows through the brain, where we worry and are anxious and afraid, flows through the intestines, where we suffer from tension.

Many men came to the Reilly Health Service in Rockefeller Center with the same complaint. "When I was in the military service, I was in wonderful shape. I felt fine all the time. Now I am out of shape and feel logy and toxic all the time. Can you put me back into the same fine shape I was in?"

I might have answered simply, "Yes, just take workouts in the gym, take an occasional steam bath along with a tonic spray and perhaps a massage, and you will be in the same good shape that regular living and regular exercise gave you when you were in the service."

But we must remember the man in service did not have to worry about a

In 1971, then-President Richard M. Nixon asked federal officials to draft a program that would make Americans the healthiest people in the world. The report revealed that although Americans spend more money for health care than any other nation, their aggregate health is worse than that of most other industrialized countries.—**H.J.R.**

Eight Enemies to Good Health

Our modern society and lifestyles hide enemies to health in the:

- air we breathe
- water we drink
- methods of modern food production
- family kitchen
- automobile
- television set
- corner drugstore
- stresses of our jobs

Less wax on the car and more peanut oil on the body should be the rule in households for a stronger, healthier population.—**H.J.R.**

raise in salary, the mood in which he might find his wife on returning home from work, the possibility of being fired, or the payment coming due on the mortgage. He did not have to make decisions; they were made for him. Therefore, he was able to relax, and the relaxation, along with the release from responsibility and tension, was partly responsible for the good physical condition in which he found himself.

The problem of putting these men into the same condition of "feeling good" is not simply one of improved nutrition and exercise. Also required is a psychological adjustment in the whole area of living—an adjustment that all people are forced to make if they are to participate in society as responsible citizens and if they are to maintain themselves and not be dependent upon other people or the state.

Everyone today, man or woman, lives as a soldier on an economic front of competition where one must constantly be on the alert to maintain security, keep the home and family, and put away something for the future.

The curious thing is that if it were not for your body, you wouldn't have to make that adjustment. If it were not for your body, you wouldn't have to conduct that lifelong fight!

If you had only a mind, and not a body, the world of economics would disappear. You wouldn't need a house, or food to put in your body, or clothes to cover it, or cosmetics to disguise it, or an automobile in which to move it around. Marriage would not be necessary, because sex would not exist in the physical sense and would not result in children. It is the body that causes economics, marriage, politics, and war.

But a fact that has amazed me all my life is that the body, which causes these elements of struggle and pressure and work, is not only neglected but also misused and abused. It would seem that the ancient Greeks, who respected and even worshiped the body, were closer to a reasonable attitude toward daily living than we are. They at least recognized that the body is the focal point of life in the world.

It is the body that causes us to be here in this three-dimensional world. It is therefore the body that must be kept in harmony and in balance—healthy, in other words—so that through the body, the parts of us that are nonphysical, but that give us our greatest pleasures and make us human beings—that is, the mind and the spirit—can function well enough to reach their greatest potential.

In modern living, we concentrate on putting the body out of balance rather than in balance. We overburden it to the point of exhaustion in our efforts to make money and achieve success. Every misused, overworked, or neglected part of the body must be accounted for in the whole condition of the body itself.

If there is one thing that the readings of Edgar Cayce prove, it is that a human being cannot be broken into parts—each with a structure and a system of its own, capable of being understood and treated without regard to the other parts.

Edgar Cayce stated over and over again that everything we do and think is directly related to what we are as complete human beings; that what we eat has an influence on what we think; that what we think has an influence on what we eat; and that what we eat and think together influence what we do, how we feel, and what we look like. I quote an example from Case 288-38, which states, " . . . what we think and what we eat—combined together—*make what we are, physically and mentally*."

In another reading (2528-2) Cayce says, "But when the law is coordinated, in spirit, in mind, and in body, the entity is capable of fulfilling the purpose for which it enters a material or physical experience."

It has been my exceptional privilege to have known and worked with Edgar Cayce. Through him, we have access to the timeless wisdom that this great human being and psychic tapped from his "universal sources" of knowledge. I think that this wisdom was never needed so urgently as we need it today in the midst of the external and internal ecological chaos that humanity, science, and technology have wrought.

The purpose of this book is to teach you how to stay well by sharing with you the natural drugless therapies, mental attitudes, and spiritual attunement that Edgar Cayce prescribed in his over 14,000 readings for some 6,000 individuals. You must bear in mind that a majority of the people who sought help from Mr. Cayce and me were medical rejects—discouraged, disheartened souls who had tried everything that orthodox and unorthodox healing had to offer. In turning to Cayce, many were appealing to a court of last resort. Cayce was able to diagnose their troubles by slipping into a trance, although he almost never saw the subject, who might have been thousands of miles away. He then prescribed the therapies to help them. Many recovered in what seemed miracle cures. Others did not. Although the method was strange and psychic, there was nothing mysterious about the therapies—which included osteopathy, correction of nutrition, exercise, massage, hydrotherapy and electrotherapy, packs applied externally, remedies and formulae based on natural foods, herbs, and occasionally even chemical medicines and surgery. It required persistence and mental and spiritual attunement to achieve results, as Cayce often explained:

> Then keep that attitude of constructive, creative forces within self. For all healing of every nature must arise within the self. For there is the ability within the physical body to re-create or reproduce itself, as well as the activities for assimilating that from which the re-creation is to be brought about. (1663-1)

> For all healing, mental or material, is attuning each atom of the body, each reflex of the brain forces, to the awareness of the divine that lies within each atom, each cell of the body. (3384-2)

In the following reading (528-9) Cayce emphasizes the importance of persistence and consistency:

> . . . the body must not, should not, lose courage to carry on, but working in patience knowing that all healing, all help, must arise from constructive think-

---

The Big Picture of Holistic Health

If there is one thing that the readings of Edgar Cayce prove, it is that a human being cannot be broken into parts—each with a structure and a system of its own, capable of being understood and treated without regard to the other parts.

Edgar Cayce stated over and over again that everything we do and think is directly related to what we are as complete human beings; that what we eat has an influence on what we think; that what we think has an influence on what we eat; and that what we eat and think together influence what we do, how we feel, and what we look like.

—H.J.R.

. . . what we think and what we eat—combined together—make what we are, physically and mentally. (288-38)

But when the law is coordinated, in spirit, in mind, and in body, the entity is capable of fulfilling the purpose for which it enters a material or physical experience. (2528-2)

For all healing, mental or material, is attuning each atom of the body, each reflex of the brain forces, to the awareness of the divine that lies within each atom, each cell of the body. (3384-2)

ing, constructive application, and most and first of all constructive spiritual inspiration. Use [body] . . . disturbances as stepping-stones for higher and better and greater understanding.

Over the last fifteen years of Edgar Cayce's life (1930 to 1945) I worked with nearly 1,000 cases that he referred to me. There seemed to be a bewildering difference in the readings from individual to individual, even when their complaints fell under the same medical classification. (In this regard, as in so many others, Cayce was far ahead of his time in recognizing the biochemical individuality of each person, a subject we will take up in detail in later chapters.) At the time, I must confess I often did not understand some facets of the therapy. But as I applied the treatments in the sequence suggested by Cayce to thousands of patients in my forty-five years of clinical experience with them, I began to recognize the underlying philosophy and the principles involved. These principles are based on the basic structure and processes of the human body, mind, and spirit.

It soon became clear to me that no matter which of the therapies or combination of therapies he was prescribing, he was aiming at four basic goals: improvement and normalization of the functions of assimilation, elimination, circulation, and relaxation. With the restoration to normal balance of these four basics, the body then proceeds to heal itself of the disorders that manifest as symptoms of disease. In fact, both Cayce and I always dealt with causes, not symptoms, and therefore his readings seldom used medical labels. As a physiotherapist, I did not diagnose, but in clinical practice I found that a large percentage of the medical diagnoses with which patients arrived dealt with symptoms of a breakdown in bodily functions. In any case, no matter what the label, when the attitude of the patient was right and the treatments were followed with persistence and consistency so that the assimilation, elimination, circulation, and relaxation were once more normal, the results were full or partial recovery and many remarkable Cayce cures.

I like to make an acronym of the vital four goals mentioned above: when you do, you come up with the word CARE. In this book I will try to share with you the principles, methods, and detailed instructions for using the Cayce CARE home handbook to better health—for I have found this the key not only for healing the sick, but for building and maintaining a buoyant, energetic, and productive state of vibrant health capable of prolonging a youthful *joie de vivre* into the middle and golden years, free of disease. No matter what trials and tribulations life holds, one is better equipped to handle them in good health than in sickness.

To me, the Cayce readings are as alive today as when Cayce was living. In the years since he died (1945), I have continued to use many of the same therapies and remedies with repeated success. The main difference is that when Cayce was alive one could get definite suggestions for individuals. One could even find out by a series of questions the reasons why different suggestions for treatment were given to various people who seemed to have had the same disease. Often even the formula for a massage ointment was specific and detailed as to the amount and the timing, and in many cases he even predicted the results that one could expect. A distinctive characteristic of the Cayce work was that each human being received an individually orchestrated composition of therapies designed to restore the harmony of the body, mind, and spirit. At other times, he just sent patients to me and left it to me to decide what they needed.

We no longer have Cayce as a personal source of information. Now it remains for those who have had the experience, educational background, scientific training, and wisdom of correct interpretation to use the readings in the best possible manner to heal the sick and to make the knowledge available to those who are well so that they can maintain their health throughout life.

The Cayce therapies and remedies are timeless—reaching back into the past over the centuries and often projecting into the future, anticipating by many years discoveries of science and research to validate them. Cayce was tapping "universal sources of intelligence" and receiving from them the natural laws of the universe. The wisdom Cayce received recognized the God–given ability of the human body, mind, and spirit to heal themselves. This is why it works as well today as it did when Cayce was alive, if interpreted properly.

The infinite wisdom contained in the Cayce readings must be continually researched, applied, and explored for the possible remedies contained therein. There is still much to learn from them that we do not fully understand, that has yet to be used. But with study, experience, and the clinical research of some forty–five years, it has been possible for me to deduce from the advice he gave to individuals certain general principles that I have found, in clinical experience, can heal the sick and serve as a guide to better health for all.

I have selected those procedures, therapies, and remedies that are suitable for home use, provided you observe the parameters described for each one and you have consulted your own or a Cayce–oriented doctor for a diagnostic analysis. As Cayce himself said, his work would first teach individuals, then groups, and finally the masses. It is our hope that *The Edgar Cayce Handbook for Health Through Drugless Therapy* will teach the fundamentals of glowing health, youthfulness, weight control, disease prevention, sexual fertility and fulfillment, and a long, happy, productive life.

The Cayce therapies and remedies are timeless—reaching back into the past over the centuries and often projecting into the future, anticipating by many years discoveries of science and research to validate them. Cayce was tapping "universal sources of intelligence" and receiving from them the natural laws of the universe.

—H.J.R.

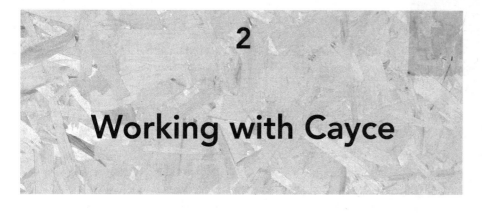

2

Working with Cayce

You will give a physical and mental reading for this body, with suggestions for the improvement of either, and you will answer the questions which I will ask you regarding these. (5439-1)

I had never heard of Edgar Cayce, but I assumed him to be one of the hundreds of medical doctors, osteopaths, dentists, chiropractors, or naturopaths who were making regular patient referrals to us for physiotherapy treatments.

—H.J.R.

Edgar Cayce came into my life on a raw wintry day in January 1930. At the Reilly Physicians' Service we were in the middle of our usual post-holiday rush. Clients were dashing about, working hard to shed their guilt and pounds to undo the damage of Christmas and New Year partying. My sister Dorothy, one of the five who worked with me, was paging me over the intercom. I was very busy and I brusquely asked her if our brother Dr. Pat couldn't take care of the matter. She was insistent that I come to the reception room.

"I have a Mrs. L.S. here with some papers for you to see. She says Edgar Cayce of Virginia Beach sent her."

I had never heard of Edgar Cayce, but I assumed him to be one of the hundreds of medical doctors, osteopaths, dentists, chiropractors, or naturopaths who were making regular patient referrals to us for physiotherapy treatments.

At that time we were located at 1908 Broadway, in New York City, on the second floor of a wooden building on the northeast corner of 63rd Street. It wasn't a fancy place—nothing like the plush Reilly Health Service in Rockefeller Center that was to become famous in later years. But it was a well-equipped gymnasium and health spa with plenty of space indoors and on the roof for exercises and a handball court. We had one of the city's most elaborate hydrotherapy departments—European-spa baths, Scotch douches, sitz baths, a variety of steam baths, massage rooms, electric cabinets, and electrotherapy equipment—everything needed for a complete physiotherapy service.

When I entered the reception room, I found an attractive, red-haired woman examining the pictures of business tycoons, labor leaders, politicians, and opera, theater, and radio stars that covered our walls, all of them inscribed to me with appreciation or a similar sentiment.

Mrs. [5439] had an air and bearing that made me think of the theater and star quality. I asked if she were an actress. She smiled a little and looked pleased. She told me that her great love was writing, especially for the theater, and that she hoped to write a good play one day. She looked much younger than her age, which I discovered was forty–two.

"Edgar Cayce of Virginia Beach sent me here," she said, holding out a sheaf of papers. "He said I was to have massage and electrotherapy."

"I never heard of him," I replied. With the arrogance of youth I casually accepted the fact that he had heard of me, whoever he was. "Let me see what you have there," I said.

The sheets of paper she handed me were headed:

This psychic reading given by Edgar Cayce at his office, 115 West 35th Street, Virginia Beach, Va., this day 11th of January, 1930, in accordance with request made by self—Mrs. [5439] (then the woman's full name was given).

Next, it read:

PRESENT—Edgar Cayce; Mrs. Cayce, Conductor; Gladys Davis, Steno. The Time of Reading 4:00 P.M. Eastern Standard Time. Mrs. [5439] of Central Park West, New York City.

Then it went on with the following instructions to Edgar Cayce given by Mrs. Cayce:

You will give a physical and mental reading for this body, with suggestions for the improvement of either, and you will answer the questions which I will ask you regarding these.

At first I thought this was some kind of joke, or that Mrs. [5439] and Cayce were crazy. Yet I was curious enough to go on reading. I was not totally hostile to the idea of a referral from a psychic, because over the years we had had a number of astrologers, psychics, palmists, numerologists, and other devotees of the occult among our clientele, and frequently we had received recommendations from them. But in all my experience I had never read a diagnosis or prescription for therapy like the one I now started to read.

When Mrs. [5439] told me that Cayce gave what she called the "reading" while he was in a trance in Virginia Beach and she was in New York, I became really intrigued. Even now, with forty–five years of hindsight, it is very difficult to explain what made me stop in the middle of one of our busiest days to read the following, but I did. Cayce said:

Yes, we have the body here, Mrs. [5439]. Now, we find the body very good in many respects, physically and mentally. There are rather conditions of which the body physical should take warning, and by correction of what is minor in the physical functioning at present, bring about a better condition in the physical and furnish the channel through which the mental and spiritual may manifest; *for the body-physical is truly the temple through which the mental and the spiritual and soul development must manifest, and in manifestation does the growth come.* [Italics added.]

I reread the phrase "for the body-physical is truly the temple through which the mental and the spiritual and soul development must manifest," finding in it an echo of my own deeply held conviction, one that I had dedicated my life to as a physiotherapist. I often reminded my patients that "the same blood that goes through your intestines and your feet goes through your brain." My words were not as poetic and spiritual as the language Cayce used, but I meant the same thing.

The diagnosis began with an analysis of the blood supply. Cayce found that the emotion of fear was creating a condition that "must be eliminated" from the system:

> . . . there are many channels through which eliminations are carried on. First, in the respiratory system. This *not* merely the deoxidization being thrown off through the breath, or through the clarifications of the bloodstream as it flows to the lungs for the oxygen necessary to carry on certain conditions . . . but also that of the whole of the exterior . . . through the various pores of the system [and that of the lymphatic circulation].
>
> Also that in the liver, or through the alimentary canal. *These,* at present, suffer the most—for as seen, the blood supply flows twice through the liver to any other portion of the system and in the left lobe or the smaller lobe of same, do we find those conditions as represent disorders as are affected by the splenic and this lobe, or portion of lobe of the liver—for the liver being both excretory and secretive in its functioning, then acts upon the system in a more than twofold manner.

The Cayce reading went on to explain how the breakdown in elimination in the woman's respiratory system, liver, and kidneys had affected her nervous systems, creating "disorders—not disease" resulting in overacidity.

> These . . . give rise to the expressions of dullness in head, fullness in throat, the misdirection in the mucus-producing tissue in bronchia, nasal cavities, antrum, and those conditions where soft tissue becomes involved. These are merely signposts not causes—not the reactions, even. Rather those *warnings* as to disorders, or distresses, as come to the physical [to the body].

After this accurate diagnosis of Mrs. [5439]'s symptoms and their cause, the entranced clairvoyant went on to a discussion of the mental forces at work on her.

> Fear [is] the greatest bugaboo to the human elements, for in fear comes those conditions that destroy that vitality of that assimilated.

His advice to her hit with uncanny accuracy her most secret desires:

> The mental developments should be in the direction of the directing play, writing play, writing book, writing song—for *these* may give an *outlet* of self

. . . for the body-physical is truly the temple through which the mental and the spiritual and soul development must manifest, and in manifestation does the growth come. (5439-1)

Fear [is] the greatest bugaboo to the human elements, for in fear comes those conditions that destroy that vitality of that assimilated.
(5439-1)

Do not lose self in the individual nor in the self-centered interest, but rather in that the body, the body mental, the body spiritual may make an ideal. (5439-1)

to *manifest* that which the body, the mental *being* may hold as ideal. *Find* an ideal. Do not lose self in the individual nor in the self-centered interest, but rather in that the body, the body mental, the body spiritual may make an ideal. Ready for questions:

(Q) What books can the body read to help improve her talents for writing?
(A) Tacitus, or Plato, or such—for the entity was associated with Plato, and the rise and fall of same would mean much.

(Q) Shall I write with someone else, or shall I write by myself?
(A) Fear enters here, when the entity attempts to write alone—but *write* alone, and keep that *near* self as the *ideal,* when doing so. Be not afraid to really express those children of the mental body as flow in, in meditation, for these—in use—will grow and will not destroy self, will they but be tendered by the love of the Creator, or of the body itself.

(Q) Is the body necessary to her husband's business? Is it advisable for her to return to the business?
(A) Would be advisable that at *least* in the advisory capacity the body see much *more* of same than it has recently; but to return to same would be to smother self's own endeavors, and self's own personality, self's own *individuality* would also suffer . . .

(Q) Will the business come back successfully without the body?
(A) With her *advice,* would come back! With her *counsel,* come back!

(Q) What attitude should she take toward her husband?
(A) Not merely of duty's tolerance, but that of helpfulness; for one is as *necessary* to the other as is that of *any* condition where there are two poles. (5439-1)

I agreed with his interpretation that the range of symptoms came from a toxic condition, brought on, at least in part, by emotional causes and by improper elimination.

Mrs. [5439] did not present an exceptional or challenging health problem, and certainly the recommended treatment of massage and electrotherapy was well within our routine therapy.

I immediately knew that when we gave her the manipulation we would increase her circulation. The drainage therapy would relieve pressure in the head. In the massage we would pay special attention to the abdomen to stimulate the liver and spleen, and we would work the legs so as to normalize and stimulate circulation in the legs, and this would stimulate circulation in the whole body.

As for the excessive mucus, that will often appear when the diet is incorrect or where there is irritation. It is nature's way of trying to heal or protect the tissues so they won't become overly inflamed. Some foods are more mucus forming than others (see Chapter 5 on diet and nutrition).

Cayce's recommended treatment called for electrotherapy with ultraviolet, infrared, Nile green, and then orange lights. We did not go in for chromo-therapy or color therapy, but we did use the infrared and two types of ultra-violet (one pure ultraviolet and the other with the complete sun spectrum produced by the use of carbon–arc lamps). I was most interested in the use of the lights, which Cayce claimed would "equalize the circulation, relieving this condition in the central nervous system."

In the reading I was intrigued by a number of concepts that not only struck a responsive chord with my own ideas but represented thinking that was not at that time generally accepted by the medical profession. Now, however, these ideas have become commonplace.

For example, a whole section dealt with Mrs. [5439]'s anxieties and fears about her husband's business. She had been working with him in what, I later learned, was a very successful business, but she was semiretired and was feeling guilty because the business had developed some difficulties. Another portion of the reading dealt with her frustrated desires to write creatively, particularly for the theater. All these tensions, fears, and emotions, Cayce indicated, were largely responsible for her physical disorders. Back in 1930, psy-

---

Dr. Reilly and the Opera Singer

I recall one amusing incident that taught me a good lesson in psychosomatic illness. For a number of years I had been taking care of Beniamino Gigli, the great Metropolitan Opera Italian tenor. When Gigli's chauffeur brought him to me, he was overweight and suffering so severely from arthritis he was forced to cancel performances. I helped him get into good shape—brought him down from 245 to a more romantic-looking 195 pounds—and after a few months he never again missed a performance. We became close friends—I went to Italy with him every two years—and he wanted me to give up my practice and just travel and work with him on exercise, massage, diet, and reinforcing his discipline.

Then one day I learned that Gigli was to give a Carnegie Hall concert and I took an advertisement covering the entire back page of the program. It read, "Why Gigli Never Misses a Performance," and then went on to summarize what I did to keep him fit. When Gigli saw the program, he became angrier than I had ever seen him. Although he had a well-known temper, his anger and moods never had lasted very long. This time, however, he raved and stormed—but worst of all, he caught a severe cold. Anger had set up a chemical condition that created the acids that made him vulnerable—and now he was sick. It was two days before the concert and he threatened to cancel it.

"What a fool you will look before the whole world—you and your ad," he taunted.

I never worked so hard in my entire life as I did in the next two days, but I did get him well in time to save two reputations.

**Types of Treatments
Cayce Recommended**

- osteopathy
- chiropractic
- exercise
- conventional medi-
  cine
- sophisticated diets
- all forms of hydro-
  therapy
- electrotherapy
- surgery
- herbs
- oils
- lights
- colors
- energy appliances

*As men and women continued
coming in with Cayce readings or
directions, I became more and
more interested in the source. How
did he get my name? How did he
know the type of treatments that
we were giving and had the facilities to give?*—**H.J.R.**

chosomatics was a novel idea. Only a few pioneering doctors connected the emotional, mental, and spiritual conditions of their patients with their state of health or dis-ease, which Cayce interpreted literally to mean just that: lack of, or disturbance of, ease.

I had arrived at the same conclusion myself. As a young man, I taught jujitsu and boxing for the army, serving both on the Mexican border with the 22nd Regiment and later in World War I. I trained soldiers and did special physical conditioning to turn them into commandos. An athlete myself, I did quite a bit of boxing and learned early what it meant to get a "fighting edge," and what effect a man's emotions and fears had on his physical condition and performance.

In the months following Mrs. [5439]'s successful treatment I received a number of other referrals from Edgar Cayce, but it was to be two years before we met face to face. Sometimes the patients arrived with the readings, sometimes with slips of paper indicating the kind of therapy to be given. Sometimes the directions were very precise, even to specifying the kind of oil or combination of oils to be used for a massage, and the precise proportion. Sometimes there were no specific directions, leaving the entire modality of treatment—or application of the therapeutic agent—to my judgment.

I have said through the years, in many of the speeches that I have given to medical and lay groups, that every type of healing has cured someone, although no type has cured everyone. My training and experience have been eclectic and I have an open mind. But never have I encountered elsewhere or seen duplicated the wide range of therapies Cayce recommended. They included osteopathy, chiropractic, exercise, conventional medicine, the most sophisticated nutrition and diet, every known form of hydrotherapy, electrotherapy, and even surgery; and he used a bewildering variety of herbs, oils, lights, colors, and original appliances that he had invented.

Where did he get his knowledge of the value of so many different therapies for different individuals—for no two were ever alike? This was uncanny, for with all my knowledge and experience, I found it practically impossible to improve on his suggestions. I also found it hard to understand how a man could go to sleep and give as good or better advice than I was able to give in my waking state.

As men and women continued coming in with Cayce readings or directions, I became more and more interested in the source. How did he get my name? How did he know the type of treatments that we were giving and had the facilities to give? My curiosity continued as, without either of us planning it consciously, a two-way traffic was growing between the Reilly Physicians' Service and Edgar Cayce at Virginia Beach.

One of my favorite patients was Clara Belle Walsh. A tall blonde of Wagnerian proportions and nearly six feet tall, Clara Belle was the heiress of a great old Kentucky family and was internationally famous as a hostess, a theater and music patron, and an intimate personal friend of England's Queen Mary.

She sponsored many great performers and artists, and I particularly remember meeting Vincent Lopez, then unknown, in her suite at the Plaza Hotel, where she held court when in New York. One day she casually informed us in a matter-of-fact voice that Lopez was the reincarnation of (according to a Cayce life reading) Leonardo da Vinci. Leonardo had been left-handed, which is why Vincent Lopez always conducted with his left hand.

Mrs. Walsh had one painful physical complaint. Her legs were elegantly slim, but the left knee was arthritic and had a spur. Occasionally the knee would hook up on the spur and cause swelling and excruciating pain. When this would happen, she would send for me, I would hasten to the Plaza Hotel, apply packs to reduce the swelling, and work to unlock the knee from the spur. This gave her immediate relief. Once I was out of town when her knee became hooked up for four or five days and developed a terrible inflammation. She had called in the doctor from the Plaza Hotel and he gave her drugs—but not even the strongest narcotic had any effect on her. She was in excruciating pain. When the Plaza's doctor called in a specialist, he suggested opening the knee or, if necessary, amputating the leg at the knee.

When I came back to town, I found a sheaf of urgent messages from Clara Belle. I hurried to the Plaza and was told by the nurse that my patient was unconscious, under anesthesia, which they had given her while they tried manipulation. The nurse wouldn't let me enter her room. I explained that I was quite familiar with Mrs. Walsh's condition and had treated her many times in the past. During this time the anesthesia wore off and she began screaming with pain. As soon as she heard my voice, she demanded that I come to her. I treated her with packs, since manipulation at that point was impossible, and after I brought the inflammation down, I was able to give her relief. I had to see her three times a day for the next three days.

After this bout, Clara Belle was worried and a bit frightened, and she wrote to Edgar Cayce, hoping to find a more permanent cure: "I have seen doctors, some who wanted to operate and others who suggested serum treatment. So far H. J. Reilly of the Reilly Physicians' Service has helped me more than any other doctor. I believe you know him as you have sent several people to him."

But I didn't know him—Edgar Cayce and I still had not met. Mrs. Walsh brought me her reading from Cayce, and the treatment he had recommended coincided with that which she was already receiving. This continuing evidence of our agreement on philosophy and therapy increased my desire and determination to meet this psychic genius from Virginia Beach, but life was crowded and time was scarce, and I had to wait longer for the great moment to happen.

My curiosity about Cayce might have been satisfied much earlier if I had known that two patrons of the Reilly Health Service, Mr. and Mrs. David Kahn, had been close friends and sponsors of Edgar Cayce for many years. David Kahn, in fact, was a boy in Lexington, Kentucky, when he first met the psychic.

David and Lucille Kahn's enthusiasm and love for, and dedication to, Edgar Cayce and his healing work became a lifelong commitment for this wonderful couple that began in the early 1900s, when David first met Cayce, and continued, in partnership, after David and Lucille married in 1927.

In turn Cayce regarded them as members of his own family. In a letter to Case 1294, Cayce wrote: "We had a lovely visit with Lucille and David [Kahn].

Since hundreds, perhaps thousands, of the readings were given in the Kahn home, David had firsthand knowledge of the many cures brought about by Cayce's unorthodox diagnostic technique and subsequent treatments.

—H.J.R.

David Kahn Meets Edgar Cayce

One day, stretched out on the massage table, David described his first encounter with Cayce, who had come to Lexington to help a paralyzed neighbor. David was selected to give the instructions that Cayce needed to receive as he went into a trance and to bring him out of it. David was only fifteen years old at that time, but he said the incident changed his life and influenced him to dedicate a good portion of his efforts to the Cayce work.

The neighbor, Mrs. William De Laney, was remarkably improved after Cayce diagnosed the source of her trouble as an old injury to the spine from a long-forgotten accident. Osteopathic treatment and a specially compounded medication were recommended and administered and Mrs. De Laney made a remarkable recovery. This "miracle" made a deep impression on the young, impressionable David.

Just hope we did not wear out our welcome, but I think of—and feel toward them—as if they were my own people, know I couldn't love them any better were they my own blood kin."

Since hundreds, perhaps thousands, of the readings were given in the Kahn home, David had firsthand knowledge of the many cures brought about by Cayce's unorthodox diagnostic technique and subsequent treatments. It must be remembered that at that time (1931–'32), when I was developing such a strong interest in Cayce, none of the bestselling books about the psychic and "sleeping prophet of Virginia Beach" had been written and the readings had not yet been coded and indexed to become such a rich storehouse of material for writers, students, scientists, and the faithful to study. Except for occasional newspaper stories, the chief source of information was word of mouth. In David Kahn, Cayce had a powerful clarion trumpeting to anyone who would stop and listen for five minutes the wonders of Cayce and his cures.

At the time I had David Kahn on the massage table, trying to relax him, he was a bustling and successful businessman, whose faith in Cayce's diagnosis, treatment, prophecies, philosophy, and spirituality were the cornerstones of his life.

It did not take much encouragement to get David Kahn to tell me Cayce's life story—a story told so well and so often that I shall not repeat it here. If, however, there are any among you who have not read Cayce's biography, I refer you to David's *My Life with Edgar Cayce* and Mary Ellen Carter's *My Years with Edgar Cayce: The Personal Story of Gladys Davis Turner,* as well as to those written by two other friends and patients: Tom Sugrue and Jess Stearn.

I learned that Cayce had cured his wife, Gertrude, of tuberculosis by having her inhale brandy fumes from an old charred oak keg and by the administration of a certain narcotic given in unorthodox dosage; how he had saved his son Hugh Lynn's eyes, burned by a photographer's exploding flash powder, with poultices of tannic acid.

Biographies of Edgar Cayce

There Is a River by Thomas Sugrue (A.R.E. Press, 1997).

Edgar Cayce: An American Prophet by Sydney Kirkpatrick (Riverhead Books, 2001).

Edgar Cayce—The Sleeping Prophet by Jess Stearn (A.R.E. Press, 1997).

Hugh Lynn Cayce: About My Father's Business by A. Robert Smith (The Donning Company, 1988).

A Prophet in His Own Country by Jess Stearn (Bantam Books, 1989).

My Life with Edgar Cayce by David Kahn and Will Oursler (Doubleday & Co., 1970).

The Lost Memoirs of Edgar Cayce: My Life as a Seer by A. Robert Smith (St. Martin's Press, 1999).

My Years with Edgar Cayce: The Personal Story of Gladys Davis Turner by Mary Ellen Carter (Harper & Row, 1972).

I learned that Cayce had cured his wife, Gertrude, of tuberculosis by having her inhale brandy fumes from an old charred oak keg and by the administration of a certain narcotic given in unorthodox dosage; how he had saved his son Hugh Lynn's eyes, burned by a photographer's exploding flash powder, with poultices of tannic acid.—**H.J.R.**

The more I heard, the more anxious I was to meet the man who—without education or training—had helped thousands of people since he began giving physical readings in 1901. I envisioned Cayce as a person of commanding presence with piercing eyes, majestic gestures, and turban-draped head. But the Edgar Cayce I finally met in 1932 was a tall, slightly stooped man with wide eyes, an open face, an extremely soft-spoken manner. He looked like a minister of some quiet country church or like the Sunday school teacher he was all his life.

We met for lunch and as soon as we were seated at the table he took out a pack of cigarettes, lit one, and drew deeply on it, obviously inhaling. He must have caught my look of disapproval and surprise, for he said, a little apologetically, "It's the natural leaf." (The readings say that the natural leaf is less harmful than the combinations ordinarily put on the market in packaged tobacco.) He added, "Besides, I just can't give up smoking."

It was the only point of real difference between us. I do not approve of smoking.

Then we ordered the meal. I noticed he did not pay much attention to the rules of diet that he himself prescribed in the readings. Cayce confessed he was not a nutritional specialist. "In fact, I have no medical knowledge at all. I am just a channel for the information that comes through in the readings."

Then we ordered the meal. I no-
ticed he did not pay much atten-
tion to the rules of diet that he
himself prescribed in the readings.
Cayce confessed he was not a nu-
tritional specialist. "In fact, I have
no medical knowledge at all. I am
just a channel for the information
that comes through in the read-
ings."—**H.J.R.**

> ### Cayce's Successful Treatments
> Cayce treated incurable psoriasis successfully with osteopathic adjustments and a simple mixture of sulfur, cream of tartar, and Rochelle salts, plus liberal dosages of mullein and saffron teas and elm water. A mysterious disease sweeping the South—later identified as pellagra—was corrected with a diet of "turnip greens"; heart disease was rediagnosed as toxemia and miraculously disappeared when the subject was given a series of colonics, sweat baths, massage, and hydrotherapy; tumors were melted away on a diet of grapes and daily applications of grape poultices; castor oil packs healed broken bones, cured liver and gallbladder ailments, and soothed epileptics; peanut oil relieved arthritis; three almonds a day were given to prevent tumors and cancer; an apple diet for three days was a Cayce cleansing routine that cleared up more sins of the body than the Garden of Eden's serpent whispered to Eve. Stony scleroderma softened and healed under the Cayce treatment. The stories of healing seemed really miracle cures.

Actually, he was being modest. Although he had never been formally trained, he had studied the readings for thirty-odd years, and by the time I met him he was no longer the uninformed country boy he had been in his youth, when he started using his remarkable gift of clairvoyance. He had learned and had come to know a great deal. So began a working partnership that has lasted now for forty-five years—fifteen wonderful years while Edgar Cayce lived on this plane—and another thirty years posthumously in my daily practice of natural, drugless therapy, from which thousands of people say they have benefited.

In November 1933, Edgar Cayce, his son Hugh Lynn, and secretary Gladys Davis (later to become Gladys Davis Turner) came to visit me at Sun Air Farm, a health farm I owned and operated at Oak Ridge, in northern New Jersey. It was the first of many such visits and, according to Hugh Lynn, his father looked forward to them and enjoyed taking long walks in the woods. Hugh Lynn Cayce reminisced about those days to my coauthor Mrs. Brod.

"Following the many sessions that Dad had, giving readings to a variety of people in New York while staying at the home of David and Lucille Kahn or occasionally some other member of the A.R.E., we would visit with Dr. Reilly at his Sun Air Farm. There were many such visits—sometimes Dad and Mother and Gladys Davis and myself; at other times whoever happened to be with him in New York at the time.

"The readings didn't tire Dad so much as the talking with people after the readings. They insisted of course in describing in detail their symptoms, which Dad really didn't want to hear about . . . He would be very tired and he enjoyed the opportunity of getting away . . . So the relationship between my father and Dr. Reilly developed.

"He particularly enjoyed the meals that Mrs. Reilly arranged. She was an excellent cook and so was her mother whom we all called Ama. They had been in the restaurant business . . . Father particularly enjoyed the biscuits, and I can still remember how big they were; they rose to prodigious heights and Dad used to enjoy them so much and cover them with gravy which was against everybody's dietary recommendations—including Dad's suggestions from the readings, Reilly's rules of diet, and even Mrs. Reilly's. Nevertheless all would enjoy the delicious meals that were served. Dad would praise Mrs. Reilly and Ama, knowing they would outdo themselves to top their latest culinary triumph, and I quickly caught on and would join him in fulsome praise of the household chefs.

"Dad also enjoyed talking with the people at Reilly's who were there for treatment . . . They didn't know he was a psychic and that suited him. Of course, in those days he wasn't as famous as he later became and they would just talk to him about their problems and business, and he loved to sit around and talk with them . . . he enjoyed long walks in the woods with all kinds of people and he loved the birch and beech trees which surrounded the lake . . . I remember him talking with many different types of people that Reilly had up there. Some of them had problems with drinking, some of them were quite famous and sometimes they would be very surprised to learn that they had been talking to a psychic."

(As Hugh Lynn recalled, his father would be exhausted after spending two or three weeks in the city giving readings and then they would go to Sun Air Farm to rest. He sometimes would have a cold or chest congestion.)

"Dad, like many psychics, had an amazing capacity for recovery," he said. "He could be very sick one moment and completely recovered the next. He had the power to give himself self-suggestion in the unconscious state or to accept suggestion in that state from someone beside him who was told to give him a suggestion to increase circulation to a certain part of the body. I have seen this happen.

"In readings up there at Sun Air Farm he would include either at the beginning or the end an instruction that the circulation of the body should be increased to remove the congestion or cold. And I could watch the color in that particular part of the body involved in the suggestion change as the blood flowed. He was an excellent subject in terms of having his unconscious accept suggestions. He could change the whole nerve energy flow."

But Cayce never changed his lifestyle to conform to his own suggestions about health. Hugh Lynn said that his father liked to eat certain foods that he had grown up with back in Kentucky. "He loved certain things that my mother would fix for him, for example, pork. He told everyone not to eat pork, but Dad enjoyed it and he particularly enjoyed pig's feet. He enjoyed wild game, and he did recommend that. He drank coffee and he recommended this in moderation. He recommended smoking in moderation. Many people have raised questions about his smoking, and I suspect that during those early years when Dad was recommending moderation, tobacco was not being treated in the same way as it is now. You must remember, Dad grew up on a tobacco farm. He was a chain smoker.

"Yes, Dad ate what he pleased and occasionally he suffered for it. He would

---

**Edgar Cayce at
Sun Air Farm**

Dad was a most unassuming person and I think this is one of the interesting facets of Dad's relationship with Dr. Reilly—meeting and seeing the unusual people that Reilly had at the Reilly Health Service in Rockefeller Center in New York—and frequently at the farm. They were name personalities. He would come back after spending a whole day up there getting everything they offered in physiotherapy; baths, fume baths, massage—sun lamp—and then when he came home he was all excited about having seen some well-known entertainer or motion picture personality. There were always a great many people from the Broadway stage there. Dad was a great admirer of the theater and so enjoyed seeing some of these people from time to time.

—Hugh Lynn Cayce

have irritation and stomach pains and congestion. But then he would go into a trance state and get up completely free of whatever he happened to have.

"Dad always insisted that if he couldn't raise his vibration over a piece of meat that there was something wrong with him."

Gladys's Dream

It was at Sun Air Farm that Gladys Davis had a remarkable psychic experience. She saw a dream come true. Gladys had more or less systematically recorded her dreams since 1924—one year after she had become Cayce's private secretary. As she tells it:

"In late January of 1934 Edgar Cayce, Hugh Lynn Cayce, and I were visitors for the weekend at the Ladd home on Long Island. They were both dear friends and Cayce followers. Late Sunday night Mrs. Ladd was telling me about her husband's financial difficulties; his job was insecure, and they were about to lose their home. As I got into bed, I remember wishing I could do something to help the Ladd family. It turned awfully cold that night and I was very uncomfortable. Early the next morning I was awakened by this dream:

"A knock on the door. I said, 'Come in.' Mr. Ladd stood there with a coal scuttle in his hand and wearing a lumber jacket. (I had never seen him in anything but a business suit.) He came in and made a fire in a little coal stove which stood in the room, saying, 'Now the room will soon be warm so you can get up.'"

Miss Davis related the dream to Mr. Cayce and Hugh Lynn on the train back to New York that morning, and she agreed with them when they attributed it to her discomfort. "Still, I remember remarking how strange it was that the room should be different from the one I was occupying, which had two radiators on opposite walls."

In early April 1935 Miss Davis was a guest at Sun Air Farm. "On Sunday morning," Gladys recalls, "when I said, 'Come in,' to a knock on the door, there stood Mr. Ladd in his lumber jacket, a coal bucket in his hand, and he said, 'I thought you'd like a little fire in your stove to take the chill off while you get dressed.' I noticed that the little room was exactly the same as I had dreamed it over a year before."

In January of that year Ladd had become manager of Sun Air Farm.

It was on his first visit to Sun Air Farm that Cayce gave me my life reading, which began at 11:50 A.M. November 12, 1933, and ended at 12:40 P.M., a very long period. My wife and daughter were present, and so were my brother Pat and his wife. The reading is too long to reproduce here, but certain observations had a bearing upon my future work. Cayce noted that "from Jupiter there are those things that gather around the body; and individuals of affluence, position, power, place, in the affairs of all walks of life," a good description of the Reilly clientele, especially those who would be patronizing the Reilly Health Service in Rockefeller Center (at that time just a hope).

The reading went on: "Hence those that are in that position of being influenced by wrath, or temper, or activities within selves that have brought about detrimental influences in their experience, will be drawn to the body's association. Not those of mental derangements, but those of mental weaknesses in and through the weaknesses of the body–physical. These, we find, will be the greater attraction towards the entity, because of the entity's ability to aid such relations, such associations . . . " (438-1)

Cayce said that among my incarnations I had been a Roman gladiator in the arena and had served with Nero's soldiers and that "the entity had the ability to be masterful in the games in the arena," which possibly explains my interest from boyhood in athletics and conditioning. I had always been puzzled by my bent, since no one in the family before me had been particularly inclined to athletics or therapy: "Hence the games of the Romans, the baths of the Romans, dress of the Romans, are to the entity in the present . . . of particular interest; and much may be gained by the entity in the present by following those lines of thought pertaining to the particular activity of the entity in the past," also a possible explanation of my early interest in hydrotherapy.

In Egypt, Cayce said, I kept the records on the arts of healing and those of music: "The entity then through these activities brought much to a disturbed people; and aided those that would be called physicians of the day in establishing places of retreat and conditions that might aid the individuals and groups in cleansing their bodies, purifying their minds, by the activities of the body, and by the classifying of the foods during the period." (438-1)

Perhaps this explains my exceptional success with musicians right down to the date of this writing.

The reading dealt with two other incarnations: one as a member of the company of Eric the Red "when the entity was among those of that company who made the first attempts for the permanent settlement in the land known as Vineland on coasts about Rhode Island and portions of the land lying north of Massachusetts. Then the entity was strong in body, in mind and in the activities both on the land and the sea and was in name Osolo Din."

Another incarnation dealt with a sojourn in Atlantis. There was much more about my character, emotions, spiritual life—all of it remarkably accurate and perceptive in describing me as I now am and the roots of my present characteristics in previous incarnations. In any case, the reading established beyond a question that I was predestined for the work of healing through physiotherapy and drugless therapy, and that I would be doing this work in many future lifetimes as I had in past lives.

In the question period I was able to ask about something that was giving me sleepless nights. I had been negotiating to get space for an enlarged Reilly Health Service Institute in Rockefeller Center, which was then under construction. David Kahn and a wealthy client who had worked closely with officials of RCA were helping me. My client had opened a line of credit for me, for I had not nearly enough money to finance the $125,000 necessary to set up such an establishment. However, we had run into snag after snag in dealing with the building's sponsors and management.

Cayce said that among my incarnations I had been a Roman gladiator in the arena and had served with Nero's soldiers and that "the entity had the ability to be masterful in the games in the arena," which possibly explains my interest from boyhood in athletics and conditioning. I had always been puzzled by my bent, since no one in the family before me had been particularly inclined to athletics or therapy.—**H.J.R.**

At the time of my life reading I had been negotiating for over two years and I was very discouraged. In fact, I was ready to drop the whole thing. I put the question to Cayce: "Is it advisable to continue my efforts to secure an establishment in Radio City?"—**H.J.R.**

I have always been deeply grateful to Cayce and I tried to express that gratitude in concrete ways. If at any time a person had secured a reading in which the type of work that was to be done at my institute was beyond the means of the patient, I would gladly give them all the necessary treatments free of charge. This commitment I honored during the life of the institute.—**H.J.R.**

At the time of my life reading I had been negotiating for over two years and I was very discouraged. In fact, I was ready to drop the whole thing. I put the question to Cayce: "Is it advisable to continue my efforts to secure an establishment in Radio City?"

"Advisable to continue," he replied. "As we find, this should culminate in the latter part of the coming year, when those influences from the efforts of others from without are attracted to the activities of the entity and bring better relationships."

There were other words of guidance and reassurance. Encouraged by the reading, I persisted. Fourteen months after the reading—in December 1934—the lease was sent to me for signing. Everything I had been working for was incorporated in it. However, during the negotiations and plans for my establishment, I found that my space needs were even greater than originally anticipated. I needed another thousand square feet of space. Should I try to change the terms of the lease or let well enough alone?

With the confidence generated by the Cayce reading, I took the long chance and asked for the extra space. The Rockefellers okayed my request, making me a very happy man and again corroborating Edgar Cayce's great gift of prophecy.

I have always been deeply grateful to Cayce and I tried to express that gratitude in concrete ways. If at any time a person had secured a reading in which the type of work that was to be done at my institute was beyond the means of the patient, I would gladly give them all the necessary treatments free of charge. This commitment I honored during the life of the institute.

In the years since my friend's passing I have tried to honor his memory by making full use of the many suggestions he gave for the body and mind. And I have insisted that anyone wishing to be treated by me become a member of the A.R.E. I do this not only because of my interest in supporting the organization but because the patient's attitude is so important. Unless the patient is attuned mentally and spiritually, results can be very disappointing. Attitude is all-important in achieving success with Cayce treatments. The key word is attunement. Cayce and I shared a common viewpoint. We do not treat diseases—we treat, care for, and teach people. I think this quotation from one of his readings sums up this philosophy of healing:

> . . . all strength, all healing of every nature is the changing of the vibrations from within—the attuning of the divine within the living tissue of a body to Creative Energies. This alone is healing. Whether it is accomplished by the use of drugs, the knife, or what not, it is the attuning of the atomic structure of the living cellular force to its spiritual heritage. (1967-1)

3
The Cayce Philosophy of Healing

The attitude of the patient is of primary importance in achieving success with the "Cayce CARE" therapy. Long before the medical profession had generally accepted the concept of psychosomatic illness, Cayce recognized the unity of body, mind, and spirit.

Some of you may remember Adelaide's famous song from the musical *Guys and Dolls*, in which she blames her cold on frustration caused by her lover. Many years before this Broadway success, Cayce told a thirty–six–year–old man: " . . . when there is the ruffling of your disposition, when there is any anger, it prepares the system so that it blocks the flow of the circulation to eliminating channels. Thus you can take a bad cold from getting mad. You can get a bad cold from blessing [cursing] out someone else, even if it is your wife." (849–75)

To be sure attitudes oft influence the physical conditions of the body. No one can hate his neighbor and not have stomach or liver trouble. No one can be jealous and allow the anger of same and not have upset digestion or heart disorder.
(4021-1)

. . . we would administer those activities which would bring a normal reaction through these portions, stimulating them to an activity from the body itself, rather than the body becoming dependent upon supplies that are robbing portions of the system to produce activity in other portions, or the system receiving elements or chemical reactions being supplied without arousing the activities of the system itself for a more normal condition. (1968-3)

Quiet, meditation, for a half to a minute, will bring strength—will the body see physically this flowing out to quiet self, whether walking, standing still, or resting. Well, too, that oft when alone, meditate in the silence—as the body has done. (311-4)

Edgar Cayce on Anger

For anger can destroy the brain as well as any disease. For it is itself a disease of the mind! (35l0-l)

(Q) Any other advice or counsel?
(A) Only as to the attitude. As indicated for most people and it is very well here: don't get mad and don't cuss a body out, mentally or in voice. This brings more poisons than may be created by even taking foods that aren't good. (470-37)

(Q) Am I working too hard for my health?
(A) If the body imagines that it is working too hard, it's working awfully hard! But if you will make play of the work [seeing] that as an opportunity, it's not so hard. (1968-6)

(Q) How can I keep from worrying so much about my wife's health?
(A) Why worry, when ye may pray? Know that the power of thyself is very limited. The power of Creative Force is unlimited. (2981-1)

*. . . the Spirit is of the Creator,
and thy body is the temple of that
Spirit manifested in the earth to
defend or to use in thine own ego,
or thine own self-indulgence, or
to thine own glory, or unto the
glory of Him who gave thee life
and immortality—if ye preserve
that life, that Spirit of Him.*

(2448–2)

Here are a few examples of Cayce's insight into the effect of emotions and attitudes on the body:

To be sure, attitudes oft influence the physical conditions of the body. No one can hate his neighbor and not have stomach or liver trouble. No one can be jealous and allow the anger of same and not have upset digestion or heart disorder. (4021-1)

For the powers within must be spiritualized. Not that the body is not spiritual-minded, but there is the necessity to be spiritual-minded and then able to gain control sufficiently over the power of mind in the body as to cause the vibrations from the atomic structures to produce health-giving forces, rather than taking the continual suggestion, "I'm sick and going to stay sick." These reactions should be brought about by suggestion as well as application. For know, as was given from the beginning, it is necessary to subdue the earth. Man is made, physically, from every element within the earth. So, unless there is a coordination of those elements of the environs in which the animal-man operates, he is out of attune—and some portions suffer. He must contain and command those elements. These are subduing, using, controlling; not being controlled by, but controlling, those environs, and influences about same. (3455-1)

. . . keep the mind in that condition through the means as has been outlined for the developing of the physical, mental and spiritual forces; keeping those contacts in that manner that brings the awakening of the physical in its ability to re-create in itself that necessary for the developing of the soul and spirit forces through the mental man; ever remembering that the physical must be kept in that way that the mental may manifest . . . (294-l0)

Dr. John A. Schindler of Monroe, Wisconsin, author of the bestseller *How to Live 365 Days a Year*, claims that between 35 to 50 percent of all sick people are sick because they are unhappy. His estimates may have to be revised upwards in the light of the important work on stress done by Dr. Hans Selye, director of the University of Montreal's Institute of Experimental Medicine and Surgery. Dr. Selye subjected rats to a variety of stresses: cold, fatigue, frustration, noise, poisons, hatred, anxiety, and fear—experiments that revolutionized medical thinking: "No matter what the nature of the stress, the same type of internal wreckage resulted. Blood pressure soared. At autopsy the rats showed gross enlargement of the all–important adrenal glands, shrunken thymus and lymphatic glands and peptic ulcers."[1]

The United States Office of Vital Statistics in the Department of Health, Education and Welfare classifies the following as psychosomatic illnesses: ulcerative colitis, hypertension, chronic constipation, headache, fatigue, arthritis, insomnia, backache, and a host of other illnesses, including asthma and allergies.

Modern and more esoteric research techniques with Kirlian photography, a process first developed by the Russians for photographing the bioenergy fields in and around a living organism (which Edgar Cayce could see and called the "aura"), now postulate scientifically that illness shows up in one's energy field before the symptoms manifest in the body.

A number of notable, respected American scientists are working on this field of research, including Dr. William Tiller, a physicist at Stanford University; Dr. Thelma Moss at UCLA; Drs. Stanley Krippner and Montague Ullman of the Dream Laboratory at Maimonides Hospital in New York City; and Drs. Gerald Jampolsky of Tiburon, California, and Gary Poock, who have developed the first Kirlian motion-picture process in the United States.

Let us now examine the means Cayce used to achieve the goals of normalizing assimilation, elimination, circulation, and relaxation. Despite his lack of formal education, when in trance, Cayce's terminology and understanding of the body processes were medically correct. His physical readings usually contained an analysis of the blood system, the nervous system, the state of the organs and their functioning, and the causes of the symptoms and prescriptions for their relief. Where mental, emotional, and spiritual problems existed, he analyzed them and related them to the physical diseases.

When asked how he could diagnose for a person thousands of miles away whom he had never seen, Cayce replied as follows:

> The information as given or obtained from this body is gathered from the sources from which the suggestion [which was given verbally to Mr. Cayce by the conductor of the reading] may derive its information.
>
> In this [trance] state the conscious mind becomes subjugated to the subconscious, superconscious or soul mind; and may and does communicate with like minds—and the subconscious or soul force becomes universal. From any subconscious mind information may be obtained, either from this plane or from the impressions as left by the individuals that have gone on before . . .
>
> Through the forces of the soul, through the minds of others as presented, or that have gone on before; through the subjugation of the physical forces in this manner, the body [Edgar Cayce] obtains the information. (3744-2)

Cayce's explanation that the correct diagnosis and the healing knowledge lies in the subconscious of the sufferer is not too far from the technique used by the practitioners of Freudian and Jungian psychoanalysis and psychiatry to treat their patients. Cayce expressed it thus:

> All healing comes from the Divine within . . . Thus, if one would correct physical or mental disturbances, it is necessary to change the attitude and to let the life forces become constructive and not destructive. Hate, malice and jealousy only create poisons within the minds, souls and bodies of people.
>
> (3312-1)

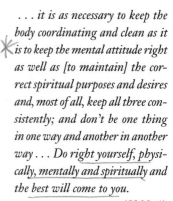

. . . it is as necessary to keep the body coordinating and clean as it is to keep the mental attitude right as well as [to maintain] the correct spiritual purposes and desires and, most of all, keep all three consistently; and don't be one thing in one way and another in another way . . . Do right yourself, physically, mentally and spiritually and the best will come to you.

(5203-1)

On the subject of the body's capacity to heal itself he said:

> . . . within each physical being [there exist] the elements whereby the organs . . . are enabled within themselves to supply what is needed for replenishing or rebuilding. (3124-1)

Each day our bodies must manufacture millions of new cells. Our health and youthfulness depend on our ability to do so. When we can no longer do this, we age and die. We can see that here again Cayce was far in advance of medical thinking of his time and right up to date with the latest cellular research.

In *Nutrition Against Disease*, Dr. Roger Williams says, "It is common knowledge that the cells in our bodies get their supply of raw materials largely from the circulating blood. It is not so generally known that each of us has a circulatory pattern of his own and that the dispensing of suitable amounts of oxygen and about forty nutrients to billions of diverse cells all over the body is a huge logistic undertaking."[2]

Since we must depend on food, water, and air to nourish these cells and the ability of our body to metabolize these elements and nourish them through the blood supply to the cells, it is easy for even the layperson to understand why efficient assimilation, elimination, circulation, and relaxation are so important to health and so interdependent.

Assimilation

Let us first consider assimilation. Cayce was far ahead of his time in understanding the importance of nutrition in the cause, cure, and prevention of disease:

> There should be a warning to ALL bodies [with respect to assimilations and eliminations] . . . for would the assimilations and the eliminations be kept nearer NORMAL in the human family, the days might be extended to whatever period as was desired; *for the system is builded by the assimilations of that it takes within,* and is able to bring resuscitation so long as the eliminations do not hinder. [Italics added.] (311-4)

In the field of diet and nutrition, Cayce has proven to be as good a prophet as he was in other more glamorous and publicized ways. Current scientific research in biology and biochemistry have confirmed the essential wisdom of many of his theories. Unfortunately, medical practice still has not caught up with current research.

Cayce was concerned with food and drink, the combinations in which they were ingested, and their chemical interaction in the digestive processes; how and where food was grown and reached the table; cooking methods to preserve nutrients; and the condition of the emotions, mind, and spirit at mealtime. He also understood the differences among diet, nutrition, and assimilation. Diet is an outline of what to eat; nutrition is the study of what happens to food in the body after you swallow it; and assimilation, as he used it, is the individual's capacity to utilize the food and the body's performance of the complicated metabolic processes of digestion and elimination of indigestible material.

While many factors are involved, your nutrition has a great effect on your personality—on whether you are Caspar or Millie Milquetoast, Superman, or Glamour Gloria.

What happens to the food after you swallow it (assimilation) depends to a large extent on the other three ingredients of the Cayce CARE package—circulation, relaxation, and elimination.

Over the years, I have treated many women and some men who developed osteoporosis in later life. Osteoporosis is a disease involving thinning of the bones, which become porous and decalcified. Many of these patients were milk drinkers all their lives and otherwise followed a good diet, but at some point—usually, for women, after menopause—they lost their ability to absorb calcium. In these cases, many have been helped by a calcium-rich diet accompanied by daily exercise and massage. The increased circulation helps them absorb the calcium. Exercise and exercise equivalents like massage and manipulation, which stimulate circulation, play a vital role in our assimilation of food, a subject that we will go into in great detail in later chapters. Cayce even specified certain exercises to be performed to stimulate assimilation (see Chapter 7).

We all recognize how important relaxation is to digestion. If we eat when we are tired, angry, excited, or under stress or other emotion, the most nutritious food will give us indigestion, and if we make a habit of it, ultimately an ulcer. Too much food, eaten too rapidly, has killed many people. I always told my clients at the institute, "An excellent way to become a widow is to serve your husband a good, well-balanced meal, well cooked and attractively served, and then argue with him or nag him while he is eating."

I would tell my many men patrons, "Don't take your business out to lunch with you. It makes a very bad companion and will give you an ulcer. And never take it to dinner—it could give the whole family ulcers or a divorce."

(Q) Why should there be difficulties with the digestion?
(A) A great many things that are easily digested, if taken when the body is angry, will be hard to digest. This doesn't matter whether [one is] a baby or 105. At any age it produces poison to eat when angry, as it does with most everything else attempted to be done under such disturbances. (3172—2)

Elimination

Cayce gave this information:

. . . clear the body as you do the mind of those things that have hindered. *The things that hinder physically are the poor eliminations. Set up better elimina-*

In the field of diet and nutrition, Cayce has proven to be as good a prophet as he was in other more glamorous and publicized ways. Current scientific research in biology and biochemistry have confirmed the essential wisdom of many of his theories. Unfortunately, medical practice still has not caught up with current research.—**H.J.R.**

The Cayce CARE Principle

- Circulation
- Assimilation
- Relaxation
- Elimination

Many people go through life taking chronic constipation casually, little realizing how serious it is and what diseases it can lead to.

—H.J.R.

tions in the body. This is why osteopathy and hydrotherapy come nearer to being the basis of all needed treatments for physical disabilities. [Italics added.] (2524-5)

The word *elimination* is a broad term. We eliminate through the intestines, through the kidneys, skin, and lungs. If you go through a number of the Edgar Cayce physical readings, however, you will find that all these channels of elimination are covered very thoroughly. In this reading he explains, with uncanny medical accuracy and comprehensiveness, how wastes are accumulated in the body:

> . . . each activity, whether the pulsation of the heart or the movement of the hand, the use of the vision, speech, walking, or *what* activity, is USING energy in the body, and this energy leaves what may be called ash—or what we have chosen to term the *drosses*. As the circulation passes through the system, the natural activity is that along the corpuscles' activity; *these [drosses] are thrown into the channels of not only the alimentary canal as the drosses from food taken into the body* . . . the nerve and muscular reaction carried into the blood supply is to be, through the activity of the liver, the lung, thrown off through one or the other of these channels . . . It is thrown off in the breath, through the liver activity—as an excretory and secretive functioning; that is, the secretions are activities from the system and as these are thrown into blood supply here, with the activity of the pancreas, gall duct, spleen, these all . . . throw out drosses, as in the rest of the system. If the eliminating channels coordinate one with another, then these are thrown off in their *regular* way and manner. [Italics added.] (480-8)

Many people go through life taking chronic constipation casually, little realizing how serious it is and what diseases it can lead to. Dr. Max Bircher-Benner, the world-famous pioneer in preventive medicine (probably known to Americans chiefly through his organic Swiss breakfast food), was fond of quoting Professor Elie Metchnikoff of the Pasteur Institute, who called the large intestines "murderer of men."

"Not only are poisons carried often to the blood," Dr. Bircher-Benner points out, "but the mucous membranes, which are a kind of barricade, allow germs to pass. This is the beginning of the accumulation of bacillus coli in kidney and bile ducts . . . Serious operations become necessary, such as the removal of the gall bladder; there is no end to the trouble."[3]

As for remedies, Dr. Bircher-Benner (and I agree) decries the use of laxatives, which has steadily increased since his death in 1939. "The quantities of laxatives which are so largely used by millions of constipated people are by no means harmless. They will never remove the dangers inherent in all constipation: autointoxication and its incurable sequels. The convenience of their use prevents doctors and patients from applying drastic measures that would really cure. Here again we may quote the words of Nietzsche: 'The seeming shortcuts always mean danger to mankind! As soon as glad tidings of this shortcut are heard, mankind leaves its path and the way is lost!'"[4]

Before describing the remedies that Cayce used to treat elimination—none of them "shortcuts," but real corrections—I would like to point out the parallel in philosophy and wisdom of the great doctor Bircher-Benner with Cayce, the simple man who gained his knowledge through his psychic ability. In both cases the men have died, but their work not only lives on but grows more alive and relevant every day.

The great health spa that Dr. Bircher-Benner founded in Switzerland to carry out his theories is more popular today than ever and the greatest celebrities of the world flock to it for rejuvenation.[5] Similarly the Cayce health and medical readings are attracting more doctors, osteopathic physicians, therapists of all kinds, and patients to the clinic in Phoenix and to Virginia Beach. And I believe that we still have a gold mine of health information buried in the readings, from which we have only extracted a few nuggets.

How did Cayce cope with the problem of elimination?

In cases of extreme toxemia he recommended a controlled fast for complete bodily cleansing—either a three-day apple diet, a four-day grape diet, or a five-day orange diet, all of which will be described with instructions in Chapter 11.

Unless contraindicated, we always give daily colonic irrigation with these diets, followed by castor oil packs to improve elimination and stimulate the gallbladder, spleen, and digestive organs. Cayce was a great advocate of colonics:

Take a colonic irrigation occasionally, or have one administered, scientifically. One colonic irrigation will be worth about four to six enemas. (3570-1)

The subject of colonics and enemas will be described and instructions given in Chapter 11.

Cayce was also very sold on all forms of hydrotherapy and massage for elimination as well as circulation:

For the hydrotherapy and massage are preventive as well as curative measures. For the cleansing of the system allows the body-forces themselves to function normally, and thus eliminate poisons, congestions and conditions that would become acute through the body. (257-254)

To promote elimination through the kidneys Cayce advised drinking water—six to eight glasses a day:

. . . there should be more water taken into the system in a more consistent manner, so that the system, especially in the hepatics and kidneys, may function more nominally [normally?], thus producing the correct manner for elimination of drosses in the system, for, as we see, there are many channels of elimination from the system. For this reason, each channel should be kept in that equilibrium or in that balance wherein the condition is not brought to an

Many patients who came to me from Cayce brought directions and instructions for "sweat" and "fume" baths. The fume bath is a light steam or vapor bath, using certain chemicals, oils, or drugs that vaporize easily.—**H.J.R.**

Diet as Therapy
We find that those food values are best that make for the eliminating forces of the body through the alimentary canal; that is, leafy vegetables will make for the better eliminations—also, as a part of the diet (in the mornings or evenings), use either stewed figs, raisins, apricots, or pears occasionally. All of these will be found to be most helpful to the body in these directions. (480-24)

accentuated condition in any *one* of the eliminating functioning conditions; not overtaxing the lungs, not overtaxing the kidneys, not overtaxing the liver, not overtaxing the respiratory system, but all kept in that equal manner . . .

The lack of this water in system creates, then, the excess of those eliminations that should nominally [normally] be cleansed through alimentary canal and through the kidneys, back to the capillary circulation . . . [This brings about, at times,] congestion and weakened condition. (257-11)

Many patients who came to me from Cayce brought directions and instructions for "sweat" and "fume" baths. The fume bath is a light steam or vapor bath, using certain chemicals, oils, or drugs that vaporize easily. We usually give it in an electric cabinet but we will give you directions for home use in Chapter 10. Cayce often recommended that Atomidine ("atomic iodine")[6], witch hazel or eucalyptus, and balsam or pine oils be used to make the vapor.

Elimination through the skin is very important, for the skin normally does about one-twentieth of the work of the kidneys. When the skin elimination is speeded up, it can take care of practically one-tenth of the work that the kidneys usually do for the body. Therefore, stimulation through the skin is important for elimination, for it can help kidney function and prevent kidneys from becoming overloaded. Fume baths are useful not only for the skin but also are used for inhalations, thus aiding elimination through the lungs.

A great deal of elimination takes place through the lungs, by means of deep breathing. When you take a good deep breath, especially if you exhale it completely, forcing the residual air out of the lungs, you bring about a complete change of air. By doing so, you not only drive oxygen down into the lower part of the lungs, but you also help to speed the elimination of carbon dioxide, which is the end product of fatigue. Protein waste is also eliminated through the lungs in the form of carbon dioxide. The bloodstream picks up some of the acid waste and turns it into gas, which is exchanged for oxygen in the lungs. Cayce placed great emphasis on deep breathing and even paralleled some of the breathing techniques used in yoga, incorporating them and combining them with stretching and bending exercises in the yoga tradition (see Chapters 6 and 7).

Circulation

The importance of good circulation is apparent even to the lay person when it is realized that cutting off blood to the brain for only a few minutes results in coma; a few minutes more (six to eight, to be exact) and the brain is permanently damaged. The frightening prevalence of atherosclerosis and its grim companions—stroke, heart attack, senility, and other death-dealing diseases—should warn us all to do everything in our power to maintain good circulation. Circulation and the glucose-carrying properties of the blood can be increased to an amazing extent by exercise, and this is what Cayce frequently prescribed—in fact, he did so in over 1,300 readings. Where serious pathology was present (and one must always bear in mind that many who went to Edgar

Cayce were seriously ill individuals who had been through the medical mill and had been dismissed as hopeless by conventional medical science), he prescribed exercise equivalents—massage, hydrotherapy, osteopathy, chiropractic, and other manipulative therapies that required a professional expert to administer. Here is what he said about a good blood supply—a state that is so dependent on good circulation:

> . . . there is no condition existent in a body that the reflection of same may not be traced in the blood supply, for not only does the blood stream carry the rebuilding forces to the body, it also takes the used forces and eliminates same through their proper channels in the various portions of the system.
>
> (283-2)

. . . [blood is] that criterion through which most any condition existent in the system may be found. (108-2)

Parenthetically, I must point out here that in discussing the blood supply, Cayce scored another bit of precognition: "The day may yet arrive when one may take a drop of blood and diagnose the condition of any physical body." (283-2)

Today, a small sample of blood is fed into computers that analyze and diagnose and return a complete range of tests as Cayce predicted.

In his explanation of his preference for osteopathy, Cayce makes clear how important circulation is:

> As a *system* of treating human ills, osteopathy . . . is more beneficial than most measures that may be given. Why? In any preventative or curative measure, that condition to be produced is to assist the system to gain its normal equilibrium. It is known that each organ receives impulses from other portions of the system by the suggestive forces [sympathetic nervous system] and by circulatory forces [the cerebrospinal system and the blood supply itself]. These course through the system in very close parallel activity in *every* single portion of the body.
>
> Hence stimulating ganglia from which impulses arise—either sympathetically or functionally—must then be helpful in the body gaining an equilibrium. (902-1)

It is interesting to note that when I studied manipulative therapy back in 1916 and 1917, I could have taken my degree in osteopathy, before going on to get my master's and doctorate in physiotherapy. However, osteopathy, which had been founded by a Kansas physician, Dr. Andrew Taylor Still, about 1878 or 1879 was so little thought of that I snubbed that degree and took my examinations and degree as a doctor of massotherapy, which was then accepted by medical doctors. Here again we see Cayce's powers of precognition at work, for today osteopathic medicine is not only recognized in most states, but both former Governor Nelson A. Rockefeller of New York and former President Richard M. Nixon have taken regular treatments from Dr. Kenneth W. Riland, a noted osteopath. Dr. Riland has traveled all over the world with his famous clients and even accompanied the former president to China and the Soviet Union.

Relaxation

. . . nerve force to the body . . . is the attribute to the mental man, same as circulation [is] to the physical [man]. (34-5)

In animals under emotional stress, fats are drawn from body deposits, emptied into the blood and deposited along artery walls. Presumably the same thing happens in man, producing those top killers, atherosclerosis and coronary-artery disease.
—Dr. Hans Selye

The strain between the physical and mental, with the spiritual attributes of the individual, finds expression not only in the brain itself, but in that of the sympathetic [nervous] system for the brain manifestation of soul forces in the body. (4566-1)

Millions of people in the so-called civilized world are suffering from "future shock." The last half-century has tremendously increased the speed, quantity, and range of sensory stimuli that strike the brain. Our senses of sight, hearing, smell, taste, and touch are assaulted by human-made pollution at every waking and sleeping moment. The increase of tension in modern life—the competitive strains in work, worry, and insecurity all adding up to stresses, even in so-called recreation and leisure—are being discussed ad nauseam with appropriate alarm in all the media, and fill the psychiatrists' offices with patients. The consequences can be observed in the increase in mental disease, drug addiction, and alcoholism, and in a population of pill-poppers living on tranquilizers, stimulants, and sleeping pills, swallowed like candy in the search for peace of mind and soul.

Dr. Hans Selye, whose studies on "stress" have won worldwide acceptance and acclaim, attributes a great many physical as well as mental ills to stress: "The body's ductless glands—mainly the pituitary and the adrenals—strive to maintain an unchanging environment inside the body. Let any threat—any stress—be applied and these glands react instantly. The response is exactly the same whether a rat is subjected to extreme fatigue or a boss bawls out his secretary. Blood pressure and blood sugar rise, stomach acid increases, arteries tighten."

In *The Stress of Life*, Dr. Selye calls this the "alarm reaction": "In animals under emotional stress, fats are drawn from body deposits, emptied into the blood and deposited along artery walls. Presumably the same thing happens in man, producing those top killers, atherosclerosis and coronary-artery disease."

Other stress diseases are skin disorders, including psoriasis and eczema; disorders of the respiratory system; sterility; diabetes, colitis, ulcers, and other gastrointestinal troubles; fall of the stomach and intestines; glandular disorders; backache and muscular aches and pains; and arthritis, to name just a few.

Although the beginning of the twentieth century—when Cayce lived and started work—seems by hindsight a quieter and more serene time, his generation did live through two world wars and the worst depression in the history of this country. He was quite sensitive to the effect of stress on people, and according to Gladys Davis Turner never dismissed anything as "just nerves." Each reading contained a detailed analysis of the two nervous systems and a great deal of importance was attributed to their delicate mechanism.

The activity of the mental or soul force of the body may control entirely the whole physical [body] through the action of the balance in the sympathetic system, for the sympathetic nerve system is to the soul and spirit forces as the cerebrospinal is to the physical forces of an entity . . . (5717-3)

Cayce often recommended in nerve conditions that rebuilding properties be carried into the system through vibration rather than through some other means, and to this end he invented (while in trance) two appliances—the wet-cell battery and the impedance device, giving precise directions for their construction:

The vibrations aid in producing that vibration necessary, not only for coordination of the glandular system, but for the ability in the nerve itself to be rejuvenated . . . This works directly upon the glandular system—the thyroid, the adrenals and the thymus, *all* the glands of the body; thus enabling them to react as assimilating forces.

For that is the process or the activity of the glands: to secrete that which enables the body, physically throughout, to *reproduce* itself. (1475-1)

The wet-cell appliance was prescribed in 609 cases for ailments such as arthritis, multiple sclerosis, paralysis, Parkinson's disease, nerve deafness, and incoordination of the nervous systems, where it was necessary for the body to rebuild tissue and restore lost body functions. The impedance device was recommended predominantly as an instrument of relaxation in cases of nervous tension, poor circulation, insomnia, neurasthenia, debilitation, etc.

It would be too complicated and take too much space to explain how they were built and operated, but suffice it to say that the wet-cell battery produced a very low electrical current that could not be felt but could be measured on a meter. It was passed through solutions that might be gold chloride, silver nitrate, Atomidine, or camphor, depending on the individual's requirement and the Cayce prescription. It was attached by plates to the body and the placement of these also varied depending on the individual's needs and complaints. Sometimes specific instructions were given for the placement and sometimes Cayce sent people to me to teach them how to use the device.

The impedance device was a gadget that had two steel poles in a small steel case lined with glass and charcoal which was to be set in ice for thirty minutes and then wired to the wrist and opposite ankle, and it stimulated circulation and relaxed the user—in fact, it usually put the person to sleep immediately. It was especially good for insomnia.

For a time, from 1933 to 1935, the appliances were made at my farm in New Jersey under the supervision of a relative of the Cayce family and then under Robert Ladd. My colleague, Betty Billings, used it with great success on her mother, who was paralyzed and suffered from degeneration of the spinal-cord nerves. Mrs. Billings had spent many years in a wheelchair and she suffered keenly from extremely cold hands and feet. The impedance device seemed to improve her circulation dramatically. "After only two days she was so warm that the family thought Mother had a fever," Miss Billings recalls.

Actually it has been very difficult to make a scientific assessment of the appliances, because we do not have enough clinical data and follow-up on them. My own feeling is that if and when the appliances are tested for research purposes, this should be done in a medically supervised research center, where the patient comes for the treatment and the treatment itself is administered by trained professionals. The answer to this Cayce therapy still lies in the future and I hope some day it will be researched.

While the theory behind this device was little understood when Cayce gave it, great advances have been made in modern times since his death in the use of electricity in healing, and scientists are finding out that there is great heal-

*The impedance device was a gadget that had two steel poles in a small steel case lined with glass and charcoal which was to be set in ice for thirty minutes and then wired to the wrist and opposite ankle, and it stimulated circulation and relaxed the user—in fact, it usually put the person to sleep immediately. It was especially good for insomnia.—***H.J.R.**

Electrosleep devices for insomni-acs have been used and marketed for a long time now in the Soviet Union, Japan, India, and West-ern Europe. Thus there is possibly something to back up the state-ment of many users of the Cayce impedance device that "it puts us to sleep."—**H.J.R.**

ing power in low-wave vibrations. Further research should be done, because it is clear that Cayce anticipated electromedicine as he did so many other medical advances.

Newsweek magazine (November 8, 1971) reported that researchers at the University of Pennsylvania have successfully used direct electrical current to accelerate the rate of healing of a patient with bone fracture.

The *Wall Street Journal* of March 27, 1972, carried a front-page report in depth on a "host of current research projects," many of them conducted with human patients involving the application of electrical signals to the nervous system in attempts to kill pain, to put insomniacs to sleep, and to relieve asthma, ulcers, and high blood pressure. According to this report, electromedicine may soon emerge as a major new approach to many diseases.

At Temple University in Philadelphia, a neurosurgeon has implanted a dorsal "column stimulator," an "electric pain killer," in the back of a salesman incapacitated by a slipped spinal disk. Dr. C. Norman Shealy of the Pain Rehabilitation Center in La Crosse, Wisconsin, and Dr. William Sweet of the Massachusetts General Hospital, who developed the device, now have research tests going on in fifteen medical centers, and they report that 85 percent of all properly selected patients are being helped "to dial their pain away." (Of course, this involves major surgery.)

Electrosleep devices for insomniacs have been used and marketed for a long time now in the Soviet Union, Japan, India, and Western Europe. Thus there is possibly something to back up the statement of many users of the Cayce impedance device that "it puts us to sleep."

Hugh Lynn Cayce told this amusing story about the impedance device and sleep. At the time this happened, it was being made by Marsden Godfrey, who was a close friend of the Cayces in Norfolk, Virginia. "One day Dad got a letter from a woman who had received one of the appliances and said, 'Mr. Cayce, I was sleeping part of the night before I got this appliance that you recommended and now I can't sleep at all. I have gotten so nervous. What should I do?'

"Well, Dad didn't know what to do either, so he suggested she send the appliance back to us, and when it arrived at Marsden's shop they decided the thing to do was to get a reading. They did that and the suggestion came that Godfrey use a magnet to remove the anger that he had built into it.

"As it turned out, Godfrey had had a violent argument with his wife at the time he was building the appliance and the vibration of their anger was picked up by the appliance. They put the magnet over the appliance and then sent it back to the woman. She subsequently reported that it worked beautifully.

"This is an incredible story, but there is a complete record of it. Of course, we could never explain to the woman what was wrong with her appliance because the explanation was harder to accept than the original malfunction."

Dr. William McGarey writes in a *Medical Research Bulletin*[7] on the work of Drs. Wheeler and Wolcott at the University of Missouri, reported in *Neuroelectric Research:*

These men have brought about remarkable regeneration of tissue in healing old chronic ulcerations of many years' standing. In their discussion of their ideas and the direction their work is taking them, they make several very interesting observations. They mention, for instance, that

> Contrary to dogma, constant electric current does not confine its physiological effects solely to the make-and-break points, but, rather is capable of causing subtle, undefined changes during a prolonged period of application.

Cayce suggested weak, electrical currents to be applied to the body in recurrent, hourly periods, and the amperage was not unlike that suggested in the University of Missouri work reported on above. His interpretation of the "subtle, undefined changes" Wheeler mentions are discussed in different terms in the following reading given for a sixty-seven-year-old woman suffering from senility and debilitation. She was told to use a wet-cell battery:

> And as the electrical vibrations are given, know that Life itself—to be sure—is the Creative Force or God, yet its manifestations in man are electrical—or vibratory.
> Know then that the force in nature that is called electrical or electricity is that same force ye worship as Creative or God in action!
> Seeing this, feeling this, knowing this, ye will find that not only does the body become revivified, but *by* the creating in every atom of its being the knowledge of the activity of this Creative Force or Principle as related to spirit, mind, body— all three are renewed. For these are as the trinity in the body, these are as the trinity in the principles of the very life force itself, as the Father, the Son, the Spirit—the Body, the Mind, the Spirit—these are one. One Spirit, One God, One Activity. Then see Him, know Him, in those influences. (1299-1)

Then, in discussing further their ideas, Wheeler and Wolcott point out that the role of biomagnetic effects in work of this kind cannot be truly separated from bioelectrical phenomena. They state further that:

> It is known, for example, that the majority of biologic processes are based on chemical reactions. The chemical properties involved in these reactions result from the arrangement and motion of electrons and atomic nuclei, which are, in turn, determined by electric and magnetic field interactions of elementary particles. As a result, the principles of chemistry are the consequence of the sciences of electrodynamics and quantum physics. In living organisms these effects are seemingly amplified by the semiconductor properties ascribed to biologic structures. It is these effects that now strongly influence our ongoing clinical and basic research.
> We believe that one of man's most human qualities is his preoccupation with the mysteries of conception, growth, disease, aging, and death. Modern technology reveals that some older intuitive hypotheses were remarkably

accurate, especially in . . . areas concerned with electricity and other physical phenomena. Therefore, part of our research is now directed toward the integration of selected products of past and present science, and toward the further development of a theoretical guide for the deeper understanding of living plants and animals.

The power of relaxation to heal has been dramatically emphasized in experiments conducted by Dr. Elmer Green, former head of the Psychophysiology Laboratory in the Research Department of the Menninger Foundation. He has used "biofeedback training" or "autogenic feedback" in training subjects to produce alpha brain waves in a meditative state of quiet relaxation. When in that state, his subjects have been able to cure migraine headaches, control their blood pressure, raise or lower the temperature of a finger, and control the involuntary bodily processes with relaxation.

Cayce frequently recommended meditation for its therapeutic as well as spiritual value. In the following case he advised a twenty–eight–year–old traveling salesman, whose disordered lifestyle resulted in digestive disorders, back trouble, head noises, and other symptoms, in the following manner:

(Q) How can I overcome the nerve strain I'm under at times?
(A) By closing the eyes and meditating from within, so that there arises—through that of the nerve system—that necessary element that makes along the *pineal* (don't forget that this runs from the toes to the crown of the head!) that will quiet the whole nerve forces, making for that—as has been given—as the *true* bread, the true strength of life itself. Quiet, meditation, for a half to a minute, will bring strength—will the body see *physically* this *flowing* out to quiet self, whether walking, standing still, or resting. Well, too, that *oft* when alone, *meditate* in the silence—as the body *has* done. (311-4)

An excellent book on Cayce's approach to meditation is *Meditation: A Step Beyond with Edgar Cayce* by M. E. Penny Baker. There are other excellent works on this subject by Cayce himself and by Elsie Sechrist. Of course, the *Search for God* books by Edgar Cayce published by the A.R.E. Press are musts for any person who wants to pursue the Cayce path to spiritual enlightenment through both prayer and meditation. The difference, I have been told, between prayer and meditation is that with prayer "you talk to God"; in meditation "you listen to God" within.

Drs. Herbert Benson and Robert K. Wallace of Harvard Medical School, who have been running tests on meditators under stringent laboratory conditions, verify the claims of enthusiasts that meditation does indeed lower oxygen consumption, decrease the heart rate, and increase skin resistance, and that other physiological changes occur that bring about complete rest. The general medical acceptance today of the benefits of meditation chalk up another precognitive hit for Cayce, who advocated it long before Americans had ever heard of yoga and other mind– and body–control exercises.

Cayce and I agree on the importance of exercise, especially in the fresh air, as an aid to relaxation. The best way to get rid of destructive emotion is to take a long walk or work off your hostility with some vigorous exercises, such as tennis, hard calisthenics, throwing a medicine ball, or punching a bag. Baths can be very relaxing or stimulating at different temperatures (see Chapter 10). And, of course, massage and manipulation can relax as well as stimulate. Cayce frequently recommended participation in a relaxing sport—not one that gets one frustrated and angry over scores—as well as music, art, theater, or the pursuit of any hobby that brings a sense of peace and fulfillment. Dr. Selye emphasizes the importance of a change of activity to relieve stress.

Above all, Cayce was a strong advocate of balance in all things, as in this letter that he wrote to me on June 3, 1933:

> I certainly do not want to take "no" for the answer regarding your being here [in Virginia Beach] on the 15th, 16th, 17th, or 18th. While I know your farm and your work at this particular time require every bit of your energy, I am sure you preach and demonstrate to those who come to you for relief that "all work and no play makes Jack a dull boy."

. . . budget the time so that there may be a regular period for sustaining the physical being and also for sustaining the mental and spiritual being. As it is necessary for recreation and rest for the physical, so it is necessary that there be recreation and rest for the mental. (3691-1)

Do not overdo same at the expense of the physical or the mental body.

The tendency . . . is to do the whole thing or nothing! Now be rather a middle-ground man once, and see how much better it will be! Work as well as you play— play as well as you work! (279-2)

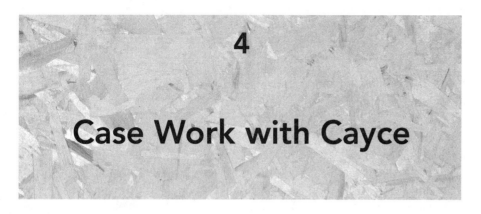

4

Case Work with Cayce

Mrs. W., a woman of about forty, of Hastings-on-Hudson, New York, was told by three specialists that she had to have her gallbladder removed because it was full of stones. In despair she turned to Cayce, who sent her to me with definite instructions: no operation—instead, colonics, drainage massage, and castor oil packs. Gradually, after about six visits, the pain subsided. Fifteen years later I met Mrs. W. and she happily told me that she still had her gallbladder but no stones.

Mrs. W. was only one of the hundreds of men and women referred to me by Cayce for drugless therapy and suffering from a wide spectrum of dis-ease. Following are several cases sent to me by Edgar Cayce that illustrate the accuracy and detail of his readings.

Case 274

Here is a classic example of the overrated value of diagnostic labels and is one of my favorite true stories. A thirty-four-year-old laboratory scientist, [274] wrote to Mr. Cayce in March of 1933, listing all the symptoms and ailments that had plagued him since childhood:

> As a child, jaundice; later erysipelas; then, from time to time, trouble of the following parts: liver, stomach, intestines, prostate, skin, throat, sinus, gums, hair falling rapidly, daily headaches, earaches, rheumatism or rheumatic aches, all of which have led me to a critical state of nervousness, of sexual weakness, of worrying, of depression affecting my mental efficiency (failing memory, restless mind and spiritual development, weak power of concentration) . . .
>
> My weight decreasing all the time. I have followed diets, chiropractic treatments, healers, health foods and what not with little success, or none at all.

Cayce's diagnosis, consisting of one word, covered the entire range of complaints listed in the letter: "TOXEMIA!"

The Readings Covered a Range of Conditions

Cayce did not put medical diagnostic labels on the patients; they came from the doctors who had previously named their conditions. My referrals included the following ailments:

acidosis	edema	obesity
anemia	epilepsy	paralysis
arthritis	endocrine glands	Parkinson's disease
asthenia	(incoordination)	pelvic disorders
angioneurotic edema	facial tics	phlebitis
aftereffects (of colds,	fibroids	poliomyelitis
operations, and	gallbladder trouble	polymyositis
accidents)	gallstones	pregnancy difficulties
back conditions	hay fever	prostatitis
blepharitis	head noises	psoriasis
blood pressure (high	heart trouble	purpura
and low)	hemorrhoids	rheumatism
brain pressure	herpes	sciatica
bronchitis	hyperacidity	scoliosis
catarrh	kidney disorders	shock aftereffects
colic	(stones, malfunc-	sinusitis
colitis	tion, and incoordi-	stricture
congestions (all kinds)	nation)	sycosis barbae
colds	liver	tremors
diabetes	lupus erythematosus	tuberculosis
dermatitis	migraine headache	ulcers
eczema	neurasthenia	and many others

The man was referred to the Reilly Health Service for the following treatment, which cleaned out his system, and his many ailments disappeared. The Cayce prescription for treatment went like this:

Begin, then (under the existent conditions) and prepare this: To a gallon and a half of distilled water, add—*in the order given*—the following:

Wild Cherry Bark	1 ounce
Sarsaparilla Root	1 ounce
Yellow Dock Root	½ ounce
Burdock Root	½ ounce
Indian Turnip	10 grains
Mayweed	¼ ounce
Dogwood Bark	¼ ounce
Prickly Ash Bark	¼ ounce

Reduce this by slow boiling, until that strained off equals to 1 quart.

Cut 2 drams Balsam of Tolu into 3 ounces of grain alcohol and add to the solution, as a preservative and to stimulate the activity.

The dose of this would be half a teaspoonful 4 times each day, before each meal and before retiring.

After this has been taken for 3 to 5 days we will then find it necessary to use high enemas for the alleviating of distresses through the alimentary canal. These high enemas (which should be taken as colonic irrigations) should be taken (after the 5 days) at first, 2 the first week—see?—one, we would say, on Monday, the other on Saturday—see?

Then skip 2 weeks before 1 or more would be taken, but continuing to take the medicinal properties throughout this period—see?

Then we would begin with the thorough *manipulations,* or the massage that would follow sweat baths which—preferably—would be medicated, see? or, as this:

Before the body goes into the cabinet for the sweat bath, massage *into* the body those properties of olive oil, tincture of myrrh and sassafras oil—equal parts (heating the olive oil and adding the other ingredients). This would be massaged *all over* the body, and especially along the cerebro-spinal system, through the shoulders over the head, and all portions of the body.

Do not raise the temperature of the cabinet other than that which creates the general perspiration, see?

The bath would be followed by a general rubdown, with the stimulation of those oils or properties combined in this manner:

Russian White Oil	1 pint
Rub Alcohol	1 pint
Witch Hazel	½ pint

This would be massaged thoroughly into all portions of the body, arms, neck, torso, legs, feet, hands—all over the body, see?

Then there should be the general rubdown following same.

These sweat baths would only be taken once a week, in the manner outlined; continuing, of course, with the medicinal properties throughout the period.

Follow this, then, for this time—and after the fifth of such treatments we would give further instructions in this direction.

During this period there shall be, of course—and *especially* when the baths are taken, or the sweats—*plenty* of water taken at all times! Drink at least six to ten glasses of water each day! This doesn't mean beer, or other things—but *water!* If other drinks are desired they would not be harmful—if taken with *meals,* but not at other times!

The diet—let this be as an outline, which may be altered or changed to suit the tastes; but this may be used as a general outline:

Mornings—first a little tea or coffee may be taken; a very small quantity, as a demitasse.

Twenty to thirty minutes later there may be taken citrus fruits or stewed fruits, or cereals; but when fruits or cereals are taken do not take the citrus fruit juices. Citrus fruit juices are *preferable* to the other two.

Following this there may be taken small cakes or dried toast (rice cakes, buckwheat cakes, or the like) with a little honey—see?

Or, occasionally, there may be taken an egg with some very *crisp* bacon. Alter these, to be sure.

This meal should be taken by seven-thirty or eight o'clock in the morning, or before.

By nine-thirty or ten o'clock take a malted milk, with *egg* in same—see? To it may be added a few drops of rum or of spirits frumenti, but not too much; just sufficient to take away the taste of the egg. Do not include the white of the egg in this, only the yolk, see?

Noons—preferably meat *juices,* or vegetable juices. With these there may be altered from time to time the whole wheat, rye, or any of the whole wheat crackers, wafers, or the like. Not those that carry white bread, nor white crackers, with *this* particular meal—especially.

Evenings—the whole vegetable dinners, which would include meats; and, at least three times each week, include among the meats those of calf's liver or of tripe—and pig knuckle. These may be altered, you see. At least three times each week these should be among, or on, the menu—in the evenings. (274-2)

Case 274 wrote to Mr. Cayce on July 8, 1933, that he was delighted and enthusiastic with his reading: "I am keeping up the suggestions, adding some light exercises under the care of Dr. Reilly. I'll be glad to let you know how I am getting along."

In the same reading he asked: "Are any laxatives necessary; if so, what special ones are best for me?"

Mr. Cayce answered, "We are preparing the system so that these will not be necessary. The laxatives will be within those properties taken as the general tonic, or for the toning of the system; with the food values and the enemas, for the *time being* . . . Let's do this first, and then we may ask more questions." (274-2)

I should like to comment on two aspects of this reading. Note that in the diet, Cayce specified that in adding the egg to the malted milk only the yolk be included—not the white. This is quite remarkable, for at the time the reading was given in 1933, research had not yet established that *raw* egg white destroys biotin, an important component of vitamin B, and this in turn affects the entire B chain of nutrition.

In answering the question on laxatives, there is a decided parallel between the Cayce reply and the opinions of Dr. Bircher–Benner, which I quoted in the previous chapter, and general medical opinion today, which decries the use of laxatives as a palliative rather than a curative measure.

We had our failures, too. Most of the patients, as I have mentioned, had tried orthodox methods without finding relief; thus we could not expect 100 percent success. In some cases, the individuals would not take the advice given in the readings or persist with the therapy.

Case 1684

I recall one case in particular. Mr. Cayce had referred the president of a large advertising agency, a man of great wealth with large property holdings in Florida, which were to make him even wealthier—the kind of person who is used to giving orders, not taking them.

He had developed dangerously high blood pressure, and the reading warned that "unless there *are* some measures taken to make the corrections, they may of a sudden cease to perform their functioning . . . or the pressure that is a part of the disturbing conditions upon the arteries may become so intense that the very walls may give way or allow seepages."

This was the remedy that Cayce proposed:

Not taking drugs, but rather activities . . . *in the open* . . . walking, golfing, riding—all such should be at some time a part of the activity; or as combined with the hydrotherapy . . . and massage, also the handball, the electric horse, the bicycle, as a part of the exercise.

In the diet keep away from fried foods, or large quantities of fats that are not easily assimilated. (1684-1)

I believe that most cardiac specialists would agree that the advice was sound. We gave him oxygen baths and light massage, as Cayce instructed.

For years he had been having very heavy massage and manipulation. He came to me four or five times and got light massage for relaxing. He protested, "I am used to having a good heavy vigorous massage. I miss that. If I can't get it here, I will have to stop coming."

I told him, "You can't get it here because I don't want to be a pallbearer, in fact, at the beginning I would only give you the hydrotherapy and light massage. You came in with a Cayce reading that warns you about that. What's the use of wasting time if you are going to seek advice and not follow it? I guess you'd better go back to your routine, but I don't know how long you are going to last."

He did go back to heavy massage elsewhere and he dropped dead of a stroke three or four months later.

Sometimes even those nearest and dearest to Cayce could not benefit from his guidance and remedies. This was so with his dearest friend, David Kahn, who probably was the source of more Cayce clients than almost any other single person. Despite his great faith in the Cayce treatments and the fact that the Kahn family and friends consulted the seer religiously, when David had a reading for what turned out to be an obstruction in the intestine, Cayce recommended surgery.

"Is there no other way?" Kahn asked.

"Yes, but you would not do what is necessary," Cayce responded while in trance.

I should like to comment on two aspects of this reading. Note that in the diet, Cayce specified that in adding the egg to the malted milk only the yolk be included—not the white. This is quite remarkable, for at the time the reading was given in 1933, research had not yet established that raw egg white destroys biotin, an important component of vitamin B, and this in turn affects the entire B chain of nutrition.

—H.J.R.

Sometimes even those nearest and dearest to Cayce could not benefit from his guidance and remedies.—**H.J.R.**

I treated Tom for years, including the time he spent writing There Is a River. *I often told him, "Tom, I doubt whether you would be the author you are if you were not forced to sit down," teasing him about his restlessness. When he took therapy regularly, he showed some improvement, and after a year and a half of three-times-a-week treatment I had his arms loosened up so that he could shave and feed himself.*—**H.J.R.**

Another example was the case of Cayce biographer Thomas Sugrue. Tom had been a classmate at college of Cayce's eldest son, Hugh Lynn, and was regarded as another member of the family. Yet, when he developed crippling arthritis, the Cayce magic was no match for the dashing young journalist's Irish impatience. The treatments Cayce recommended were long and arduous, and in addition to daily manipulation, exercise, and hydrotherapy, included the wet-cell appliance, which sends low-voltage electrical impulses into the system. Cayce said that the wet-cell battery could take seven years to completely change the system.

Instead, Sugrue tried the new and experimental high-fever therapy, which burned out all his nerve endings, leaving him paralyzed and immobile for the rest of his life. Later he tried cortisone treatments, and the prolonged use of the drug undermined his kidneys.

I treated Tom for years, including the time he spent writing *There Is a River.* I often told him, "Tom, I doubt whether you would be the author you are if you were not forced to sit down," teasing him about his restlessness. When he took therapy regularly, he showed some improvement, and after a year and a half of three-times-a-week treatment I had his arms loosened up so that he could shave and feed himself.

I didn't like him to miss treatments, and when he received an assignment from *Harper* to go to Israel, I said I would train someone to continue the treatments on the trip. The publisher was sending one of their young editors along with Tom, and I taught Tom's companion-to-be to give the massage and manipulation and passive exercises that kept him from stiffening up again. Unfortunately, the young editor was a diabetic and on the way over he went into shock on the ship and had to be sent home. Tom went on alone. In an incredible adventure, he had himself pushed in his wheelchair between the Israeli and Arab armies to arrange his interviews. The Arabs thought the wheelchaired man was a booby trap and it's a wonder that they didn't shoot him on sight. Despite his handicap, the trip was very successful and resulted in his book *Watch for the Morning,* the story of Israel's struggle to achieve independence. Tom had previously written *Starling of the White House* and *Stranger in the Earth.*

Cayce had sent Tom to live in Clearwater Beach, Florida, where the gentle sea water seemed to help him. Tom tried cobra venom—a treatment quite new then—to no avail, and he chafed with impatience. Although he was productive, Tom wanted, more than anything else, to be free of the wheelchair. He heard of a new operation, experimental at that time, which entailed implanting a new hip. I was fearful that he could not stand the operation, for his kidneys had been weakened by the cortisone therapy. But I said nothing, because I did not want to put any negative thoughts into his head. Tragically, his kidneys did not function properly after the operation and he died of uremic poisoning. He was only forty-six years old.

Case 1511

This involved a twenty-eight-year-old woman suffering from a tilted stomach and incoordination of the nervous systems, who had recently had a miscarriage. She apparently also had a bad "allergy," which affected her head, nose, throat, and sinuses. In her reading on January 5, 1932, Cayce prescribed osteopathic adjustments and general dietary advice.

In 1938, the woman's mother wrote to Cayce that her daughter had been suffering for four years from "what we call hay fever for want of a better name."

However, unlike seasonal hay fever, her allergy persisted throughout the year and plagued her with early-morning attacks of sneezing that sometimes lasted for hours. She had been sent from one doctor to another, without relief.

Cayce replied that she should "go to Dr. Reilly for a few treatments . . . [he] has had several cases that he has handled and I'm sure he would give . . . what she is looking for, real help." The reading recommended osteopathic treatments, massage, cleansing, and a changed diet. The woman spent two weeks under my care. I treated her through elimination and the Cayce diet—and her mother again wrote Cayce, "My daughter was much benefited by following the instructions . . . given her [on April 10, 1938]."

She improved enough to carry through a successful pregnancy.

Sometimes there is no follow-up on patients, which is frustrating and makes it difficult to keep research records. In the thirties, a man, suffering from what had been diagnosed as leukemia, came to us about half a dozen times for treatment with ultraviolet light through green glass. He kept improving with each treatment despite everyone's skepticism about the value of the therapy, but as soon as he felt better, he left for places unknown.

Sometimes there is no follow-up on patients, which is frustrating and makes it difficult to keep research records. In the thirties, a man, suffering from what had been diagnosed as leukemia, came to us about half a dozen times for treatment with ultraviolet light through green glass. He kept improving with each treatment despite everyone's skepticism about the value of the therapy, but as soon as he felt better, he left for places unknown.—**H.J.R.**

Case 4873

Mrs. B.B.S. wrote to Cayce, "I have bleeding piles . . . Also I have been told by surgeons . . . that I broke a little piece off the bone of my right ankle . . . five months ago, thinking it was only a bad sprain; I find it has knitted onto a nerve."

For piles, Cayce said, "a very helpful exercise . . . would be the bending exercise with the hands raised high above the head, bending forward to bring the hands as close to the floor as possible. Do this for two or three minutes morning and evening." (4873-1)

He also gave detailed directions for preparation of the massage mixture—tincture of myrrh and olive oil—to be used in treating the injured ankle.

To relieve the tendency for contraction where there has been the disturbance of the structural portions in the right lower portion of the femur, or the shin bone, use a massage with equal parts tincture of myrrh and olive oil. This will cause the absorbing of the greater amount of the tissue that has been thickened by nature attempting to adjust itself under the unusual conditions. With this it will be found unnecessary for the removal by operation. (4873-1)

In a follow-up letter, Cayce repeated directions given in the first reading:

The activities of the massage should be once each day. Heat the myrrh and add the oil. This doesn't mean boiling, but heat and mix together for this will make for more of an ointment (while the other would remain in a different solution entirely). (4873-1)

Case 3558

Cayce had heartwarming success with children. Bobby F. N. was a five-year-old boy suffering from incoordination of the nervous system. This showed up in crossed eyes, defective hearing, retarded growth, insomnia, and extreme susceptibility to colds and coughs and bouts of chorea (also known as St. Vitus's dance).

Cayce recommended osteopathic treatments, hot baths followed by cocoa-butter massages, and a controlled diet consisting of whole grains, plenty of silicone, and plenty of vegetables.

The mother brought the boy to me and expressed anxiety over the financial strain on the family. I told her I would treat the lad twice a week and charge only five dollars for one treatment. She was so concerned about following Cayce's instructions to the letter that she wrote to him to check out my offer with him. Mr. Cayce replied in the following letter, dated August 16, 1944:

> I think it is most fortunate that you can get such wonderful cooperation from Dr. Reilly under the circumstances. I feel sure that your son needs the treatments, and if it is a hardship on you and your husband, you are most fortunate in getting these treatments and of course I will agree most heartily, if Dr. Reilly is willing to carry on, we will do the best we can to help.
>
> It is wonderful that he has shown improvement, and I do hope that with following through, you will get real, real results . . .

The treatments continued for one year and eight months. Improvement was gradual but steady. Years later his mother replied to a follow-up questionnaire sent by Gladys Davis Turner: "The first and very important result of the treatments right from the start was his ability to fall asleep at a reasonable hour for a child of that age [7:00 or 7:30 P.M.]. Before that it was 11 or 12 P.M. before he was asleep although he was in bed at the usual time.

"His eyes are perfect now. Vision is perfect, too . . . his hearing is completely normal.

"[He] is now a senior in high school, is an excellent scholar, plays basketball on the team, is 6 feet 4 inches tall and weighs 185 pounds. He's in good health except that he catches cold easily. If I said more . . . it would sound like boasting."

Case 448

One of my earliest cases from Cayce involved a man in his middle forties whose left side was paralyzed. Cayce described the cause of the condition this way:

> As to the *nerve system,* here we find the seat or the cause of the disorders that exist . . . In times back . . . when under great physical and mental strain, the body lost control of the activity of the muscular forces by a cell's reaction in

the blood stream to brain's activity, but lodgment in the right portion in the brachial centers caused the *left* portion of the body to become desensitized to its normal activity. Hence the paresis, or paralysis . . . began in first the upper, then the lower portions and the whole left side has suffered under the strain. (448-1)

Cayce's treatments prescribed the use of the radioactive appliance, manipulation, and passive exercise. The massage mixture was bizarre: one–half gallon of straight gasoline, one–half ounce of camphor gum, one ounce of oil of cedar, and one–fourth ounce of oil of mustard. But by this time I was so impressed with Cayce's remarkable abilities that I followed all his instructions to the letter.

To one of the questions put to him at the reading, Cayce replied as follows:

> Be faithful; be patient, keep in the attitude of expectancy. Do not make the applications as rote, but rather with the expectancy and the knowledge that with the applications is coming relief from the source of *all* supply—God.
>
> (448-1)

Mr. B., the patient, wrote to Mr. Cayce, "Dr. H.J. Reilly showed my wife just the places to massage . . . Although I cannot see any change, I feel it has improved my condition and in the end will work as stated." Six weeks later Mr. B. wrote again: "There have been many minor signs of improvement."

Case 1030

Another paralysis case was that of a twenty–eight–year–old woman with paralysis of an arm. An operation had been advised by a number of doctors. When the woman questioned Cayce about this, he replied in a reading for her that an operation would be harmful rather than helpful.

The treatment for which he referred her to my institute was as follows:

> . . . general massage . . . over the whole of the system, *specifically* in those areas along the cerebrospinal system, *following* some heat (not too great a heat) from a sweat and a rubdown.
>
> The general massage, following the sweat and shower and rubdown would be with oils, preferably for *this* body combined in this way and manner: to 4 ounces of Russian white oil as the base, add—*in the order named*—
> * 1 ounce olive oil;
> * 1 ounce oil of wintergreen;
> * 1/2 ounce of compound tincture benzoin; and
> * 1 ounce of rosewater.
>
> Then would follow a rubdown with grain alcohol (not rubbing alcohol, but *grain* alcohol). This would be along the cerebrospinal system and over the abdomen, and especially across the diaphragm area.
>
> Such a treatment would be given about four times each week for three weeks, then rest from same for a week and a half to two weeks. Then it would begin again. (1030-1)

Later the woman wrote Cayce, "When Dr. Reilly gave me my first therapy, he was sure (he told me later) that I was going to have a nervous breakdown. Now I'm so much better that he doesn't fear that any more."—**H.J.R.**

The above cycle of treatments was to be alternated during the rest periods with diathermy treatments given twice each week:

> We would have the diathermy treatments; that is, the electrical forces to make for the stimulation to the body itself in the areas as indicated by the massages.
> And we should find, by the second or third period or round of these treatments, these conditions will be almost entirely eliminated. (1030-1)

Case 5288

A forty-three-year-old woman wrote Cayce in desperation after three hospitals and many doctors had been unable to diagnose her "baffling disease." One doctor had said that the symptoms came nearer to resembling disseminated lupus erythematosus than anything else and the only treatment was rest and keeping out of the sun. She had been doing that for months, she said, and the disfiguring skin eruption was still all over her face and neck.

Cayce correctly described all the symptoms she was experiencing along with the rash—nausea, headache, weakness, poor elimination, and disturbances with the sensory organs.

The trouble, Cayce said, came from a breakdown of the normal channels of elimination, and poisons that should be eliminated through the respiratory system or kidneys were coming out though the skin.

Treatment included application of shortwave electrical appliances to empty the gallbladder and stimulate central forces in the kidneys, and twice-a-week gentle, relaxing massage. She should take internally once a day three to five drops of elixir of lactated pepsin in half a teaspoon of milk of bismuth in one-half to three-quarters of a glass of water.

Later the woman wrote Cayce, "When Dr. Reilly gave me my first therapy, he was sure (he told me later) that I was going to have a nervous breakdown. Now I'm so much better that he doesn't fear that any more."

There was a large element of emotional and mental strain in her illness. Her husband had been in prison and she had made great sacrifices to get him home. Then, when he returned, he was mentally ill.

"The worry, the strain, the constant watching resulted, I am sure, in my becoming ill with what the doctors considered an unknown disease. Not one doctor of all those that treated me had ever asked me if I were worried or had any problems," she wrote.

Today, medical practitioners would immediately look for psychosomatic causes in a skin disease, but not that many years ago. But Cayce was treating the whole person, not symptoms, and already preaching the doctrine that "healing begins in the mind."

Case 3040

Mrs. "EMA," Garden City, New York, was a fifty-two-year-old woman who had had so many operations, there seemed scarcely anything left of her normal bodily functions. Over the years, to try to relieve severe low spinal pain, frequent attacks of indigestion, and severe headaches, doctors had removed her appendix and right ovary, gallbladder, the fundus of the uterus (due to large tumors), and her tonsils. She had undergone operations for suspension of the uterus and suspension of the right kidney, and a septum operation, but all to no avail. She was getting weaker and losing weight; had become allergic to many foods and materials, which caused intense pain and pressure over the eyes, lasting for days; had lost fingernails; and had suffered arthritic condition of the joints, recurring spastic colitis, indigestion, distension, and gallbladder–like attacks.

The treatment that Cayce prescribed was as follows:

First, then:

As demonstrated first at Reilly's, we would use the ultra-violet with green light projected—doing this about twice each week—for twenty minutes. This would necessitate that the light be at least several feet from the body—eight to ten feet, but the green light only about eighteen or twenty inches from the body, and this moved to include the area from the throat and lungs to the end of the spine—that is, so as to cover the whole spinal area during the twenty minutes, see? (For this particular body, do not use the ultra-violet *without* the green glass between same and the body.)

Once each week, immediately following such a light treatment, have a thorough rubdown with an equal combination of Peanut Oil and Witch Hazel. It is best that these be mixed just as they are to be used on the body, or just before they are to be used, see? Massage this combination into the spine, all the body will absorb. And then, not too roughly, but gently, knead this into the activities of the alimentary canal—that is, by the gentle kneading so that there will be an aid to the general peristaltic movement through the alimentary canal. Hence knead the abdomen, you see, which would include the stomach itself—gently.

Then, be careful as to diets. Do not mix too much starches, ever. There should be taken considerable of the fruit juices, and do include in same a great deal of watercress and beets and beet tops.

These as we find, if they are followed, would be the better forces for this body.

For the general glandular system—we would take internally one drop of Atomidine in half a glass of water each morning for five days—before the morning meal, you see. Then leave it off five days. Then take again. Keep repeating this procedure for at least several months. (3040-I)

This case was interesting because it was one where I could not follow the language of the directions given in the reading without some danger to the patient, and I used my own judgment in interpreting and modifying the reading. When the patient wrote to Cayce, Cayce sustained my judgment and the exchange of letters illustrates the growth of mutual confidence between us.

The difference involved was the timing and the placement of the lights. Mrs. "EMA" [3040] wrote this to Cayce:

I have been to Dr. H.J. Reilly for the massage with the peanut oil and witch hazel, but he says that it would be impossible to have the light 8 to 10 feet away from the body and the green glass close (18 to 20 inches) from the body. He put it about two feet away with the green glass directly in front of the ultra-violet light. What do you think—will this be just as beneficial [?]

Dr. Reilly mentioned that usually it is suggested how many times one should have these treatments. In your reading, it is suggested that I have the light 20 minutes, but I received it only 3 minutes as he was afraid it might burn my skin . . .

Mr. Cayce responded on June 22, 1943:

Have yours of the 18th. I do hope you will be able to obtain the Atomidine. As for the light treatment let Dr. Reilly direct that. If he is not able to have light far away he is correct in the short time, for a burn would be very bad and that long a period close would burn, am sure. Feel sure you will get the benefits, but do keep trying to find the Atomidine.

On January 27, 1959, Mrs. "EMA," in a letter to Gladys Davis, wrote, "Many years ago I had a reading in which I had been advised to use 1 drop of Atomidine for 5 days and then not take same for 5 days. It was marvelous the way it cleared up the bad condition of my fingers and fingernails. Have taken it periodically whenever I seemed to need it."

On April 9, 1968, she wrote again to Mrs. Davis, asking her help in procuring Atomidine: "Many years ago I had a reading in which Atomidine was recommended . . . This was most beneficial for my eyes." Now apparently, Mrs. "EMA" was still living and functioning. ***Atomidine should never be taken except under a doctor's supervision.*** It is quite safe and beneficial if used externally.

Case 3274

L.R., Bayshore, L.I., was a fifty–year–old woman who had four strokes before asking Cayce for help. She had no remaining paralysis but was suffering from diabetes, high blood pressure, menopause problems, extreme edema, pain in her left arm, phlebitis in her left leg, and film over her eyes.

In her letter to Cayce she said doctors did not agree on what was causing her pain and so far no one had been able to help: "The medical doctors said the pain in my arm was a coronary condition of the heart. Another said it was either neuritis or a form of rheumatism. So far no doctor has been able to reduce the swelling nor the intense pain. I sit up a good part of each night. Cannot lie down as the pain gets worse . . . have to take sedatives for the pain."

Cayce outlined a diet for the diabetes, with plenty of Jerusalem artichokes (a natural source of insulin), and colonics with salt and soda, followed with Glyco–Thymoline to correct the "prolapsus in the colon" that Cayce found as one of the core causes of her illnesses, and "gentle massage or osteopathic relaxing of those tensions in the third cervical and through the upper dorsal [which] should reduce the blood pressure to near normal in six to eight weeks, and we should find the rest of the body responding—the disturbances through the alimentary canal, kidneys, bladder . . . will be overcome by the purifying of the system." (3274-1)

We did succeed in bringing down her blood pressure from 230 to 150. She wrote Cayce, "No medical doctor has been able to do this." We were also able to reduce the edema and the phlebitis. Pain continued in her arm. Since we did not see the patient after some months we cannot report on her progress, but in years ahead we were to have great success over and over again reducing high blood pressure with Cayce therapy and controlling edema with massage.

Case 3032

Cayce's success in curing psoriasis has received considerable publicity because this disfiguring skin disorder is usually considered incurable by the medical establishment. Although I personally make it a rule not to treat patients with skin disorders (largely because of the prejudices of the clientele in a large institute), I did accept one case and did considerable research on the Cayce approach to this puzzling and baffling aberration.

Although there has never been an officially designated medical cause of psoriasis, Cayce's theory was that it stemmed from the thinning of the intestinal walls and that usually a lack of lymph circulation through the alimentary canal is involved.

In Case 5016 a twenty-five-year-old woman asked: "Is psoriasis always from the same cause?" Cayce replied:

> No, but it is more often from the lack of proper coordination in the eliminating systems. At times the pressures may be in those areas disturbing the equilibrium between the heart and liver, or between heart and lungs. But it is always caused by a condition of lack of lymph circulation through alimentary canal and by absorption of such activities through the body.

The treatment embodied all the principles of the Cayce CARE program—and used all the modalities discussed in this book: diet, elimination by internal cleansing and the use of special herb teas and waters, osteopathy, hydrotherapy, stimulation of circulation through massage, and in some cases electrotherapy.

The following excerpt from Case 5016-1 is fairly typical of the cases of psoriasis and the recommended treatment.

A distracted mother wrote in early 1944: "I have a daughter who has had a skin condition for some years. No physician so far has helped her and not we either. We are licensed naturopathic physicians . . . I would like you to please give her a reading soon, so that I can follow your instructions during summer months and she will be cured by September before going back to college. Her trouble was so bad that she had to stop her school work . . . " Cayce replied:

*Cayce outlined a diet for the diabetes, with plenty of Jerusalem artichokes (a natural source of insulin), and colonics with salt and soda, followed with Glyco-Thymoline to correct the "prolapsus in the colon" that Cayce found as one of the core causes of her illnesses . . .—**H.J.R.***

*We did succeed in bringing down her blood pressure from 230 to 150. She wrote Cayce, "No medical doctor has been able to do this." We were also able to reduce the edema and the phlebitis.—**H.J.R.***

Cayce's success in curing psoriasis has received considerable publicity because this disfiguring skin disorder is usually considered incurable by the medical establishment. Although I personally make it a rule not to treat patients with skin disorders (largely because of the prejudices of the clientele in a large institute), I did accept one case and did considerable research on the Cayce approach to this puzzling and baffling aberration.

*—**H.J.R.***

While there is the thinning of the walls of the small intestines and there are poisons absorbed through the system that find expression in the attempt to eliminate through superficial circulation, we find that there are pressures also existing in the areas of the 6th, 7th dorsal that upset the coordination of circulation through the kidneys and the liver. These contribute to the condition, causing the abrasions which occur as red splotches or spots at times, and at other times there is the forming of blackheads apparently, or black points on the abrasions, you see, or in the abrasion areas.

. . . Then, in making applications for corrections here we would first through osteopathic adjustments correct those subluxations upon the right side at the 6th and 7th dorsal and then coordinate the 3rd cervical, the 9th dorsal and through the lumbar, with such corrections. There should only be required about twelve adjustments, if properly made, coordinating the muscular forces in areas where the sympathetic and cerebrospinal systems coordinate in the greater measure.

We would have these twice each week for the first six of the treatments. The others may be spread out longer.

After the first six osteopathic adjustments have been made (not before), begin taking internally a compound prepared in this manner:

Sulfur	1 tablespoonful
Rochelle Salts	1 tablespoonful
Cream of Tartar	1 tablespoonful

Mix these very thoroughly, as with mortar and pestle. Take a teaspoonful every morning, either in water or dry on tongue, until the whole quantity has been taken.

Then begin with Yellow Saffron Tea, a pinch of the American Saffron in a cup of boiling water—or put in a cup and fill with boiling water, allow to stand for thirty minutes, strain and drink, each evening when ready to retire.

Occasionally, about two to three times a week, drink elm water—a pinch of ground elm (between thumb and forefinger) in a cup, filled with warm water (not boiling water). Stir thoroughly and let set for 30 minutes. Drink this preferably of morning rather than at the period when the Saffron is taken.

Eliminate fats, sweets and pastries from the diet. Do have a great deal of fruits and vegetables.

The thinning of the intestinal walls of the intestinal tract would permit toxins to leak into the circulatory system and into the lymph flow of the skin. Then when the blood and lymph systems are unable to eliminate these poisons, the inflammatory skin reaction known as psoriasis is produced. A study of the Cayce readings indicates that the initial cause that triggers this malfunction could be emotional, nervous, improper functioning of the kidneys, liver, and any or all portions of the elimination systems of the body, so that the emunctory systems are unable to eliminate toxins as fast as they are absorbed; thus, the circulation becomes overburdened and the toxins find their way into the lymph flow of the skin in sufficient quantity to produce congestion and the inflamed reaction which is characteristic of the red, scaly, itchy patches on the skin.

In other readings, Cayce emphasized the need to alkalinize the system through diet:

> In the diet we would keep rather to the non-acid foods, that is, keeping rather the *alkaline-reacting foods;* letting one meal each day consist of *raw vegetables wholly.* With such there may be used an oil or salad dressing. (745-1)

In the diet we would keep rather to the non-acid foods, that is, keeping rather the alkaline-reacting foods; letting one meal each day consist of raw vegetables wholly. With such there may be used an oil or salad dressing. (745-1)

The herbal remedies such as the yellow saffron, mullein, and chamomile teas were designed to promote healing of the lesions in the intestinal wall.

Elimination was stressed through colonics, enemas, the Rochelle salts–sulfur-cream of tartar compound and the occasional use of vegetable laxatives such as a fusion of senna pods, saline laxatives, mineral laxatives such as milk of magnesia and, of course, the ever-present castor oil packs.

However, in general, Cayce preferred to stimulate elimination through the use of proper foods.

Massage with olive oil and peanut oil, and hydrotherapy—particularly fume baths—were encouraged to aid circulation and elimination, and the use of violet ray was recommended in some cases.

For external relief and treatment of the lesions he frequently mentioned the application of Resinol and Cuticura ointments.

> In the evenings when the bath is taken, we would apply Cuticura Ointment followed by Resinol—both applied, you see, one following the other. Apply these especially over the areas of the abrasions. Do not apply it in the hair, but around the edges—and on all other portions of the body where the skin is irritated. If we rid the condition from the system, then these disturbances should be eliminated. (2455-2)

I had my first psoriasis case from Cayce in the early 1940s. This woman had suffered from psoriasis for twenty-two years, since she was a girl of thirteen. Usually Cayce recommended a series of osteopathic treatments for patients suffering from psoriasis before starting the other therapies. For some reason, in this case he started her with colonics prepared with "a level teaspoonful of table salt and half a teaspoonful of baking soda to each half gallon of water . . . In the last rinse water, put a tablespoonful of Glyco-Thymoline as the intestinal antiseptic." (3032-1) The rest of the treatment included showers, thorough rubdown, saffron tea, milk of bismuth, and elixir of lactated pepsin in water. After three months of this, violet-ray treatments began.

The patient wrote to Mr. Cayce: "I went to see Dr. Reilly . . . already I feel less fatigued and considerably more ease of body. It is wonderful! . . .

"There are times when words fall so short of our feelings and in wanting to thank you, Mr. Cayce, I find this is one of those times."

I often find my own feelings echoing those of this grateful patient. As the years go by, I never cease to get a thrill when I learn of another Cayce-inspired cure and receive this reassurance that his work and his goodness live on. It doesn't matter whether this occurs in my own practice or elsewhere.

Last summer, my co-author, Mrs. Brod, returned from a statewide meeting of the New Jersey Society of Psychical Research, thrilled over an interview she had had with the parents of a young girl who had been cured of psoriasis by the Cayce treatment just described. The girl and her family were transfigured by this extraordinary experience.

The child had developed psoriasis at about eight years of age and had been covered from head to foot with lesions of the disease. She was taken from doctor to doctor without relief or improvement. She was so disfigured that it was not possible for her to lead any sort of normal life. Her performance in school and her personality were affected, and her life and her family's life were completely dominated by this tragedy.

One day, when the girl was about eleven years of age, her parents were opening a new bookstore in a New Jersey town when a woman rushed in and asked for a copy of a book she had heard discussed on a radio talk show the night before. She did not know the name of the book, nor much about it, except that it contained a cure for psoriasis given by a psychic named "Casey." The alerted parents traced the book down. It was *Edgar Cayce—The Sleeping Prophet* by Jess Stearn. They wrote to the A.R.E. immediately, joined the organization, and got the file on psoriasis. It took a lot of hard and persistent effort for them to find an osteopath who would follow the treatment, and they did not know how to procure the herb teas—particularly the mullein—which is an ordinary roadside wild weed. However, they persisted and were more than rewarded when after the first series of osteopathic treatments no new lesions appeared. After the Rochelle salts combination was taken, the lesions faded from red to pale pink, and within three months the child, now a beautiful teenager, was cured and has never had a reoccurrence of the disease. (See source of supply at the back of this book for help in procuring the necessary herbs and Rochelle salts mixture.)

Case 2924

Another patient who received relief from a longstanding condition was E.D.G., a fifty-year-old man who lived in Massachusetts. He had suffered ill effects from working in very cold conditions, making hive equipment in the dozen years he had been a beekeeper.

"I think I eventually got a permanent condition of cold in my back and this seemed to have considerable influence on my bearing," he wrote. Besides back-aches, he suffered affected heart action, breathlessness, headaches, and loss of memory. A medical doctor's treatments had taken care of the trouble for two years, but the man was apprehensive that it might return, so he appealed to Cayce.

Cayce prescribed hydrotherapy treatments, including mild, dry heat, then a fume bath, preferably with witch hazel, followed by thorough massage and at least two colonics two weeks apart.

The patient came to New York so that I could get him started on the treatment and help him to locate a fume-bath device for home use. His wife wrote Cayce, "We are now carrying on the treatment the best we can at home, and we are delighted with the good results even in this short time."

Case 3286

The case of [3286], in which I was only slightly involved, is a dramatic example of the importance of patience and persistence in achieving one of Cayce's miracles. It took twelve years to come about. This is the story:

The young woman, severely handicapped by poliomyelitis since infancy, was twenty-five when she received her first Cayce reading (October 11, 1943). He prescribed the daily use of the wet-cell appliance carrying gold, silver, and iodine alternately. This was to be followed by massage with a combination of these oils: Russian white oil, oil of pine needles, olive oil, peanut oil, and sassafras oil. "Be persistent, be consistent, be instant [insistent] in prayer," he told her.

Cayce sent her to me for instruction in the use of the appliance and massage. I saw her twice.

In November 1955, Cayce's devoted secretary, Gladys Davis Turner, was making a survey of cases. She wrote Miss [3286] asking for a report on her experience with the wet-cell appliance.

The reply came back: the wet-cell appliance and massage had been used faithfully for over a year, but "as to the overall results of the reading . . . I have absolutely nothing to say one way or the other. If you have information on others who were helped from the results of polio, I would be most happy to know about it."

Gladys wrote back relating the story on file of a thirty-year-old woman [2778] whose legs had been paralyzed by polio when she was a year old. She used huge, clumsy braces and crutches in order to walk. Her reading from Mr. Cayce prescribed the use of the wet-cell appliance, massage, and heat cabinet. In three months' time she could stand alone and in two years' time she was using braces from the knees down and a cane to help her keep her balance. "On the basis of her progress alone I would certainly encourage you to take out your readings again and follow the treatments," Gladys wrote Miss [3286].

In time, [3286] replied that as a result of Gladys's letter she had bought an appliance and supplies and started in again, this time with her mother and sister giving the massage. "I'm getting straighter, I'm told. My spine seems to be straightening out . . . I believe I can raise my left arm higher than I did . . . I have gotten up out of the wheelchair . . . from a slightly lower height than usual."

Case 2966

To a fifty-five-year-old woman suffering from uterine tumors and insomnia, Cayce recommended twenty to twenty-five hydrotherapy treatments under my direction:

Gladys wrote back relating the story on file [2778] of a thirty-year-old woman whose legs had been paralyzed by polio when she was a year old. She used huge, clumsy braces and crutches in order to walk. Her reading from Mr. Cayce prescribed the use of the wet-cell appliance, massage, and heat cabinet. In three months' time she could stand alone and in two years' time she was using braces from the knees down and a cane to help her keep her balance.—H.J.R.

Hydrotherapy should include the steam baths . . . fumes, alternately, one time Atomidine and the next time Witch Hazel . . . followed with a thorough rubdown . . . following the hot and cold water spray . . . For the thorough massage we would use a combination of 2 parts Russian White Oil . . . to one Pine Oil. And use the regular Pine Oil, not pitch, not pine needles, but Pine Wood Oil, see?

Have sufficient exercise in the open each day. Walking is the better exercise, besides that which will be attained in taking the hydrotherapy and massage. (2966-1)

He said the tumors did not necessarily require an operation since they "as we find, are lymph accumulations." Two months after the April 1943 reading she wrote, "The operation is now behind me . . . My recovery has been excellent. I attribute this in goodly measure to the seventeen treatments that I managed to get in at Reilly's."

Case 2774

A forty–eight–year–old woman suffering from glaucoma was being given Cayce treatments by both Dr. George N. Coulter, an osteopathic physician, and by me in hydrotherapy and massage.

Dr. Coulter wrote, after [2774] returned to him from my physiotherapy treatments, that "her improvement was astounding. Her pain was greatly relieved and she acted like a different person."

Case 1841

A fifty–three–year–old woman was advised by a surgeon to have a major operation (hysterectomy) immediately. David Kahn prevailed on his friend to consult Cayce for a reading first before surgery.

The reading, in March 1939, diagnosed her disorder as "glandular disturbances [which] . . . produce the forming of lymph globules . . . in the pelvic or digestive areas . . . " No operation was necessary if she followed the treatments, Cayce said, which included two periods of Atomidine taken for seven days, "for cleaning the system," omitted for five days and taken again for seven. After the Atomidine the patient was to start with a pine–oil fume bath and full massage and some osteopathic adjustment for six or eight weeks. He also recommended pelvic douches and a diet that avoided fried food, white bread, potatoes, and red meat.

Mr. Kahn wrote Cayce a few months later, "You no doubt have heard from Mrs. [1841] that she is 100 percent improved and cured . . . "

The woman never had that "urgent" operation.

Case 4020

A thirty–eight–year–old New York policeman, suffering for years from a painful back (sacroiliac joint) and pain down the leg, had sought relief from many doctors, hospitals, and even the Mayo Clinic.

After his return from Rochester, Minnesota, he wrote an anguished letter to

Cayce. "At the Mayo Clinic," he said, "doctors say that my symptoms and certain laboratory tests all point to one condition but the X-rays show nothing . . . They told me to return in six months or a year if the condition became aggravated.

" . . . I am married and have a nineteen–month–old daughter. I write to you now in more of a desperate mood than a despairing one. My job is in jeopardy. There is a strong possibility that I may be retired on an annual pension of only a thousand dollars. That is entirely inadequate to support my family . . .

"Mr. Cayce, would you employ your marvelous gift in order to help me?"

Cayce would and did. He recommended a hydrotherapy treatment once a week to include short wave and fume baths and thorough massage.

Cayce wrote him:

Do by all means see Dr. Reilly himself or Mr. Eigen and show them the reading. They are quite familiar with the work and have handled quite a number of people with marvelous results. I am sure if you don't already know them, you will find them most accommodating and very lovely men to deal with.

Part II

Your Home Health and Beauty Spa

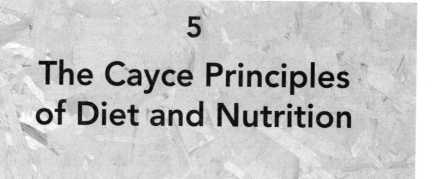

5
The Cayce Principles of Diet and Nutrition

The wagon drew up before the office of Dr. Wesley Ketchum in Hopkinsville, Kentucky. It was filled with straw and on it lay the inert figure of Homer Jenkins, a man who worked in the local brickyard.

"He just keeled over in a faint," the wagon driver told the doctor. "One minute he was working . . . the next . . . there he was stretched out on the ground. We thought down at the brickyard that you had better look at him."

Dr. Ketchum did look and listen with his stethoscope. He probed and thumped and questioned and tested in his best diagnostic manner. He could find nothing organically wrong with the man. It was a puzzle.

Dr. Ketchum placed a call to his friend and secret colleague, Edgar Cayce, and told him about the case. "I'd like you to see what you can do with it," he told Cayce. "I can't figure out what's wrong with him."

Cayce loosened his collar and tie, lay down, stretched out, and received instructions from Dr. Ketchum as he slipped into trance.

"The body is suffering from malnutrition," he told Dr. Ketchum, "too much hominy, hog, and grits." The treatment consisted of changing the diet and adding lots of greens such as turnip greens.

Reporting the case in *Edgar Cayce–The Sleeping Prophet*, Jess Stearn wrote, "It was the first case of pellagra that Ketchum had ever seen, and it helped him diagnose and treat other cases which had been puzzling local doctors.

"Again Cayce did not get the credit. One of the Hopkinsville doctors whose patients had been helped by the Cayce 'turnip green diet' read a paper on his diagnosis of pellagra to the Kentucky Medical Society, but he didn't mention Cayce, or Ketchum for that matter."[1]

In 1924 the Cayces were living in Dayton, Ohio, and were invited by David Kahn's future bride, Lucille Kahn (they coincidentally both bore the same last name), to attend a performance at a local theater of *Sancho Panza*, in which she was playing opposite Otis Skinner. They did and enjoyed the play.

"Now you have seen our show, I would like to attend yours," Miss Kahn told

Lucille watched Cayce slip into a trance state and was startled to hear him diagnose the condition of the baby. But when he came to the treatment and advised the parents to put the child on an "all-banana diet," she was appalled.
                                    —H.J.R.

Over the years, I have had the privilege and joy of witnessing many equally remarkable recoveries emanating from Cayce's principles of diet combined with other therapies. For example, the Cayce apple and grape diets have produced many improvements . . .
                                    —H.J.R.

Mr. Cayce. She had been hearing about the great Edgar Cayce ever since she had first met David, who was one of the "Judge's" closest friends and greatest fans, but Lucille had never seen him do a reading. The Cayces were delighted to extend the hospitality of their home to the charming, petite actress who had captivated David's heart.

The reading was for an infant dying of malnutrition because he could keep nothing in his stomach.

Lucille watched Cayce slip into a trance state and was startled to hear him diagnose the condition of the baby. But when he came to the treatment and advised the parents to put the child on an "all-banana diet," she was appalled.

"Are you really going to tell the parents to feed that baby bananas?" she asked incredulously. In those days, it must be remembered, bananas were regarded as a very hard-to-digest food—absolutely poisonous for infants.

"I was so worried about that baby that even after we left Dayton to continue our tour, I had to inquire some time later about the child and how it was getting along," Lucille confessed. "I was surprised when I was told that the parents had reported a great improvement."

Of course today, the all-banana diet pioneered by Dr. Valentine Haas is a standard medical treatment for celiac children.

Over the years, I have had the privilege and joy of witnessing many equally remarkable recoveries emanating from Cayce's principles of diet combined with other therapies. For example, the Cayce apple and grape diets have produced many improvements equal in drama to the two stories I have just related. However, since these are used in conjunction with the colonics, castor oil packs, and a variety of hydrotherapy techniques for a total recycling program, I will discuss them in Chapter 11, "Internal Cleansing." In this present chapter we will learn some of Cayce's ideas on what he termed "normal diet"—that which would be good for everybody—and the best way to use food to build better health.

Of course, it is not possible to go into every detail of Cayce's wisdom on nutrition and diet in this chapter. However, we hope to give you the highlights in this overview of the Cayce diet and nutrition ideas.

 . . . what we think and what we eat . . . *make* what we *are*; physically and mentally. (288-38)

This simple sentence uttered by Edgar Cayce many years ago crystallizes much of the wisdom and knowledge that has been accumulated in the last sixty years through chemical, biological, nutritional, and medical research. At the time the few words embodied some pretty revolutionary concepts. It must be remembered that Cayce treated pellagra with turnip greens around 1909–10. Little was known and far less was medically accepted of the relationship of food to health, and the word *psychosomatic* had not yet been invented.

Recommended Books on Diet and Nutrition

Visionary Medicine by Simone Gabbay (A.R.E. Press, 2003).

Nourishing the Body Temple: Edgar Cayce's Approach to Nutrition by Simone Gabbay (A.R.E. Press, 1999).

Edgar Cayce on Healing Foods for Body, Mind, and Soul (revised edition) by William A. McGarey, M.D. (A.R.E. Press, 2002).

Edgar Cayce Encyclopedia of Healing by Reba Ann Karp (Warner Books, 1999).

An Edgar Cayce Encyclopedia of Foods for Health and Healing compiled by Brett Bolton (A.R.E. Press, 1998).

Physician's Reference Notebook by William A. McGarey, M.D. (A.R.E. Press, 1991).

Edgar Cayce's Diet and Recipe Guide by the Editors of A.R.E. Press (A.R.E. Press, 1991).

An Edgar Cayce Home Medicine Guide by Gladys Davis Turner (A.R.E. Press, 1983).

Edgar Cayce on Diet and Health by Anne Read, Carol Ilstrup, and Margaret Gammon (Warner Books, 1969).

In correlating nutrition with health and diet deficiency with disease, Cayce was far ahead of his time. The importance and validity of his nutritional theories unfold and gain with every passing year as laboratory research confirms the information he was receiving from his "Higher Sources." It is significant to me that nearly every one of the over 9,000 physical readings contain advice and guidance on diet as part of the overall therapy.

Cayce considered diet such an important feature of therapy that he frequently outlined entire menus for a patient. It is important to keep in mind when drawing general principles from readings that specific diets were recommended for an individual with highly individualized nutritional needs and pathology. Then, too, diet was only a part of the general therapy, which might include osteopathy, massage, exercise, hydrotherapy, electrotherapy—and, as he himself indicated, these could bring about changes in the nutritive value and degree of assimilation in the body. Here again, Cayce was anticipating the most advanced research in nutrition.

In correlating nutrition with health and diet deficiency with disease, Cayce was far ahead of his time. The importance and validity of his nutritional theories unfold and gain with every passing year as laboratory research confirms the information he was receiving from his "Higher Sources." It is significant to me that nearly every one of the over 9,000 physical readings contain advice and guidance on diet as part of the overall therapy.

—H.J.R.

From the practical standpoint we cannot neglect the facts of biochemical individuality. Of necessity, for reasons involving inheritance, every individual has nutritional needs which differ quantitatively with respect to each separate nutrient from his neighbors. Some individuals in the case of specific nutrients may need from two to ten times as much as others.—**Dr. Roger J. Williams**

The most basic weapons in the fight against disease are those most ignored by modern medicine: the numerous nutrients that the cells of our bodies need. If our body cells are ailing—as they must be in disease—the chances are excellent that it is because they are being inadequately provisioned . . .

—Dr. Roger J. Williams

Dr. Roger Williams, author of *Biochemical Individuality* and *You Are Extraordinary*, has done extensive research to prove that human beings are not carbon copies of each other. As he writes in another one of his books: "From the practical standpoint we cannot neglect the facts of biochemical individuality. Of necessity, for reasons involving inheritance, every individual has nutritional needs which differ quantitatively with respect to each separate nutrient from his neighbors. Some individuals in the case of specific nutrients may need from two to ten times as much as others."[2]

Dr. Williams also says, "Speaking of the onset of disease, I propose the motto, 'If in doubt, try nutrition first.'"[3]

"The most basic weapons in the fight against disease are those most ignored by modern medicine: the numerous nutrients that the cells of our bodies need. If our body cells are ailing—as they must be in disease—the chances are excellent that it is because they are being inadequately provisioned . . . Cellular malnutrition, which is the basis of all malnutrition, is probably *at the roots of ten times as many disease conditions as the clinically defined deficiency diseases* listed above.

"*Since every cell and tissue in our bodies needs nourishment, and each part may be subject to the nutrition which is faulty in varying degrees, the number of human ills that may arise because of imperfect nutrition is very large.* Faulty cellular nutrition of one type or another may be a basic cause of most of the noninfective diseases—diseases that are at present poorly controlled by medical science."[4]

"Clinical nutrition is not even taught in most medical schools," N. S. Scrimshaw of M.I.T. reminds us, "and not really adequately done in any of them."

"It is only to be expected that this woefully weak clinical nutrition education," Dr. W.H. Sebrell of Columbia points out, "should produce in the words of Dr. Frederick Stare of Harvard, 'physicians who are not well trained to identify malnutrition except for gross under- and overweight and this anyone can do.'"

Criticisms and dire warnings about the dangerous state of nutrition in this country are not coming solely from food faddists or the nonestablishment doctors who have been preaching the gospel of pure, unadulterated, natural food for over a century. Perhaps their almost fanatical zeal and the conflicting claims of one cult over another have undermined the credibility of their ideas. In any case, their combined efforts have been no match for the giant corporate manufacturers with their multimillion-dollar advertising budgets.

We spend $125 billion a year for food. Are we then the best-fed nation in the world? We have the greatest supermarkets, brimming over with the widest variety of foods available to any peoples of the world. Does this mean we are well nourished?

In December 1972 Senator Richard S. Schweiker (R.-Pa.) chaired a series of hearings of the Senate Select Committee on Nutrition and Human Needs. After listening to the testimony of leading doctors and nutritionists, he charged that "Americans have turned into a nation of nutritional illiterates."

Dr. Jean Mayer of Harvard University, French-born nutrition adviser to presidents of the United States, told the committee that America's white-bleached dough products would not even be called bread in his native land.

Dr. Mayer called for the public and private sectors together to spend at least $100 million a year on public-nutrition education. He pointed out that such an expenditure would be only one percent of total food expenditures and would be much less than is now spent on food advertising which, he said, "too often represents a massive threat to nutrition education."

Dr. Mayer and the other expert witnesses testified further that "there is extensive malnutrition in America today. Only some of it is attributable to poverty (although if food costs continue to rise at present rates, this will be a growing problem). Even among those who can afford to eat properly, there is unhealthy overuse of fats, sugar and alcohol."

Advertising has "glorified out of proportion to their nutritional contribution, some processed foods," said Robert Choate, a noted critic of "empty-calorie" products and their merchandising.

The hearings charged that children have been converted through television ads into "in-the-home hucksters of junk food."

Dr. George Christakis of the Mount Sinai School of Medicine in New York called for nutrition education in schools and for doctors, dentists, and other health professionals.

The food industry was exhorted to live up to the responsibility to produce nutritious foods.

Manufacturers are more concerned with the "shelf life" of food than its ability to nourish "human life," and the thousands of chemical additives to "dead food" that will not sustain the life of bug, weevil, or rat cannot be expected to sustain the life and energy needs of human beings.

In another session before the committee, Dr. Abraham E. Nizel of the Tufts University School of Dental Medicine and a group of other dental and nutritional experts testified that tooth decay is the country's most prevalent disease. The toll in yearly dental bills alone is $5 billion and the biggest single cause of the problem is sugar.

Dr. George M. Briggs, professor of nutrition at the University of California, executive editor of the *Journal of Nutrition Education*, and an adviser to the National Institutes of Health, said, "The typical American diet is a national disaster. If I fed it to pigs or cows, without addition of vitamins and other supplements, I could wipe out the livestock industry." Dr. Briggs, who has served since 1962 as a member of the Research Advisory Committee of the National Livestock and Meat Board and was a delegate to a White House Conference on Food, Nutrition, and Health, added the following on the American diet:

"It shows up in many different ways—hunger and outright nutrient deficiencies, high incidences of anemia, increased infections, underweight and overweight, severe dental problems, reduced growth, needless problems in pregnancy, and with infants, shortened life spans, and even in behavioral and mental problems in children and older people.

"Diabetes, heart disease, alcoholism, absenteeism, and other great problems are related in part to poor nutrition. This is very costly to our nation, costing us as much as $30 billion per year—nearly 50 percent of our total health care costs."

Dr. Briggs cited U.S. Department of Agriculture statistics showing that in 1970 we ate more "empty-calorie foods than traditional foods or those containing more of the proper nutrients." Empty-calorie foods include:

- table sugar
- fats and oils, such as margarine
- shortening, lard, butter
- cooking and salad oils
- white flour
- corn sugar
- milled rice

Consumption of such foods totaled 264 pounds for each person.

In the same period, the USDA figures show the average American consumed only 259 pounds of the twelve types of food that could help keep one physically sound, mentally alert, sober, disciplined, and hard at work, according to Dr. Briggs.

"These twelve traditional food types include meat, poultry, fish, eggs, milk, cheese, ice cream, all fruits, potatoes and other vegetables, whole cereals, and peanuts and beans that contain the forty-five essential nutrients. Instead today over half the calories we eat come from sugar, fat, and white flour," Dr. Briggs concluded.

Miss Betty Billings, in a speech delivered at a "Week of Attunement" lecture in Virginia Beach in August 1973, pointed out that "Cayce almost always advocated whole grain breads and cereals." In reading 826-5, which was given in July 1935, Cayce said:

> . . . as is generally known and seen, in each land there is that prepared—as it were—by nature or the creative forces—to make for the body-development of those within that particular environ. And in how many lands is *wheat?* It is the greater portion, and should be the greater portion of that which is to supply not only body-heat but body-development for an equal balance in the mental influences upon the physical forces of man in his activity . . . (826-5)

> Take whole grain cereals or citrus fruit juices though not at the same meal.
> (1523-17)

> Rolled or crushed or cracked whole wheat . . . not cooked too long so as to destroy the whole vitamin force . . . this will add to the body the proper proportions of iron, silicon, and the vitamins necessary to build up the blood supply that makes for resistance in the system. (840-1)

He considered whole grains so important that if a person had ulcers of the stomach or anywhere in the digestive tract, they were told to cook the whole grains and then strain them; or if the condition was not too acute he would have the cereals cooked, uncovered, for a long period of time; this, he said, would break down the cellulose (or fiber). One can assume that it was very necessary for the person for whom the following reading was made to have adequate bulk in the diet:

> In the matter of diet . . . [eat] more of the well balanced that carry more of
> the irons in their reaction—as will be found in those of all the vegetable forces
> . . . [take] those of the wheat or oaten, preferably in the whole grain rolled—
> not soured before rolled, but rolled—and made in a gruel. *These* would be
> well for the body, but should be *well* cooked . . . at least three to four hours—
> in double boilers *preferably not* aluminum. (505-1)

Some time ago a very distinguished British surgeon and cancer researcher, Dr. Denis T. Burkitt, addressed a group of 200 doctors in Los Angeles. He stunned them by saying: "During my twenty years of practicing surgery in Africa I did not encounter a single case of inflammation of the colon known as diverticulitis, no appendicitis, no obesity, no diabetes, no hernias, no colonic polyps. These conditions commonly seen in the United States are almost unknown among rural African natives. This is no freak of geography either, because Africans who live in cities and eat Westernized diets soon begin to have as much bowel pathology as do the Englishmen who live in these cities and who eat a strictly Western diet."

Dr. Burkitt found that Africans eat a diet high in roughage. They grind their grain between two stones without removing any part of it. I might add here that if they were familiar with the composition of the different stones used they could add many minerals to their diet at the same time. For example: the late Dr. Michael Walsh found that the Mexican Indians had a calcium intake equivalent to eight quarts of milk daily. This calcium was obtained from the soft limestone used in grinding corn for tortillas. To get back to the research, it also said, "There is no refined sugar in the diet of these rural Africans." He believes in the possibility that very large amounts of refined carbohydrates which Westerners eat play a crucial role in triggering cancer of the colon.

An article in the *Wall Street Journal* on October 26, 1973, headlined the importance of this research: "New Research Indicates the Diet Is a Villain in U.S.'s No. 1 Cancer." The subhead read: "Beef, Fat, and Refined Flour Cited in Different Studies of Colon–Rectal Sickness."

The article goes on to say that the "malignancy [colon–rectal cancer] is already the most common major cancer in the U.S., topping in incidence both lung cancer and breast cancer, and is second only to lung cancer in the number of cancer deaths.

"If preliminary estimates are correct, 99,350 Americans will develop the malignancy next year, up from 86,000 new cases five years ago. Deaths from the disease will reach 48,000, up from 44,400 five years ago. This is due to more than the population increase. The colon–rectal cancer rate has climbed to 46.8 per 100,000 Americans from 43 per 100,000 in 1968 and 39.3 per 100,000 in 1947."

The British authority Dr. John Yudkin, who now heads the Department of Nutrition at London's St. Elizabeth's Hospital, warns that refined sugar is as dangerous and addictive in humans as heroin. Americans are now eating a

The British authority Dr. John Yudkin, who now heads the Department of Nutrition at London's St. Elizabeth's Hospital, warns that refined sugar is as dangerous and addictive in humans as heroin. Americans are now eating a yearly average of 120 pounds of sugar and sweeteners a year, a frightening increase in sugar consumption.—H.J.R.

Sugar, along with fats, is now conceded to be a prime factor and suspect in the higher levels of cholesterol and triglycerides found in the more industrialized nations, leading to cardiovascular disease and diabetes.—H.J.R.

Do not use bacon or fats in cooking and vegetables . . . (303-11)

Beware of white potatoes, fats of any kind, and greases. No meat save fish, fowl or lamb. No fried foods. No white bread. Not too much of pastries. (2415-2)

. . . keep away from too much grease or too much of any foods cooked in quantities of grease—whether . . . of hog, sheep, beef or fowl . . . But rather use the lean portions and those [meats] that will make for body-building forces . . . (303-11)

yearly average of 120 pounds of sugar and sweeteners a year, a frightening increase in sugar consumption.

Dr. Yudkin says, "Biologically, man has not had time to change into a sugar eater. Refined sugar was introduced into man's diet only 200 years ago. But the average American consumes about twenty-five times as much sugar in two weeks as our ancestors ate (in fruit and other natural forms) in a year."

Sugar, along with fats, is now conceded to be a prime factor and suspect in the higher levels of cholesterol and triglycerides found in the more industrialized nations, leading to cardiovascular disease and diabetes.

The U.S. Department of Agriculture says that per capita sugar consumption had jumped from 77.4 pounds in 1911 to 101.6 pounds in 1971 and is higher today (125 pounds annually). Moreover, the experts testifying before the Schweiker committee reported that Americans today are shaking only half as many spoonfuls of sugar on their food but are eating even more sugar, mainly in "fun foods" such as soft drinks, chewing gum, candy, pastries, ice cream, and sugared cereals. But even more dangerous, these scientists point out, is that sugar may be found in the most unlikely foods, such as canned corn, beef hash, and ketchup—in nearly all canned and prepared foods. The amount of sugar used in processed foods has increased 50 percent in just one four-year period in the 1960s.

Dr. Mayer told the Senate committee that the promotion of high-sugar cereals, snacks, and soft drinks also "may be a factor in increasing the likelihood of diabetes in genetically vulnerable subjects." He pointed out that many persons are eating sugar unknowingly, including diabetics and persons who would develop it by eating sugar.

Cayce's dietary "dos and don'ts" would have won approval from the American Heart Association, the cancer researchers, the low-fat-cholesterol advocates, and the entire medical establishment alarmed about excessive fats, sugars, and starches in the American diet. He also cautioned against the use of too much red meat, ham, rare steak, or roasts.

Edgar Cayce on Meats

The meats taken would be preferably fish, fowl and lamb . . . Breakfast bacon, crisp, may be taken occasionally. (1710-4))

. . . no raw meat, and very little ever of hog meat. Only bacon. Do not use bacon or fats in cooking the vegetables . . . (303-11)

Plenty of fowl, but prepared in such a way that more of the bone structure itself is [used] . . . [so that the assimilation of] calcium through the system is obtained . . . Chew chicken necks, then. Chew the bones of the thigh. [Also] have the marrow of beef . . . (1523-8)

Keep away from heavy foods. Use those which are body-building [such] as beef juice, beef broth, liver, fish, lamb, all may be taken but never fried foods.

(5269-1)

Any wild game is preferable even to other meats, if these are prepared properly. [In cooking] rabbit—be sure the tendon in both left legs is removed for this is the part which might cause a fever. (2514-4)

At least once or twice a week the sea foods may be taken, especially clams, oysters, shrimp, or lobsters . . . (275-24)

Beware of all fried foods. No fried potatoes, fried meats, fried steaks, fried fish or anything of that nature. (926-1)

. . . those that are boiled, roasted or broiled are much better than any fried meats of any kind.

(416-6)

Cayce's readings reveal his preference for the natural sugars from fruits, honey, raw sugar, and sometimes he even recommended saccharin in specific cases. When and if table sugar was used, Cayce preferred beet to cane sugar. Although we do not know the reason for this latter preference, we can speculate that it may have been because he was precognitively aware that in the future there would be a new importance attached to the presence of zinc in the diet and sugar beets are high in zinc.

Edgar Cayce on Starches and Sugars

Beware in the diet of sugars, starches, or those that produce same. (119-1)

Do not combine *any* of starches with any quantities of sweets. Do not take food values that cause great quantity of alcoholic reaction. This does not refer to alcohol, but sweets *and* certain starches produce a character of fermentation that is alcoholic that makes for excess of fatty portions for the body. (1125-2)

For in all bodies, the less activities there are in physical exercise or manual activity, the greater should be the alkaline-reacting foods taken. Energies or activities may burn acids, but those who lead the sedentary life or the non-active life can't go on sweets or too much starches—but these should be well-balanced. (798-1)

(Q) What is particularly wrong with my diet?
(A) The tendencies for too much starches, pastries, white bread should be almost entirely eliminated . . . They are not very good for the body in any form.
(416-18)

Do be careful that there are no quantities of pastries, pies, or candies, especially chocolate, or carbonated waters. These, as we find, will be hard on the body.
(5218-1)

(Q) Suggest best sugars for body.
(A) Beet sugars are the better for *all,* or the cane sugars that are not clarified.
(1131-2)

Keep the body from too much sweets—though [have] *sufficient* of sweets to form sufficient alcohol for the system; that is, the kind of sweets, rather than sweets. Grape sugars—hence jellies, or [sweets] of that nature—are well. Chocolates that are *plain,* not those of any brand that carry corn starches should be taken—or not those that carry too much of the cane sugar. Grape sugar, or beet sugars, or [sweets] of that nature, may be taken. (487-11)

Saccharin may be used. Brown sugar is not harmful. The *better* would be to use beet sugar for sweetening. (307-6)

(Q) What type of sweets may be eaten by the body?
(A) Honey, especially in the honeycomb; or preserves made with *beet* rather than cane sugar. Not too great a quantity of any of these, of course, but the forces in sweets to make for the proper activity through the action of the gastric flows *are* as necessary as body-building [elements]; for these become body-building in making for the proper fermentation (if it may be called so) in the digestive activities. Hence two or three times a week the honey upon the bread or the food values would furnish that necessary in the whole system. (808-3)

Cayce was a strong advocate of fresh vegetables:

Include in the diet often raw vegetables prepared in various ways, not merely as a salad but scraped or grated and combined with gelatin. (3445-1)

Do have often raw vegetables such as celery, lettuce, carrots and watercress. Prepare these often . . . with gelatin. Do not throw away the juices when grating or preparing any of these, but include the juices also in the gelatin for the greater amount of the vitamins necessary. (3413-1)

[Do not eat] too much of potatoes, but more of the skins. Plenty of onions, raw as well as cooked. Plenty of [the legumes] . . . peas, beans and the like.
(480-52)

Detailed instructions are given for the preparation of vegetables to conserve their vitamins.

Have at least one meal each day that includes a quantity of raw vegetables, such as cabbage, lettuce, celery, carrots, onions and the like. Tomatoes may be used in their season.
   Do have plenty of vegetables [grown] above the ground; at least three of these to one below the ground. Have at least one leafy vegetable to every one of the pod vegetables taken. (2602-1)

Normal diet . . . use at least three vegetables that grow above the ground to one that grows under the ground. (3373-1)

. . . vegetables will build gray matter faster than will meat or sweets!
(Q)   Would it be well for me to eat vegetables such as corn, tomatoes, and the like?
(A)   Corn and tomatoes are excellent. More of the vitamins are obtained in tomatoes [vine-ripened] than in any other *one* growing vegetable! (900-386)

Cayce was right on the beam with the best thinking in modern nutrition in his awareness of the role of the vitamins, minerals, and enzymes in building and maintaining health. He seldom prescribed them in the form of supplements except in severe illness, pregnancy, or other special situations; he much preferred that people obtain them from foods—especially fresh, sun–ripened, raw fruits and vegetables, whole grain cereals and breads, lean meats, fish and poultry, and dairy products.
   Let us examine some of his comments on vitamins and minerals. It is interesting to note that he frequently used food as medicine and he usually prescribed a wide variety of foods, which most nutritional experts suggest is our best protection, since all nutrients form a "chain of life" and need each other in order to do their work.

Include in the diet often raw vegetables prepared in various ways, not merely as a salad but scraped or grated and combined with gelatin. (3445-1)

Do have often raw vegetables such as celery, lettuce, carrots and watercress. Prepare these often . . . with gelatin. Do not throw away the juices when grating or preparing any of these, but include the juices also in the gelatin for the greater amount of the vitamins necessary. (3413-1)

(Q)   What relation do the vitamins bear to the glands? Give specific vitamins affecting specific glands.

(A)   You want a book written on these!

They are food for same. Vitamins are that from which the glands take those necessary influences to supply the energies to enable the varied organs of the body to reproduce themselves. Would it ever be considered that your toenails would be reproduced by the same [gland] as would supply the breast, the head, or the face? Or that the cuticle would be supplied from the same source as would supply the organ of the heart itself? These [building substances] are taken from glands that control the assimilated foods, and hence the necessary elements or vitamins in same to supply the various forces for enabling each organ, each functioning of the body to carry on in its creative or generative forces, see?

These begin with A—that supplies portions to the nerves, to bone, to the brain force itself; not all of [the supply to] this [area], but this is a part of [the function of] A.

B and B$_1$ supply the ability of the energies, or the moving forces of the nerve and of the white blood supply, as well as the white nerve energy in the nerve force itself, the brain for itself, and the ability of the sympathetic or involuntary reflexes through the body. Now this includes all [such energy], whether you are wiggling your toes or your ears or batting your eye, or what! In these [B vitamins] we have that supplying to the chyle that ability for it to control the influence of fats, which is necessary (and this body has never had enough of it!) to carry on the reproducing of the oils that prevent the tenseness in the joints or that prevent the joints from becoming atrophied or dry, or to creak. At times the body has had some creaks!

In C we find that which supplies the necessary influences to the flexes of every nature throughout the body, whether of a muscular or tendon nature, or a heart reaction, or a kidney contraction, or the liver contraction, or the opening or shutting of your mouth, the batting of the eye, or the supplying of the saliva and the muscular forces in face. These are all supplied by C—not that it is the only supply, but a part of same. It is that from which the [necessary supplies for] structural portions of the body are [taken and] stored, and drawn upon when it becomes necessary. And when . . . [lack of C] becomes detrimental, or there is a deficiency of same—which has been for this body; it is necessary to supply same in such proportions as to aid; else the conditions become such that there are the bad eliminations from the incoordination of the excretory functioning of the alimentary canal, as well as the heart, liver and lungs, through the expelling of those forces that are a part of the structural portion of the body.

G [B$_2$ in modern usage] supplies the general energies, or the sympathetic forces, of the body itself.

These are the principles. (2072-9)

In the matter of the diet throughout the periods [of convalescence] we would constantly add more and more of vitamin B$_1$, in every form in which it may be taken: in the bread, the cereals, the types of vegetables that may be prepared for the body, the fruits, etc. Be sure that there is sufficient each day of B₁ for the adding of the vital energies. These vitamins are not stored in the body as are A, D and G, but it is necessary to add these daily. All of those fruits and vegetables, then, that are yellow in color should be taken; oranges, lemons, grapefruit, yellow squash, yellow corn, yellow peaches—all of these and such as these; beets—but all of the vegetables cooked in their own juices, and the body eating the juices with same. (2529-1)

Cayce preferred natural food over human-made sources of vitamins:

So, keep an excess of foods that carry especially vitamin B, iron and such. *Not take the concentrated form, you see, but obtain these from the foods.* These would include all fruits, all vegetables that are yellow. [Italics added.] (1968-7)

As to the diet: Add to the diet more of those foods that carry vitamin B₁. In conjunction with the applications we have suggested for improvement, it is preferable that this be done by *taking an excess of foods carrying same than by taking the vitamins in concentrated form as in tablet or capsule.* [Italics added.] (2564-1)

There is no supplementary to green foods in the real way or manner; though if there are the periods when there is not the ability to obtain or have the green foods . . . these others may be used, but rather as extremities than as a regular activity in same, see? (1158-11)

To another question from a menopausal woman about certain vegetable tablets recommended by her physician, Cayce gave this advice:

These [referring to vegetable supplements] may be taken if there is a lack of those activities from the raw salad [she found it difficult to arrange one daily meal of raw salad as she had been advised by Cayce]; but they do not, *will* not, supply the energies as well or as efficaciously for the *body* as if there were the efforts made to have at least one meal each day altogether of raw vegetables or two meals carrying a raw salad as a portion of same—each day. (1158-18)

Cayce occasionally did prescribe extra vitamins in certain cases, but he warned that these should not be continued indefinitely:

All such properties [as vitamins] that add to the system are more efficacious if they are given for periods, left off for periods and begun again. For if the system comes to rely upon such influences wholly, it ceases to produce the vitamins even though the food values may be kept normally balanced.

And it's much better that these be produced in the body from the normal

On Calcium

Keep plenty of those foods that supply calcium to the body. These we would find especially in raw carrots, cooked turnips, and turnip greens, all characters of salads—especially as of watercress, mustard, and the like. These are especially helpful taken raw, though turnips should be cooked—but cooked in their own juices and not with fat meats. (1968-6)

On Phosphorus

The phosphorus-forming foods are principally carrots, lettuce (rather the leaf lettuce, which has more soporific activity than the head lettuce), shell fish, salsify, the *peelings* of Irish potatoes (if they are not too large), and things of such natures . . . Citrus-fruit juices, and plenty of milk—the Bulgarian [buttermilk is] the better, or the fresh milk that is warm with the animal heat which carries more of the phosphorus and more of those activities that are less constipating, or [that are capable of] acting more with the lacteals and the ducts of the liver, the kidneys and the bowels themselves. (560-2)

development than supplied mechanically, for nature is much better yet than science!

This we find then, given twice a day for two or three weeks, left off for a week and then begun again, especially through the winter months, would be much more effective with the body. (759-12)

(Q) Please give the foods that would supply these [minerals].
(A) We have given them; cereals that carry the heart of the grain, vegetables of the leafy kind, fruits and nuts as indicated. *The almond carries more phosphorus and iron in a combination easily assimilated than any other nut.* (1131-2)

Acid-Alkaline Balance

One of the most important hallmarks of the Cayce philosophy of nutrition is the necessity of keeping the system alkaline by maintaining a ratio of 80 percent alkaline–reacting foods to 20 percent acid–reacting foods as a protection against colds and infection. The fact that antacid nonprescription preparations are the number–one sales item in drugstores today is some measure of the need and usefulness of this Cayce theory, which in application can avoid many gastrointestinal disorders and colds. In many readings Cayce was asked:

(Q) What causes colds? Can you give me a formula or method of preventing them or curing them?
(A) Keep the body alkaline! Cold germs do not live in an alkaline system. They do breed in any acid or excess of acids of *any* character left in the system.
(1947-4)

Again in case 3248–1, Cayce says, "As we have just indicated, by keeping the body alkaline. Only in acids do colds attack the body."

How was one to achieve this desirable alkaline state? Cayce was quite specific in defining not only the foods but the combinations of foods that produce either the alkaline or acid condition in the system in the process of assimilation.

Acidity

(Q) What foods are acid-forming for this body?
(A) All of those that are combining fats with sugars. Starches naturally are inclined for acid reaction. But a normal diet is about 20 percent acid to 80 percent alkaline-producing. (1523-3)

The acidity was produced by taking too much sugar in the system in candies and in those properties as were taken before the stomach was filled with foods; and then overloading the system at such times . . .
(Q) What properties were referred to as being taken into the system before food was taken?

(A) Candies—and smoking. (294-86)

Alkalinity

The diet should be more body-building; that is, less acid foods and more of the alkaline-reacting . . . Milk and all its products should be a portion of the body's diet now; also those food values carrying an easy assimilation of iron, silicon, and those elements or chemicals—as all forms of berries, most all forms of vegetables that grow under the ground, most of the vegetables of a leafy nature. Fruits and vegetables, nuts and the like, should form a greater part of the regular diet in the present . . .

Keep closer to the alkaline diets; using fruits, berries, vegetables particularly that carry iron, silicon, phosphorus, and the like.

(Q)   Can immunization against them [contagious diseases] be set up in any other manner than by inoculations?
(A)   If an alkalinity is maintained in the system—especially with lettuce, carrots and celery, these in the blood supply will maintain such a condition as to immunize a person. (480-19)

Acid-Alkaline Food Combinations

Cayce stressed the value of certain food combinations and the harm in others in relation to the acid–alkaline balance. Many of his theories have been validated by important research since he advanced them. Others seem to work, although just why they do is a job for further research. Here are a few examples:

(Q)   What foods should I avoid?
(A)   Rather it is the combination of foods that makes for disturbance with most physical bodies, as it would with this . . . Do not combine the (alkaline) reacting acid fruits with starches, other than *whole wheat bread*. That is, citrus fruits, oranges, apples, grapefruit, limes or lemons or even tomato juices. And do not have cereals (which contain the greater quantity of starch than most) at the same meal with the citrus fruits. (416-9)

This, as you will see, radically alters the usual pattern of the American breakfast. It suggests that citrus juice–such as orange juice–should be taken between meals or at least one to two hours before breakfast. However, it can be combined at breakfast with an egg and toast, not cereal.

While we are still talking about breakfast, it would be well to point out that Cayce felt very strongly about coffee, which he suggested was a food when taken alone, but should never be taken with milk or cream and sugar, since the milk transformed itself into a leathery curd blocking the digestive process. The research of British scientists has confirmed this.

Coffee, taken properly, is a food; that is *without* cream or milk. (303-2)

On Iron
Let the iron be rather taken in the foods [instead of from medicinal sources] as it is more easily assimilated from the vegetable sources . . . [Foods with iron include spinach, lentils, red cabbage, berries, raisins, liver, grapes, pears, onions, asparagus.]
(1187-9)

One of the most important hallmarks of the Cayce philosophy of nutrition is the necessity of keeping the system alkaline by maintaining a ratio of 80 percent alkaline-reacting foods to 20 percent acid-reacting foods as a protection against colds and infection.
—H.J.R.

Alkaline-Forming Foods
All fruits, fresh and dried
Except large prunes, plums, and cranberries, with this exception: "The prune or pieplant juices [rhubarb] of course are acid but with cereals [whole grain] are more alkaline reacting."
(305-2)
All vegetables, fresh and dehydrated
Except legumes (dried peas, beans, and lentils).
All forms of milk
Buttermilk, clabber, sour milk, cottage cheese, and cheese.

Acid-Forming Foods

Animal fats and vegetable oils
Large prunes, plums, cranberries, and rhubarb.

All cereal grains
Plus other such products, as bread, breakfast foods, etc., rolled oats, corn flakes, corn-meal mush, polished rice, etc. (brown rice is less acid-forming).

All high-starch and protein foods
White sugar, syrups, syrups made from white sugar (starchy foods in combination with fruits or proteins are acid combinations and should be avoided).

Nuts
Peanuts, English walnuts, pecans, filberts, and coconut.

Legumes
Dried beans, dried peas, and lentils.

Meats
Beef, pork, lamb, and veal.

Poultry
Chicken, turkey, duck, goose, guinea hen, and game.

Visceral meats
Heart, brains, kidney, liver, sweetbreads, and thymus.

Egg whites
Yolks are not acid-forming.

If coffee is taken, do not take milk in same. If tea is taken, do not take milk in same. This is hard on the digestion . . . (5097-1)

(Q) Is [the use of] tea and coffee harmful to the body?
(A) Tea is more harmful than coffee. (303-2)

Citrus Fruits Should Be Mixed with Lemon or Lime Juice

Four parts orange juice should be combined with one part lime or lemon. Grapefruit juice may be prepared the same way.

To the question, "Is the quart of milk a day, and orange juice, helpful?" Cayce answered, "Orange juice and milk are helpful, but these would be taken at opposite ends of the day; not together." (274–9)

Avoid Eating Meat and Starch at the Same Meal

Rather is it the combination of foods that makes for disturbance with most physical bodies . . .

. . . avoid combinations where corn, potatoes, rice, spaghetti or the like are taken all at the same meal . . . all of these tend to make for too great a quantity of starch—especially if any meat is taken at such a meal . . . for the activities of the gastric flow of the digestive system are the requirements of one reaction in the gastric flow for starch and another for proteins, or for the activities of the carbohydrates as combined with starches of this nature . . . Sweets and meats taken at the same meal are preferable to starches and meats. (416-9)

Combinations of Vegetables

Have at least three vegetables that grow above the ground to one that grows under the ground.

Have at least one meal each day that includes a quantity of raw vegetables such as cabbage, lettuce, celery, carrots, onions, and the like. Tomatoes may be used in their season. Have at least one leafy vegetable to every one of the pod vegetables taken.

Do include often in the diet raw vegetables, prepared in various ways, not merely as a salad, but scraped or grated and combined with gelatin.

Milk

Cayce often advised people to leave milk alone.

I agree with him on this, because milk is hard to digest, and I do not think it is a very good food for adults. It makes a great deal of mucus and, when we train athletes who have to have good wind like boxers, runners, swimmers, we always cut milk out of the diet. Milk is also constipating and should be taken alone at body temperature and chewed well. It should take five to ten minutes to drink a glass of milk.

However, Cayce and I do favor milk in its predigested forms, such as yogurt, or acidopholus, and buttermilk, especially if these are made from raw certified milk rather than the pasteurized variety.

> . . . and raw milk [is good]—provided it is from cows that don't eat certain types of weeds or grass grown this time of year. (2752-3)

To the question "Is buttermilk good?" he answered, "This depends upon the manner in which it is made. This would tend to produce gas if it is the ordinary kind. But that *made* by the use of the Bulgarian Tablets is good, in moderation, not too much." (404–6)

Special Foods

Cayce had some highly individualistic ideas about certain foods. Although Dr. William McGarey, other doctors, and I have had clinical experience and good results with them, additional research should be undertaken under control conditions.

Almonds

For example, Cayce was enthusiastic about almonds:

> And if an almond is taken each day and kept up, you'll never have accumulations of tumors or such conditions through the body. An almond a day is much more in accord with keeping the doctor away, especially certain types of doctors, than apples. For the apple was the fall, not the almond—for the almond blossomed when everything else died. Remember all this is life!
>
> (3180-3)

In another reading in answer to a question he said, "The almond carries more phosphorus *and* iron in a combination easily assimilated than any other nut." (1131–2)

NOTE: Almonds contain the right proportion of calcium, phosphorus, and iron: 245 mg of calcium to 475 mg of phosphorus and 4.4 mg of iron.

Usually, Cayce recommended that one eat two or three almonds each day.

> . . . those who would eat two to three almonds each day need never fear cancer. Those who would take a peanut oil rub each week need never fear arthritis." (1158-31)

Dr. William McGarey at the A.R.E. Clinic in Phoenix is trying to launch a nationwide clinical research project on almonds in cooperation with the many

There is no supplementary to green foods in the real way or manner; though if there are the periods when there is not the ability to obtain or have the green foods . . . these others may be used, but rather as extremities than as a regular activity in same, see? (1158-11)

Cayce often advised people to leave milk alone.

I agree with him on this, because milk is hard to digest, and I do not think it is a very good food for adults. It makes a great deal of mucus, and when we train athletes who have to have good wind like boxers, runners, swimmers, we always cut milk out of the diet.—**H.J.R.**

. . . and raw milk [is good]—provided it is from cows that don't eat certain types of weeds or grass grown this time of year. (2752-3)

And if an almond is taken each day and kept up, you'll never have accumulations of tumors or such conditions through the body. An almond a day is much more in accord with keeping the doctor away, especially certain types of doctors, than apples. For the apple was the fall, not the almond—for the almond blossomed when everything else died. Remember all this is life! (3180-3)

physicians, osteopaths, and others who are exploring the Cayce therapies.

The Research Department of the Rothschild Municipal Hospital in Haifa began to test the therapeutic properties of almonds after observing that heavy smokers among the Arabs and Jews chewed them to alleviate heartburn or stomach pain (*Medical Tribune*, March 27, 1969). Professor Julius J. Kleeberg, head of the Research Department, reported that peeled sweet dried almonds are effective in the treatment of heartburn and peptic ulcers.

We would welcome the investigation of independent researchers in this as in other aspects of the Cayce work.

One grateful almond fan, Mrs. H.B. of Long Island, New York, wrote the following on October 28, 1970:

"I inadvertently discovered that my eating three almonds a day cleared up a chronic case of hemorrhoids. I recommended the almonds to others with a similar condition and they met with equal success. One case in particular was extremely severe and due for surgery. Now they won't even go on vacation without the almonds. I'm reluctant to tell them that the source of my information was a famous psychic—they'd never understand. In humble gratefulness I thought I'd pass this on."

This case would seem to indicate that the relief experienced by a friend who knows nothing of Mr. Cayce was not due to faith or suggestion.

Another unsolicited testimonial came from Mrs. [5009]:

In July 1957, my mother was operated on for a malignant mass in the intestines. The surgeon removed a segment of bowel to which was attached a polyp, as well as the mass. He told my brother and me that he would have liked to have removed also a further segment on which two or three more polyps (benign of course) were located but he feared she could not have stood that much nerve shock. He said he wished to watch closely by X-ray the polyps every three months. Subsequently, I urged Mother—as soon as she was out of the hospital—to eat several raw almonds a day—whether she believed in them or not (and although she tends to discount and negate a lot she was scared enough to heed me!). In three months the X-ray picture showed the remaining polyps "somewhat smaller"—the doctor reported. In another three months the doctor said he couldn't discern any polyps at all in the X-ray pictures and was so pleased that he changed her periodic X-ray pictures from every three months to every six months. In another year—he changed to X-ray photos only once yearly. It has almost been three-and-a-half years now since her surgery and there has been no return of any trouble or of any polyps (and her last X-ray photos were of her entire body-torso as well as of the abdominal region). So, this is a good report for "the Almond."

Jerusalem Artichokes

The Jerusalem artichoke, a tuberous root with a top like sunflower, was recommended because of its high insulin content to patients with diabetes or a tendency to diabetes. Dieters are probably familiar with the products such as bread sticks, rusks, and pastas made from the flour of the Jerusalem artichoke, which is lower in starch and calories than white flour. It is very popular in fashionable health and beauty spas. The vegetable has the texture of a Chinese water chestnut and is excellent raw in salads and as an hors d'oeuvre. It can be eaten raw or cooked like potatoes.

Cayce most frequently recommended it steamed in Patapar paper [parchment paper].[5] There is an interesting report on the use of Jerusalem artichokes that I have been able to use with the obese and those with craving for sweets. A woman who had had a hysterectomy at thirty-eight years of age and was menopausal suffered from insomnia and neurasthenia and was overweight brought her problem to Cayce.

> (Q) [What about my] craving for sweets?
> (A) This is natural with the indigestion and the lack of proper activity of the pancreas. Eat a Jerusalem artichoke once each week, about the size of a hen egg. Cook this in Patapar paper, preserving all the juices to mix with the bulk of the artichoke. Season to taste. This will also aid in the disorder in the circulation between liver and kidneys, pancreas and kidneys and will relieve these tensions from the desire for sweets.
> Do not take chocolate in any form, especially as it is prepared in the present.
> (3386-2)

The Jerusalem artichoke, a tuberous root with a top like sunflower, was recommended because of its high insulin content to patients with diabetes or a tendency to diabetes. Dieters are probably familiar with the products such as bread sticks, rusks, and pastas made from the flour of the Jerusalem artichoke, which is lower in starch and calories than white flour.
—H.J.R.

Gelatin

There has been a great deal of medical and nutritional controversy over gelatin because it lacks certain amino acids and thus is an incomplete protein. Cayce frequently recommended that raw vegetables be taken with gelatin in a salad (recipe included in this chapter). However, it was recommended not for its vitamin or protein value, but for its enzymatic action in aiding the assimilation of the vegetables.

> It isn't the vitamin content [in gelatin which is important], but its ability to work with the activities of the glands, causing the glands to take from that absorbed or digested the vitamins [otherwise inactive] . . . if there is not sufficient gelatin in the body. See, there may be mixed with any chemical that which makes the rest of the system . . . able to use that needed. It becomes then, as it were, "sensitive to conditions." Without it [the gelatin], there is not the sensitivity [to vitamins]. (849-75)

To the question "What will help the eyesight?" he replied in this way:

> If gelatin will be taken with raw foods rather often (that is, prepare raw vegetables such as carrots often with same)—grate them, eat them raw, we will help the vision. (5148-1)

In another case involving eyesight he again repeated:

> Do add to the diet about twice as many oranges, lemons and limes as is a part of the diet in the present. These also supplement with a great deal of

Add to the diet the Irish potato peel, but not the pulp a great deal. It would be better if the nice potatoes are cleansed, peeled and only the peelings cooked and eaten! Throw the other part away, or give it to the chickens, or distribute it in some other manner besides eating it! (1904-1)

carrots, especially as combined with gelatin, if we would aid and strengthen the optic nerves and the tensions between sympathetic and cerebrospinal systems. (5401-1)

NOTE: Cayce also used a variety of packs for the eyes, including those made from raw organic potatoes (see Chapter 11).

In another reading in which he recommended gelatin salad with raw vegetables for improving eyesight, Cayce made an interesting observation that has been confirmed by modern nutrition:

> Do include, when these are prepared, carrots with that portion especially close to the top. It may appear the harder and the less desirable but it carries the vital energies, stimulating the optic reactions between kidneys and the optics. (3051-6)

Potatoes

> Add to the diet the Irish potato *peel,* but not the pulp a great deal. It would be better if the nice potatoes are cleansed, peeled and only the *peelings* cooked and eaten! Throw the other part away, or give it to the chickens, or distribute it in some other manner besides eating it! [Also see raw potato packs in Chapter 11.] (1904-1)

NOTE: Irish potatoes here refer to *all* white potatoes as distinguished from sweet potatoes.

Beef Juice

> Beef juice would be excellent for the body taken as medicine, or as doses—teaspoonful at a time, or as improvement is shown, tablespoonful at time may be taken. Those properties of the juices also of vegetables will be better than too much of the pulp itself . . . [The recipe is in this chapter.] (5522–1)

Oyster Plant (Salsify)

Cayce set great store by the merits of the oyster plant (also known as salsify). It would be well for home gardeners to cultivate it, since it is not readily available in supermarkets. Cayce said of it, referring to the need for calcium in a female of thirty-five years of age with back trouble:

> Those as we find in . . . the oyster plant and those of such natures should be a portion of the diet. (903-25)

> All of those that carry a great deal of iron and silicon, and things of that nature; that is . . . oyster plant. (538-66)

> . . . [have] green vegetables . . . Also those foods that carry sufficient elements of gold and phosphorus; which are found partially from the . . . veg-

etable forces—as in . . . the oyster plant. (951-2)

Cayce believed that gold from natural foods was important in preserving
youthfulness and had anti–aging properties:

Salsify [oyster plant] . . . are those that carry the vitamins necessary for body-
building with *this* body. (578-5)

Acclimatization

Cayce was very concerned about the freshness of food and a concept he
called "acclimatization."
He answered a question as follows:

[Retention of food values] depends upon preparation of same, the age, and
how long [since] gathered. All of these have their factors in the food values.
As it is so well advertised that coffee loses its value in fifteen to twenty to
twenty-five days after being roasted, so do foods or vegetables lose their food
values after being gathered—in the same proportion in hours as coffee does
in days. (340-31)

Have vegetables that are fresh and especially those grown in the vicinity where
the body resides.
   Shipped vegetables are never very good. (2-14)

Do not have large quantities of any fruits, vegetables, meats that are not
grown in or come from the area where the body is—at the time it partakes of
such foods.
   This will be found to be a good rule to be followed by all. This prepares the
system to acclimate itself to any given territory. (3542-1)

(Q)   Is a diet composed mainly of fruits, vegetables, eggs, and milk the best
diet for me?
(A)   As indicated, use more of the products of the soil that are grown in the
immediate vicinity. These are better for the body than any specific set of
fruits, vegetables, grasses, or what not.
   We would add more of the original sources of proteins. (4047-1)

Of all the vegetables, tomatoes carry most of the vitamins, in a well-balanced
assimilative manner for the activities in the system. Yet if these [tomatoes] are
not cared for properly, they may become very destructive to a physical organism; that is, if they ripen *after* being pulled, or if there is contamination
with other influences. (584-5)

[Eat] more of the vegetables that are *raw.* These may be made into salads with salad dressings, especially with as much of the olive oil as is palatable and that will be assimilated with the character of foods. This would include lettuce, turnips, cabbage and all of those . . . Tomatoes, if they are *ripened on the vine;* otherwise, those that are canned *without* preservative—or especially benzoate of soda. (Do not use such as use that as preservatives.) (135-1)

. . . tomatoes—these are *well* for the body . . . only when well ripened on the vine; not as gathered green and ripened afterward. (894-4)

Cooking Methods

Cayce was strongly opposed to fried foods and the excessive consumption of fats:

Beware of all fried foods. No fried potatoes, fried meats, fried steaks, fried fish, or anything of that nature. (926-1)

The preferable way to prepare such [the vegetable] juices would be through cooking the vegetables after tying them in Patapar paper; not putting them in water to boil, but cooking either in the Patapar paper or in a steam steamer, so that only the juices from the vegetables may be obtained—and no water added in the cooking at all . . . A little later the body may begin with stewed chicken, or broiled chicken or broiled fish . . . Even . . . the chicken or fish would be better cooked in the Patapar paper or a steam cooker. (133-4)

The cooking of condiments, even salt, *destroys* much of the vitamins of foods. (906-1)

(Q)   Consider also the steam pressure for cooking foods quickly. Would it be recommended and does it destroy any of the precious vitamins of the vegetables and fruits?
(A)   Rather preserves than destroys. (462-14)

(Q)   Is food cooked in aluminum utensils bad for this system?
(A)   Certain characters of food cooked in aluminum are bad for any system, and where a systemic condition exists . . . a disturbed hepatic eliminating force, they are naturally so. Cook rather in granite, or better still, in Patapar paper. (1196-7)

(Q) Considering the frozen foods, especially vegetables and fruits that are on the market today—has the freezing in any way killed certain vitamins and how do they compare with the fresh?
(A) This would necessitate making a special list. For some are affected more than others. So far as fruits are concerned, these do not lose much of the vitamin content. Yet some of these are affected by the freezing. Vegetables—

much of the vitamin content of these is taken [by freezing] unless there is the re-enforcement in same when these are either prepared for food or when frozen. (462-14)

Assuming that by now you are convinced and enthusiastic about improving the nutrition of your family, what can you do about it?

Obtaining Fresh Vegetables

If you live in the suburbs or in any situation where you have access to even a small plot of ground, start growing your own vegetables. There are many excellent books available on organic gardening. Many cities are converting parcels of parkland into small garden plots.

Betty Billings, in her talks, often suggests that groups of citizens in cities interested in obtaining foods with the least amount of chemicals band together and take turns driving out into the country to purchase vegetables and fruits in season when they are at the peak of freshness and nutritional value. The surplus may be frozen or home canned for winter use.

Sprouts

"In the winter, whether you live in the city, suburb, or country," Miss Billings says, "you can sprout seeds and have a delicious new crop of fresh, live food available every three or four days without having to do any composting, spraying, or worrying about weeds, bugs, plant diseases and weather. Sprouts are the ideal solution for the city dweller, for even if you live in a one-room efficiency you can easily grow this delicious, nutritious food which can supply so many of the vital nutrients for your diet eaten raw or cooked."

Sprouts may be used as food by anyone, even someone with a health problem, for the starch and protein they contain are easily digested with the help of the enzymes also present in high quantities in sprouts. Research has shown that such protein is equal to animal protein; their vitamin B–complex content makes them a fine food for the baby, child, or adult. All sprouts contain vitamins A, B, and C equivalent to that found in fruit. Alfalfa sprouts are also rich in vitamins D, E, G [B$_2$], K, and U. Soybean and mung sprouts are high in protein. Many sprouts, including soybean, mung, lentils, peas, wheat, rice, and corn, are high in vitamin E. They are also easy on the pocketbook, since one pound of sprouts grows to six to eight pounds of fresh food and can cost as little as twenty–five cents a day.

Space does not permit an extensive and exhaustive discussion here of the vast amount of research carried on all over the world on the value of sprouts. The interested student can pursue the subject in Cathryn Elwood's excellent book, *Feel Like a Million.*[6]

Many different seeds can be sprouted: every kind of bean, especially mung and soybeans, which are almost equal to meat in protein value; peas, lentils, wheat, rye, oats, corn, barley, millet, alfalfa, clover, parsley, sunflower, sesame,

The cooking of condiments, even salt, destroys much of the vitamins of foods. (906-1)

In the winter, whether you live in the city, suburb, or country, you can sprout seeds and have a delicious new crop of fresh, live food available every three or four days without having to do any composting, spraying, or worrying about weeds, bugs, plant diseases, and weather. Sprouts are the ideal solution for the city dweller, for even if you live in a one-room efficiency you can easily grow this delicious, nutritious food which can supply so many of the vital nutrients for your diet eaten raw or cooked.—**Betty Billings**

Many different seeds can be sprouted: every kind of bean, especially mung and soybeans, which are almost equal to meat in protein value; peas, lentils, wheat, rye, oats, corn, barley, millet, alfalfa, clover, parsley, sunflower, sesame, and others too numerous to mention here.—**H.J.R.**

and others too numerous to mention here.

According to Miss Elwood, "The sprouted seeds may be used in salads, soups, casseroles, eggs, fruit and yogurt desserts, loaf bread, chop suey, and chow mein. And here is some good news—the nourishment which develops as the sprouts grow is very stable and can be frozen or dried for future use if you should have an extra supply. I am not advocating that one should sprout to dry or freeze, but if there are some extra ones don't throw them out."

An acknowledged authority on sprouts, Miss Elwood states in her book her preference for the length of different sprouts in the following manner.

- Wheat sprouts—the length of the seed
- Mung bean sprouts—1½ to 2 inches
- Pea and soybean sprouts (good either short or long)
- Lentil sprouts—1 inch
- Sunflower seed sprouts—the length of the seed[7]

The vitamin value of the seeds continues to increase as the sprout grows and lengthens, but some sprouts are not as delicious tasting when permitted to grow too long. Many people dislike the extreme sweetness that wheat develops when it is long. The taste of mung beans and alfalfa improves with length and some sprouts, when exposed to the sun grow tiny leaves, which add to their delicate flavor.

Recipes

Mummy Food

For those not familiar with the origin of the recipe for "mummy food," Edgar Cayce had a dream (12/2/37) concerning the discovery of ancient records in Egypt in which a mummy came to life and helped to translate these records. The mummy, he dreamt, gave directions for the preparation of a food that she required (see 294-189, R-2). Thus the name "mummy food."

Other readings for particular individuals recommended this same combination. One such was as follows:

And for this especial body, [a mixture of] dates, figs (that are dried) cooked with a little corn meal (a very little sprinkled in), then this taken with milk, should be almost a spiritual food for the body . . . (275-45)

More detailed instructions were:

. . . equal portions of black figs or Assyrian figs and Assyrian dates—these ground together or cut very fine, and to a pint of such a combination put half a handful of corn meal, or crushed wheat. These cooked together . . .

(275-45)

"Half a handful" is, of course, a rather indefinite amount, and the amount of water is not given. The following has been tried and found satisfactory:

Methods of Sprouting

There are a number of ways of sprouting seeds, some of which seem to work better than others, depending on the size of the seed to be sprouted. We do advise against using the paper-towel method or sprouting in plastic containers, for chemical contamination may result.

The best containers to use are glass, ceramic, earthenware, and enamel. Wide-mouthed glass jars can be covered with cheesecloth, a clean piece of nylon stocking, wire mesh, or a perforated lid (although we do not advise contact with metal). Some people use flower pots or just clean Turkish towels.

The important thing to remember about the equipment is that it should provide for easy drainage (so that the sprouts won't sour), some way of retaining moisture, proper warmth, and good ventilation. Most health-food stores sell special sprouting equipment that is not too expensive, but you can get along just as well with glass jars.

Seeds for sprouting are usually available in health-food stores. When you wash them, the dead seeds will rise to the top and are poured off with the wash water. If you find too many dead seeds, get a better source of supply.

Basic Method

1. Use about cup of mung or soybeans or any of the larger seeds, like those of chickpeas, lentils, or sunflowers; 2 or 3 tablespoons of alfalfa, sesame, or any of the small seeds will do. They will swell and become quite large when soaked.
2. Place in jar or other container and wash well in warm (about 70 to 80 degrees), pure, nonchemical water. The dead seeds will rise to the top. Pour off as you change the wash water. Then cover seeds with about 2 or 3 times as much warm, pure water. Cover the container with cheesecloth, nylon, or other top that permits drainage, fasten with rubber band or string, and soak the seeds. Six to 8 hours is about right for summer soaking and 12 to 16 hours for winter soaking. Store in a warm, dark place.
3. Wash seeds well after soaking in warm water until the water becomes clear. Cover container and invert so that drainage continues. Some people place their sprout jars to drain in their empty dishwasher. Rinse sprouts two or three times a day. The seeds must be kept damp, so if you are using the Turkish-towel method, you may need to rinse and sprinkle with water more often. Remember, if you are using glass, to keep the jar in the dark or you will lose vitamin C, which evaporates with light.
4. The sprouts are ready to eat when they attain the desired length as described earlier, which takes from 60 to 90 hours. If you want them to develop chlorophyll, expose the sprouts to the light after they have attained the right length and been removed from the sprouting container.

Alternate Method

"Another method that can be used especially with small seeds is to scatter the seeds on a damp bath towel after washing. Roll the towel loosely and sprinkle as necessary to keep damp. When the sprouts are of the desired length put in large bowl, wash, and store in refrigerator in crisper or plastic bag."[8]

COMBINING FOODS

Food types	Agrees well with:	Does not agree well with:
Starches, including all foods made from grain, potatoes, rice, breads, macaroni, spaghetti, and winter squash; freshly picked sweet corn is considered as a starch; one starch only at a meal is a good rule.	Raw leafy green vegetables; cooked root vegetables; cooked green vegetables; vegetable salads and salad greens generally	Milk, tart fruits, meats, eggs, cheese, nuts
Fresh meats, sea foods, fish, fowl, cheese, cured meats, eggs, nuts	Cooked or raw root and leafy vegetables, tomatoes, salads	Starches, milk, sweet fruits, sweet desserts
Vegetables and salads	All foods	
Dairy products: butter, milk, cheese, etc.	Most cooked or raw vegetables; all cooked or raw fruits; salads	Concentrated starches, potatoes, etc.; meats of all kinds, fish, fowl. Milk may be used after a starch meal, not with it.
Fruits fresh (sweet)	Starches, salads, raw or cooked vegetables; all dairy products, nuts	Meats, fowl, fish, sea foods, fats, eggs
Fruit salad	All foods except starches	Starches
Fruits fresh (tart); dried sweet and tart fruits follow same rules. Fresh and dried fruits are best not eaten together; the same applies to sweet and tart fruits. Melons do not agree with any food, are best eaten alone. Avoid unripe bananas.	All dairy products; meats, fowl, fish, sea foods, nuts, eggs	Starches, bread, toast

If vinegar is used, use only apple cider vinegar.
Lemon juice is better than vinegar, and combined with olive oil or honey makes a delicious dressing.

Mummy Food

½ cup chopped pitted dates   1½ cups water
½ cup chopped dried black figs   1 rounded tbsp. cornmeal

Cook over low heat, stirring frequently, for ten minutes or longer. Serve with milk or cream. Serves 2–4.

Basic Recipe for Gelatin–Vegetable Salads

1 tbsp. gelatin (unflavored, as Knox)   ¼ tsp. salt, if water is used
½ cup cold water   ¼ cup lemon juice
1 cup boiling water or light–colored stock   1 tbsp. onion, grated
2–4 tbsp. honey   2 cups diced or shredded vegetables

Soak gelatin in cold water and dissolve thoroughly in boiling water or stock. Add honey, salt, lemon juice, and onion if desired. Chill. When about set, add vegetables, and chill until set firmly. Serve on lettuce leaves with mayonnaise.

Fresh Vegetable–Gelatin Salad

2 envelopes unflavored gelatin   ⅔ cup ripe olives, pitted and
                                              diced
½ cup cold water   1½ cups cabbage, shredded
2 cups hot water   ¾ cup celery, diced
⅓ cup honey   ¾ cup carrots, shredded
1¼ tsp. salt   ¼ cup green pepper, chopped
¼ cup lemon juice   2 tbsp. pimiento, diced

Soften gelatin in cold water, add hot water, and stir until dissolved. Stir in honey and next 2 ingredients; cool. Add olives and remaining ingredients; mix well. Pour into 1¼ qt. ring mold or 8 x 8 x 2 cake pan. Chill until firm. Cut into squares. Garnish with crisp greens and serve with mayonnaise. Serves 10–12.

Fresh Fruit Salad

Use all your favorite fresh fruits (except pineapple and apples) with unflavored gelatin.

1 envelope unflavored gelatin   1 cup hot water
¼ cup cold water   ½ cup grapefruit juice
¼ cup honey   1 tbsp. lemon juice
1/8 tsp. salt   Fresh fruit, cut up

Soften gelatin in cold water, add honey, salt, and hot water. Stir until dissolved. Add grapefruit and lemon juice. Mix well. Pour 1 cup mixture into a mold that has been rinsed in cold water. When it begins to thicken, arrange fruit in it. Chill remaining gelatin until it begins to thicken, then whip until frothy and thick and pour on the gelatin mixture. Chill until firm. Serves 6.

Gelatin Fruit Salad

1 envelope unflavored gelatin	2 tbsp. banana, cut fine
½ cup boiling water	2 tbsp. pineapple, unsweetened
1½ cups pineapple juice, unsweetened	1 tbsp. orange, cut fine
1 tbsp. lemon juice	1 tbsp. coconut, finely grated

Dissolve gelatin in boiling water. Place on stove and let boil for 1 minute, stirring constantly. Add pineapple and lemon juice. Set aside to cool, and when it is half set, add the mixed fruit and coconut. Pour into molds; it will set in approximately 20 minutes.

Beef Juice

Beef Juice should be taken regularly, as a medicine; a teaspoonful four times a day at least, but when taken it should be sipped. (5374-1)

Beef juice is not a broth but a juice extracted from the meat through the process of heat. It is prepared as follows:

Take about one pound of round steak preferably. Cut off the fat, leaving the muscle and pieces of tendon. Cut this then into half-inch cubes, and put it into a glass jar without water in it. The jar should be covered but not tightly. Then put the jar into a pan with water in it, the water coming about ½ or ¾ of the way toward the top of the jar. Put a cloth on the bottom of the pan to prevent the jar from cracking. Let the water then simmer for 3–4 hours. Then strain off the juice which has accumulated in the jar, and the remaining meat may be pressed somewhat to extract the remainder of the juice. The meat will then be worthless. Place the juice in a refrigerator, but never keep it longer than three days. The quantity made, then, depends upon how much and how often the juice is taken.

It should be taken 2–3 times a day, but not more than a tablespoon at a time—and this should be sipped very slowly, taking perhaps 5 or 10 minutes to use the whole amount.

It may be seasoned to suit the taste of the individual. It would be well also to use a whole wheat or Ry-Krisp cracker at the same time to make it more palatable.

"Normal" Diets

While Cayce often gave dietary recommendations for people who were ill, he also suggested diets for healthy people. Following are seven "normal" diets that were suggested to healthy people in order to maintain their good health.

BASIC DIET #1

MORNINGS:

Citrus fruit juices or dry cereals with milk, but do not eat the cereals and the citrus fruit juices at the same meals; else we will find we change the activity of citrus fruit juices with the gastric juices of the stomach, by combining those that are acid and those that are alkaline reacting but of an acid nature. Crisp bacon, brown toast of whole wheat. Graham crackers, coddled egg, stewed fruit, fresh fruit; all of these are well, but not all at one meal, to be sure.

NOONS:

Preferably a green and fresh green vegetable salad; as tomatoes, celery, lettuce, peppers, radishes, carrots, and the like. These should be grated together or chopped very fine. An oil salad dressing may be used.

EVENINGS:

A general vegetable diet, well balanced with three vegetables above the ground to one grown below. Well-cooked and well-seasoned vegetables. And the meats should only include lamb, fowl, or fish. Do not take shellfish, but the fresh water fish would be preferable to the salt fish, see? Mackerel, and the like, don't take; but the fresh water fish will be much better for the body. Some little condiments may be taken at this meal, if so desired. Be mindful that not too much sweets are taken, but sufficient that there may be created a balance with the green vegetables for a sufficient fermentation in the proper proportion and nature. Hence tarts or fruit pies, or rolls, or the like; but not just cake alone, for this is not so well. Coffee and tea in moderation. (549-1)

BASIC DIET #2

This would be given as an outline (of the day's foods); not as the only foods, but as an outline:

MORNINGS:

Whole grain cereals or citrus fruit juices, though not at the same meal. When using orange juice, combine lime with it. When using grapefruit [juice], combine lemon with it—just a little. Egg, preferably only the yolk, or rice or buckwheat cakes, or toast, or just any one of these would be well of mornings.

NOONS:

A raw salad, including tomatoes, radish, carrots, celery, lettuce, watercress—any or all of these, with a soup or vegetable broth, or seafoods . . .

EVENINGS:

Fruits, as cooked apples; potatoes, tomatoes, fish, fowl, lamb, and occasionally beef but not too often. Keep these as the main part of a well-balanced diet.

(1523-17)

BASIC DIET #3

MORNINGS:

In the matter of diet itself, we would have this an outline, though—to be sure—this may be altered from time to time to suit the tastes of the body.

At least 3 mornings each week we would have the rolled, crushed or cracked whole wheat, that is not cooked too long so as to destroy the whole vitamin force in same, but this will add to the body the proper proportions of iron, silicon and the vitamins necessary to build up the blood supply that makes for resistance in the system. We at other periods would have citrus fruits, citrus fruit juices, the yolk of eggs (preferably soft-boiled or coddled—not the white portions of same), browned bread with butter, Ovaltine or milk, or coffee, provided there is no milk or cream in same. Occasionally have . . . stewed figs, stewed raisins, stewed prunes or stewed apricots. But do not eat citrus fruits at the same meal with cereals or gruels or any of the breakfast foods.

NOONS:

Preferably raw fresh vegetables; none cooked at this meal . . . tomatoes, lettuce, celery, spinach, carrots, beet tops, mustard, onions or the like (not cucumbers) that make for purifying of the *humor* in the lymph blood. We would not take any quantities of soups or broths at this period.

EVENINGS:

Broths or soups may be taken in a small measure at this meal; but let it consist principally of vegetables that are well cooked and a little of the meats such as lamb, fish, fowl—these are preferable. No fried foods . . . (840-1)

BASIC DIET #4

MORNINGS:

This is not all to be taken, but as an outline: citrus fruit juices. When orange juice is taken add lime or lemon juice to same; four parts orange juice to one part lime or lemon. When other citrus fruits are taken, as pineapple or grapefruit, they may be taken as they are from the fresh fruit. A little salt added to same is preferable . . .

Whole wheat bread, toasted, browned, with butter. Coddled egg, only the yolk of same. A small piece of very crisp bacon if so desired. Any or all of these may be taken.

But when cereals are taken, *do not* have citrus fruits at the same meal! . . . Such a combination produces just what we are trying to prevent in the system!

When cereals are used, have either cracked wheat or whole wheat, or a combination of barley and wheat—as in Maltex, if these are desired; or Puffed Wheat, or Puffed Rice, or Puffed Corn—any of these. And these may be taken with certain characters of fresh fruits; as berries of any nature, even strawberries if so desired. (No, they won't cause any rash if they are taken *properly!*) Or peaches. The sugar used should only be saccharin or honey. A cereal drink may be had if so desired.

NOONS:

Only raw fresh vegetables. *All* of these may be combined, but grate them— don't eat them so [hurriedly] that they would make for that [unbalanced condition resulting from improper] mastication. Each time you take a mouthful . . . it should be chewed at least 4 to 20 times . . . each should be chewed so that there is the . . . opportunity for the flow of the gastric forces from the salivary glands well mixed with same. Then we will find that these will make for bettered conditions.

EVENINGS:

Vegetables that are cooked in their *own* juices . . . each cooked alone, then combined together afterward if so desired by the body, see? These may include any of the leafy vegetables or any of the bulbular vegetables, but cook them in their *own* juices! There may be taken the meats, if so desired by the body, or there may be added the proteins that come from the combination of other vegetables . . . in the forms of certain character of pulse or of grains. (3823-3)

BASIC DIET #5

MORNINGS:

Citrus fruits, cereals or fruits . . . or citrus fruits, and a little later rice cakes, or buckwheat or graham cakes, with honey *in* the honeycomb, with milk . . . *preferably* the raw milk *if* certified milk!

NOONS:

Rather vegetable juices than meat juices, with raw vegetables as a salad or the like.

EVENINGS:

Vegetables, with such as carrots, peas, salsify, red cabbage, yams or white potatoes—these [potatoes should be] the smaller variety, with the jackets the better; using as the finishing, or dessert . . . blanc mange or jello, or jellies, with fruits—as peaches, apricots, fresh pineapple or the like. These, as we find, with the occasional sufficient meats for strength, would bring a well-balanced diet.

Occasionally we would add those of the blood-building, once or twice a week. The pig knuckles, tripe and calves' liver, or those of *brains* and the like.

(275-24)

BASIC DIET #6

MORNINGS:

Citrus fruit juices *or* cereals, but not both at the same meal. [Use with other cereals] at times dried fruits or figs, combined with dates and raisins—these chopped very well together. And for this especial body, dates, figs (that are dried) cooked with a little corn meal (a very little sprinkled in), then this taken with milk, should be almost a spiritual food for the body; whether it's taken one, two, three or four meals a day. But this is to be left to the body itself.

NOONS:

Such as vegetable juices . . . and a combination of raw vegetables; but not *ever* any acetic acid or vinegar or the like with same—but oils, if olive oil or vegetable oils, may be used with same.

EVENINGS:

Vegetables that are of the leafy nature; fish, fowl or lamb preferably as the meats or their combinations. These of course are not to be all, but this is the *general* outline for the three meals for the body. (275-45)

BASIC DIET #7

MORNINGS:

Whole wheat toast, browned. Cereals with fresh fruits. The citrus fruit juices occasionally. But do not mix the citrus fruit juices *and* cereals at the same meal.

NOONS:

Principally (very seldom altering from these) raw vegetables or raw fruits made into a salad; not the fruits and vegetables combined, but these may be altered. Use such vegetables as cabbage (the white, of course, cut very fine), carrots, lettuce, spinach, celery, onions, tomatoes, radish; any or all of these. It is more preferable that they *all* be grated, but when grated do not [discard the juices] . . . these should be used upon the salad itself, either from the fruits or the vegetables. Preferably use the *oil* dressings; as olive oil with paprika . . . Even egg may be included in same . . . [Work the yolk of a hard-boiled egg] into the oil as a portion of the dressing. Use in the fruit salad such as bananas, papaya, guava, grapes; *all* characters of fruits *except* apples. Apples should only be eaten when cooked; preferably roasted and with butter or hard sauce on same, with cinnamon and spice.

EVENINGS:

A well-balanced cooked vegetable diet, including principally those things that will make for iron to be assimilated in the system. (935-1)

Dietary Reference Intakes (RDIs)

Source: Food and Nutrition Board - National Academy of Sciences, 1998

Food and Nutrition Board, Institute of Medicine - National Academy of Sciences
Dietary Reference Intakes: Recommended levels for individual intake (a)

Life-Stage Group	Calcium (mg/d)	Phosphorus (mg/d)	Magnesium (mg/d)	Vitamin D[bc] (ug/d)	Fluoride (mg/d)	Thiamin (mg/d)	Riboflavin (md/d)	Niacin[d] (mg/d)	Vitamin B-6 (mg/d)	Folate[e] (ug/d)	Vitamin B-12 (ug/d)	Pantothenic Acid (mg/d)	Biotin (ug/d)	Choline[f] (mg/d)
Infants														
0-6 mo.	210*	100*	30*	5*	0.01*	0.2*	0.3*	2*	0.1*	65*	0.4*	1.7*	5*	125*
7-12 mo.	270*	275*	75*	5*	0.5*	0.3*	0.4*	4*	0.3*	80*	0.5*	1.8*	6*	150*
Children														
1-3 y	500*	460	80	5*	0.7*	0.5	0.5	6	0.5	150	0.9	2*	8*	200*
4-8 y	800*	500	130	5*	1*	0.6	0.6	8	0.6	200	1.2	3*	12*	250*
Males														
9-13 y	1,300*	1,250	240	5*	2*	0.9	0.9	12	1	300	1.8	4*	20*	375*
14-18 y	1,300*	1,250	410	5*	3*	1.2	1.3	16	1.3	400	2.4	5*	25*	550*
19-30 y	1,000*	700	400	5*	4*	1.2	1.3	16	1.3	400	2.4	5*	30*	550*
31-50 y	1,000*	700	420	5*	4*	1.2	1.3	16	1.3	400	2.4	5*	30*	550*
51-70 y	1,200*	700	420	10*	4*	1.2	1.3	16	1.7	400	2.4 (g)	5*	30*	550*
> 70 y	1,200*	700	420	15*	4*	1.2	1.3	16	1.7	400	2.4 (g)	5*	30*	550*
Females														
9-13 y	1,300*	1,250	240	5*	2*	0.9	0.9	12	1	300	1.8	4*	20*	375*
14-18 y	1,300*	1,250	360	5*	3*	1	1	14	1.2	400 (h)	2.4	5*	25*	400*
19-30 y	1,000*	700	310	5*	3*	1.1	1.1	14	1.3	400 (h)	2.4	5*	30*	425*
31-50 y	1,000*	700	320	5*	3*	1.1	1.1	14	1.3	400 (h)	2.4	5*	30*	425*
51-70 y	1,200*	700	320	10*	3*	1.1	1.1	14	1.5	400	2.4 (g)	5*	30*	425*
> 70 y	1,200*	700	320	15*	3*	1.1	1.1	14	1.5	400	2.4 (g)	5*	30*	425*
Pregnancy														
< 18 y	1,300*	1,250	400	5*	3*	1.4	1.4	18	1.9	600 (i)	2.6	6*	30*	450*
19-30 y	1,000*	700	350	5*	3*	1.4	1.4	18	1.9	600 (i)	2.6	6*	30*	450*
31-50 y	1,000*	700	360	5*	3*	1.4	1.4	18	1.9	600 (i)	2.6	6*	30*	450*
Lactation														
< 18 y	1,300*	1,250	360	5*	3*	1.5	1.6	17	2	500	2.8	7*	35*	550*
19-30 y	1,000*	700	310	5*	3*	1.5	1.6	17	2	500	2.8	7*	35*	550*
31-50 y	1,000*	700	320	5*	3*	1.5	1.6	17	2	500	2.8	7*	35*	550*

Footnotes

(a) Recommended Dietary Allowances (RDAs) are presented in bold type and Adequate Intakes (AIs) in ordinary type followed by an asterisk (*). RDAs and AIs may both be used as goals for individual intake. RDAs are set to meet the needs of almost all (97% to 98%) individuals in a group. For healthy breast-fed infants, the AI is the mean intake. The AI for other life-stage and gender groups is believed to cover needs of all individuals in the group, but lack of data or uncertainty in the data prevent being able to specify with confidence the percentage of persons covered by this intake. Source: The Natural Academy of Sciences, Copyright 1998.

(b) As cholecalciferol. 1 μg cholecalciferol = 40 IU vitamin D.

(c) In the absence of adequate exposure to sunlight.

(d) As niacin equivalents (NE). 1 mg niacin = 60 mg tryptothan; 0 to 6 mo = preformed niacin (not NE).

(e) As dietary folate equivalent (DFE). 1 DFE = 1 μg food folate = 0.6 μg folic acid (from fortified food or supplement) consumed with food = 0.5 μg synthetic (supplemental) folic acid taken on an empty stomach.

(f) Although AIs have been set for choline, there are few data to assess whether a dietary supply of choline is needed at all stages of the life cycle, and it may be that the choline requirement can be met by endogenous synthesis at some of these stages.

(g) Because 10% to 30% of older people may malabsorb food-bound vitamin B-12, it is advisable for those older than 50 years to meet their RDA mainly by consuming foods fortified with vitamin B-12 or a supplement containing vitamin B-12.

(h) In view of evidence linking folate intake with neural tube defects in the fetus, it is recommended that all women capable of becoming pregnant consume 400 μg synthetic folic acid from fortified foods and/or supplements in addition to intake of food folate from a varied diet.

(i) It is assumed that women will continue consuming 400 μg folic acid until their pregnancy is confirmed and they enter prenatal care, which ordinarily occurs after the end of the periconceptional period—the critical time for formation of the neural tube.

Note to Cooks

You can obtain nutrient charts and further information in the U.S. Department of Agriculture publication "Nutritive Value of Foods," Home and Garden Bulletin 72 (HG–72). HG–72 is available to download in PDF format at http://www.nal.usda.gov/fnic/foodcomp/Data/HG72/hg72.html. The publication can also be purchased in printed form from the Government Printing Office, stock number 001-000-4703-5; $14.00 (U.S.) or $19.60 (non-U.S.).

Helpful information can also be found in:

Nourishing the Body Temple: Edgar Cayce's Approach to Nutrition by Simone Gabbay, published by A.R.E. Press, 1999.

Edgar Cayce's Diet and Recipe Guide, compiled and published by the A.R.E. Press, 1991.

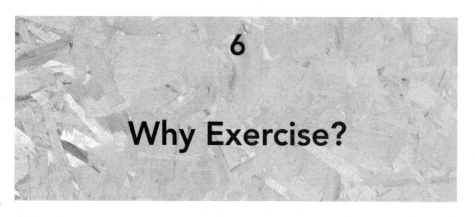

6

Why Exercise?

Take more outdoor exercise, that—brings into play the muscular forces of the body. It isn't that the mental should be numbed, or should be cut off from their operations or activities—but make for a more evenly, a more perfectly balanced body—physical and mental . . . (341-31)

The best way to acquire the correct amount of pep is to take the exercise! (288-38)

It's well that each body, everybody, take exercise to counteract the daily routine activity so as to produce rest. (416-1)

In the evolution of the human race, we humans had to exercise to survive. We had to be able to run from an enemy, catch our food, climb trees and mountains, and ford rivers; every moment of life was purchased with physical effort. Our ancestors had no need of an exercise program; the physical struggle to stay alive was exercise enough. The body that we have today is the end product of a process of survival—of thousands of years of genetic selection, and during all that long and exciting history survival was associated with physical labor and movement.

As civilization advanced and we moved into an age of mechanization and push–button ease, we found less and less need to use our bodies in our daily lives. Yet our need to move has in no way diminished. Our muscles, glands, organs, mind, and spirit still require daily movement to function properly.

Our 600–odd muscles must have tone and the ability to expand and contract. Each of them requires daily movement—exercise—to retain elasticity, power, youthfulness, and vigor. The muscles must hold the organs in position so they can function properly. Exercise is essential to keep the glands performing their complicated tasks, to maintain sexual vigor, to keep the blood circulating, and to fight the pull of gravity that produces protruding, sagging middles, dropped stomachs, sluggish livers, blood–starved hearts, clogged arteries, and unsightly fat—to mention just a few of the evil consequences of inactivity. Postural weaknesses and improper development and use of muscles result in over seven million cases a year of back trouble and other orthopedic aches and pains, which have now superceded colds as the major cause of absenteeism from work.

Humankind has always had to develop and maintain the physical capacity necessary for the body to be adequate to support the rest of life's activities— thinking, creating, carrying the responsibilities of business, profession, social and community life, and procreating and child–bearing. And to those who would attain spiritual as well as intellectual and material heights, I quote the

Best that every individual budget its time. Set so much time for study, so much time for relaxation, so much time for labor mentally; so much time for activity of the physical body, so much time for reading, so much time for social activities . . . each of these activities make for the creating of a better balance. (440-2)

We know that muscles can atrophy through lack of exercise—witness hospital patients who eat perfectly balanced meals and get out of bed too weak to walk. The reason is that muscles are nourished by thousands of miles of hairlike capillaries, which transport food and carry off wastes.—**H.J.R.**

good advice that Edgar Cayce often gave in his readings, of which so many were devoted to restoring health.

Then, be a well-rounded body. Take specific, definite exercises morning and evening. Make the body physically, as well as mentally, tired, and those things which have been producing those conditions where sleep, inertia, poisons in the system from non-eliminations, will disappear. And so will the body respond to the diets. (341-31)

Exercise is one of the most powerful preventive medicines in staving off the disabilities of middle and old age, as well as an important therapeutic tool in repairing the ravages of disease. It is an absolute essential to the maintenance of health, beauty, reproductive ability, weight control, longevity, mental equilibrium, and spiritual harmony.

In controlling weight, exercise is fully as important as diet. Dr. Roger J. Williams, the eminent biochemical researcher in nutrition, in his excellent book, *Nutrition Against Disease*,[1] reported on laboratory experiments in which rats, which otherwise have no tendency to become obese, were kept in a warm room in a very small cage where they could move very little; they invariably became obese. They may eventually weigh two or three times as much as rats that are allowed to exercise by having a larger cage. If the animals are kept in very small cages in a cool room, they get enough exercise by wriggling and shivering to prevent extreme obesity.

"Get plenty of exercise," Dr. Williams admonishes, "is therefore good advice to give those who wish to prevent obesity."

"Lack of sufficient exercise constitutes a serious deficiency comparable to vitamin deficiency," warns famed physiotherapeutic authority Dr. Hans Kraus.[2] "Physically inactive persons (those who do not exercise) age earlier, die younger, and are more prone to backaches, ulcers, lung cancer, appendicitis, prostatic disorders, psychiatric (mental) illness, cirrhosis of the liver, and hemorrhoids. Death from coronary heart disease occurs twice as often among the physically inactive," adds Dr. Kraus.

We know that muscles can atrophy through lack of exercise—witness hospital patients who eat perfectly balanced meals and get out of bed too weak to walk. The reason is that muscles are nourished by thousands of miles of hairlike capillaries, which transport food and carry off wastes.

In the sedentary adult, large numbers of these capillaries are collapsed, and hardly ever function briskly. Exercise alone can open them up and provide better muscle nutrition.

In past years, Dr. Lawrence A. Golding, director of the Applied Physiology Research Laboratory in the Kent State University School of Health, Physical Education and Recreation, conducted an experimental exercise program for adult men as part of a twenty-year research study into the effects of daily exercise in relationship to coronary heart disease.

In 1975 the study reached the halfway mark. Dr. Golding reported that preliminary test results have proven that daily exercise does reduce blood pressure, cholesterol, and obesity in adult men between thirty and sixty years of age.

An article in the *New York Times* (August 22, 1973) headlined this fact: *"Backaches Multiply, But Country Takes Threat Lying Down."* The article, by Virginia Lee Warren, went on to say, "It appears likely that plain, old-fashioned ailment, the backache, will be the most common leveler of Americans in about three years, replacing the common cold."

"It's the curse of our time," states Dr. Howard Rusk, head of the Institute of Rehabilitation Medicine. "This condition is already causing more discomfort, loss of time from work, and disability than any other."

If you wish to avoid ending up one day with an aching back, a daily exercise program is absolutely essential. Posture, correct body movement or body mechanics, abdominal muscle tone, hip and lateral muscles, the extensor muscles of the spine, and leg muscles are all involved in keeping a back strong and out of trouble.

Physical fitness does not apply only to muscular and athletic efficiency, but also to the activation of nutrients in your body—to making them work.

"Exercise stimulates body tone, sending minerals to your muscles, skin, organs, blood vessels, and other body parts," writes Carlson Wade in *Magic Minerals: A Key to Better Health.*[3] Exercise causes minerals to help keep your body properly hydrated, to get rid of waste materials properly, and to keep you operating at optimum level with little fatigue or loss of quality.

When minerals are stimulated by exercise, they work to help pass food along your digestive tract, to enable you to inhale air into your lungs, and to regulate blood-vessel action when more pressure is needed in an emergency.

Minerals that are activated via exercise will speed up circulation to furnish more oxygen to the billions of your body cells, helping them remove waste material. The faster minerals bring oxygen to your cells, the better you feel. You "come alive." The increased mineral activity brings more blood to your brain, too, making you more alert—an aid to a powerful personality!

The faster mineral action of the circulatory system also helps the functioning of the internal organs. Your heart becomes stronger and steadier. Your lungs are fed by minerals and are now capable of taking in more oxygen. Elimination of body wastes is properly regulated. *Without exercise, minerals may remain inert and lazy, and so will you!* In most cases, people grow tired because minerals cannot be sent moving to various body parts. This causes a gradual deterioration of the entire body and mind. So you can appreciate the value of movement by exercise.

Some years ago, at the Lyndon Johnson Space Center in Houston, Texas, scientists made an important and still-mysterious discovery about potassium losses in astronauts during space flights. (Potassium, a natural element, is the most abundant electrolyte in the cells of your body and is critical to the reactions necessary for all muscle contraction, including your heart muscle, which pumps blood throughout your body.)

In space, the astronaut's "weightlessness" has profound repercussions. Blood, which normally accumulates in the legs, is redistributed throughout the body.

When minerals are stimulated by exercise, they work to help pass food along your digestive tract, to enable you to inhale air into your lungs, and to regulate blood-vessel action when more pressure is needed in an emergency.—**H.J.R.**

One of the ways that the POWs of the Vietnamese war, particularly those captured by the Vietcong, sustained themselves throughout their ordeal—which exerted great pressure physiologically as well as psychologically and emotionally—was that they exercised a lot. One of the prisoners set a record of 300 pushups and 600-700 knee bends.—**H.J.R.**

Movements and work are easier because the astronaut no longer has to lift things—only direct them—thus decreasing the normal exercise work. This results in serious potassium depletion.

Potassium is normally plentiful in the fluid portion of the circulating blood. However, under certain conditions its excretion in urine is increased. Prolonged immobility in the case of the astronauts resulted in the excretion of excessive potassium. Hence special space-type exercises were prescribed for the astronauts to help protect them from potassium loss. (Incidentally, the amount of exercise prescribed for the astronauts has been substantially increased between the first and second Space Station flights.)

Potassium deficiency manifests itself in muscle weakness, slow reflexes, and mental confusion. It also produces degeneration and death of heart fibers.

About 90 percent of the body's potassium is located in cells. Barely 8 percent is found in blood plasma and lymph, but this extracellular potassium cannot be decreased without causing heart problems.

It appears that physical exercise activates the expulsion of potassium from the cells and increases plasma potassium, which is used by the heart.

Basically, any muscular activity helps, provided it is done regularly without unnecessary strain.

The psychological benefits of exercise have been well validated by research and experience. An experiment at the University of Wisconsin revealed that anxiety decreased in both normal and neurotic people after they exercised.

One of the ways that the POWs of the Vietnamese war, particularly those captured by the Vietcong, sustained themselves throughout their ordeal—which exerted great pressure physiologically as well as psychologically and emotionally—was that they exercised a lot. One of the prisoners set a record of 300 pushups and 600–700 knee bends.

They kept themselves sustained because they found that even if they were in small cells they were still able to get some amount of exercise through posture changes. They exercised for two or three hours a day and found that it was one of the things that helped them keep their sanity.

So next time you feel overwhelmed or defeated by problems—exercise!

It is quite possible to counteract the many negative aspects and impacts of life by stimulation of the circulation and the vital forces of the body organs. If we maintain the right physical condition, the "worry throw-off" effect of a vigorous workout can border on the miraculous. Even prolonged negative pressure can be diminished by that technique. But even if you are not in condition for a good workout, you can make use of such exercise equivalents as hydrotherapy, electrotherapy, and manipulation. Many of these you can do by yourself. If you like the luxury of having someone skilled do them for you, the cost need not be great. It might be a lot less expensive than a breakdown or dragging around half alive. These exercise equivalents can, in the elimination of toxins from the system, increase and stimulate the circulation and vital forces, and relax the nerves. When a lack of good physical condition makes a real exercise workout impractical or impossible, exercise equivalents furnish relief or retreat from the pressures and tensions of modern living. These exercise equivalents, or "EEs" as I term them, are fully explained in other chapters of this book.

Writing this chapter reminds me of an experience I had back in the early years of the Great Depression. In conjunction with my city establishment I was conducting a health farm. One day we had a visitor—a man in his middle fifties and a very popular and well-known figure in the vaudeville and entertainment field. In the course of our conversation I learned that he had amassed a fortune of $300,000 and in the crash of 1929 had lost over two-thirds of it. I noticed his head and shoulders were bobbing and weaving as he talked, and he dipped up and down on one leg as he walked. He twitched and weaved and "dry washed" his hands when he spoke. He had more nervous tics than a dog has fleas. He couldn't eat, sleep, or do many other things. The loss of the greater part of his savings had taken away, in addition to his money, his spirit and feeling of security, and now his sense of humor and his health were on their way out. After we chatted a bit, he asked if I could help him. I said I could if he would agree to obey orders, give me his full cooperation, and arrange to stay for at least three weeks. This he promised and we were ready to start.

Although nervous and in a very run-down condition from worry and lack of sleep (the sedatives and sleeping pills he had been taking for a long time were no longer even temporarily effective), his heart and the basic condition of his arteries were found satisfactory upon medical checkup. The first day of conditioning was really difficult. It was hard for him to concentrate on anything for long, and we really had a difficult chore in making him exercise and do his work therapy. I felt like Svengali by the end of the day.

Along with his physical activity we made certain that he had plenty of complete rest periods. At the end of the day he was also given some fatigue-relieving and relaxing hydrotherapy and massage. This helped to ease his tired muscles and relax him in general. He had little appetite that first day and slept little the first night. He said he just felt too tired to sleep. When I asked him what he was thinking about during this sleepless first night, he replied, "I was too darned tired to even think, but it was nice just not having to do anything—just lying in bed and resting this tired, old body—that felt mighty good."

The next day we gave him exercise and occupational therapy (sawing wood, digging in the garden, clearing paths through the woods, etc.), finishing with hydrotherapy and massage. After a light dinner he quickly went to bed. That night we know he slept, for we could hear him snoring. By the third day his appetite was picking up, and the fourth day he was competing with all of us in eating and sleeping.

After my friend had been with this conditioning program for about two weeks, he told me he would like to call New York City. "You know," he said, "I'm starting to feel pretty good, and I thought I might like to have my agent come up to visit me for the weekend. I think I have some ideas for a new act and would like to check with him.

"You know, Reilly, I have over $50,000 left from the crash. That's still a lot of money. In another few weeks I'll finish the skit I showed to my agent, and I think it's going to knock them into the aisles." He did make a comeback and

It is quite possible to counteract the many negative aspects and impacts of life by stimulation of the circulation and the vital forces of the body organs. If we maintain the right physical condition, the "worry throw-off" effect of a vigorous workout can border on the miraculous.—**H.J.R.**

Physical conditioning had relieved the tension and nervous tics, and restored normal eating and sleeping habits. Best of all, it had given him a vigorous and optimistic outlook on life and the capacity to enjoy what he had and not get into the deadly postmortem routine of what he had lost.—H.J.R.

Exercise can be a very effective therapeutic tool whether the disturbances are psychosomatic or physiological.—H.J.R.

was "knocking them in the aisles" for many years after that.

Physical conditioning had relieved the tension and nervous tics, and restored normal eating and sleeping habits. Best of all, it had given him a vigorous and optimistic outlook on life and the capacity to enjoy what he had and not get into the deadly postmortem routine of what he had lost. Yes, if we were to lose all our possessions but retained good health and physical fitness, we would be far from defeated. We would still possess the intelligence and drive that made for success in the first place, and we would have an added advantage of experience. Only the handicap of being physically inadequate would retard our comeback. To feel fully adequate in a changing world we must have some basic security. For many this can be found in religion and philosophy. The addition of health and physical fitness will strengthen and intensify all other securities.

Exercise can be a very effective therapeutic tool whether the disturbances are psychosomatic or physiological.

A number of my most spectacular cures have been with stars of the music world whose careers were seriously threatened by physical disabilities.

B.H. is a six-foot-two bass-baritone, whose imposing stage presence and voice have brought him acclaim on the opera stages of Israel, Europe, and Puerto Rico, and on the concert and light-opera stage in America, where he has been appearing for some years with a Gilbert and Sullivan company. When B.H. came to see me, he was suffering from a severe case of thrombophlebitis and was in fact scheduled for a surgical operation to relieve this extremely painful condition. The surgeon was just waiting for the swelling to subside to operate for the removal of the outer veins of the legs, which had caused the condition. This tall man—young and vital—was like a hobbled giant unable to walk or stand on his affected legs.

B.H. in an interview told Mrs. Brod, "Dr. Reilly told me that if I did have the veins taken out that it was very possible that within a year the inner veins, having to take over the work of the outer veins as well as their own function, might become so overtaxed that they could also get varicose and then they would have to be removed and then I would wind up being crippled for life. He said that if I promised to do special exercises faithfully two or three times a day, have special massage on the buttocks and feet (not on the legs), and the right kind of food and sitz baths, I could get the valves to start working again in the outer veins and not have them removed.

"The main feature of the diet was getting a lot of rutin—all the citrus fruits, green peppers, mustard greens, dandelion greens . . . were easy to get. I gave up the coffee as Dr. Reilly instructed me to do and substituted herb teas, which I really now like and enjoy. I never liked meat that much, I prefer seafood, so that wasn't hard to readjust, although he allowed me a little lamb or chicken.

"He gave me five different exercises. I started with six each and am now doing sixteen of each twice a day. It takes about thirty-five minutes and I rest in between and I do breathing in between them. [The exercises will be found in Chapter 7.]

"After the evening exercises, when the body is well-warmed up, I take a cold sitz bath—for about sixty to ninety seconds.

"I went once a month for checking and massage. Dr. Reilly watched me do the exercises. He thought that one of them was bad for my voice because it caused a strain on the vocal chords and he told me not to do it. He has a remarkable understanding of those things that go into performing. [The exercise here referred to was the double-leg circles, described in Chapter 7.]

"After the first month I got fantastic results. The veins went back to inside the leg. They were all sticking out before and when I went back to the specialist, he had to look twice to see which was the bad leg—they were both bad, but the left one was worse than the right. The surgeon examined me and said he thought the veins would still have to come out and he wanted to set an appointment for the operation. I told him I would call him and let him know. I just never called back.

"The leg is completely normalized now.

"Even before the first month was up and I went back to see Dr. Reilly, I knew that I was going to continue the exercises, because I already had so much extra energy that I knew this was something that I was going to do the rest of my life.

"I still want to take the sitz baths because I sleep so much better than I ever did—it is a great preventive, too. I always had poor blood circulation, because every winter I suffered terribly. I couldn't get warm no matter how many sweaters and coats I was wearing. I was always cold. And after I started on the Reilly regimen and did the exercises—I went through the entire winter, December, January, February, without having a cold or suffering from the cold.

"I had read many books about Cayce and I was quite prepared to accept the treatments. However, it was nice to hear Dr. Reilly tell me: 'You realize that you did it yourself. All I can do is tell you what exercises and baths are good for you, but you have to have the will and purpose to do it and to heal yourself.'"

I have always believed that in the end the patient has to heal him- or herself. My standard prescription is a daily dose of "RIP" (resolution, information, and perseverance). "Take this every four hours," I tell my patients. "When you get up in the morning—exercise; before each meal—eat the right food and don't overeat; and before retiring—exercise, and you will not have to worry about the 'RIP' ('Rest in Peace') you see on tombstones for many, many years."

B.H. was a good example of the healing virtues of RIP. It is even more dramatically illustrated in the case of F.L., a famous concert cellist, who could visit me only twice before leaving for Europe. He suffered from muscular tension at times that made it difficult for him to keep up his grueling schedule of practice and concerts while on tour. I taught him the arm-and-shoulder exercises (see Chapter 7), prescribed Epsom salt soaks, showers—letting water as hot as possible run on his shoulders—and self-massage with peanut oil. He followed the regimen with resolution and persistence entirely under his own discipline while in Europe.

"The tension and cramps in the shoulder subsided," F.L. told Mrs. Brod. "I felt light and free. I could play for hours, and I was able to perform during my entire European concert tour."

A Daily Dose of "RIP"

I have always believed that in the end the patient has to heal him- or herself. My standard prescription is a daily dose of "RIP":

- *Resolution*
- *Information*
- *Perseverance*

"Take this every four hours," I tell my patients. "When you get up in the morning—exercise; before each meal—eat the right food and don't overeat; and before retiring—exercise, and you will not have to worry about the 'RIP' ('Rest in Peace') you see on tombstones for many, many years."

—H.J.R.

cataracts

Ruth Hagy Brod was told by an eye specialist that she had the beginning of a cataract over her left eye. After practicing the Cayce head-and-neck exercises and Reilly eye exercise, she returned to the doctor. He admitted he was surprised. The cataract not only had not increased, it had partially dissolved. Further, she didn't need stronger glasses. —**H.J.R.**

Bleeding Hemorrhoids

emphysema

The noted American composer–conductor Alan Hovhaness suffered for years from crippling bursitis and arthritis. Finally, the stiffness in his arms threatened to end his conducting career. But a few weeks after he came to me he was a new person. The massage and manipulation helped, but what really saved Hovhaness was what he did for himself in my prescribed stretching and bending exercises. (See Chapter 7.) "It brought new life to my arms and legs," the composer told author Jess Stearn, who wrote about it in *Edgar Cayce—The Sleeping Prophet*.

Some time later Hovhaness wrote to me: " . . . as I always think of you and do your exercises every day, without ever missing one day, and always spending about twenty minutes to half an hour or more. Your wonderful help has given me years of the greatest success and activity in my musical career, and I want to thank you for it . . .

"We wish you great success with your new book and hope you are well and prospering in every way. Many thanks for all you have done for me . . . "

Mrs. E.P., an interior decorator in a large department store, had to leave her job because of bleeding hemorrhoids so severe that she was confined to her bed for six weeks. After a series of colonics, the use of hot compresses, and above all daily performance of the Cayce hemorrhoids exercises, she was able to return to work.

Dr. H.R.D., the headmaster of a Connecticut private school, was referred to us by another patient, who was the president of Queens College in New York. Both men were golfers and suffered from arthritis, which impaired their movement and activity. The headmaster was placed on a graduated program of physical exercises similar to the ones you will find in the next chapter, and a correct diet. He had some massage and manipulation, since his visits to me were limited. Some months later, he reported back to us that his golf game had improved so much everyone wanted to know what he was doing. More significantly, his doctor told him that the exercise program had given him three or four years of physical activity beyond what the X–rays indicated would have been the case.

Ruth Hagy Brod was told by an eye specialist that she had the beginning of a cataract over her left eye. After practicing the Cayce head–and–neck exercises and Reilly eye exercise, she returned to the doctor. He admitted he was surprised. The cataract not only had not increased, it had partially dissolved. Further, she didn't need stronger glasses.

Mrs. H.H., a New Jersey housewife, had been coming to me regularly for some time for help for her deformed hip. One day she complained of difficulty in breathing and a medical examination confirmed the fact that she was developing emphysema. When I gave her some balloons to blow up and told her to take them home and keep blowing on them several times daily, she thought I was joking. Actually this is a very effective exercise for asthma, emphysema, and other disorders of the lungs and breathing mechanisms. In addition, I taught her daughter to give her mother a "cupping" massage, which is very effective in breaking up chest and back congestion. (This type of massage, so useful in chest colds, is described in Chapter 8.)

Which Exercises?

A television interviewer once asked me, "Which are the best exercises?" My reply was, "The ones you do."

From time to time, in my sixty years of experience, I have seen exercise fads come and go: the best "daily dozen," the "serious seven," the "Royal Canadian," isometric, isotonic, aerobic, jogging, rope-skipping, yoga—I have no objection to any of them. They are all good if done regularly and correctly, with the proper preparation after a good medical examination has described the parameters of your personal limitations. The next important thing is to exercise regularly every day. There are no Sabbaths in exercise.

I do have reservations about isometrics, which oppose one muscle against another or against an immovable object, and I am glad to see others speaking out against them, such as Dr. Charles B. Mullins of the University of Texas Southwestern Medical School at Dallas, who said: "Isometric exercises don't help your cardiovascular system. Such exercise elevates blood pressure and could be dangerous for people with heart trouble," he cautions. "The heart is made to pump volume. With isometrics, the heart doesn't pump much more volume, but has to work against higher pressure."

With general exercise you pump a lot more blood with only a little more pressure.

Cayce told a thirty-three-year-old woman, "Walking is the best exercise, but don't take this spasmodically. Have a regular time and do it, rain or shine." (1968-9)

In fact, he prescribed walking in 280 of the 1,469 cases in which exercise was part of the general therapy.

In the case (1530-2) of a fifty-year-old woman whose ailments included arthritis, poor circulation, hypertension, neuritis, rheumatism, and toxemia, he said, "Well that the body take each day a certain amount of exercise, or as much as possible in the open. Walking is the best exercise, but this—though—in the *open* when at all practical."

To a man suffering from nervous tension, which had produced a great many physical complications, Cayce, when asked, "What exercise is best?" answered (277-1), "A general exercise, but—as stipulated—a great deal of the exercise would be *given* the body, that makes for a better balancing in the system. The better is walking or rowing."

Cayce also frequently recommended swimming, bicycling, horseback riding, tennis, badminton, and any exercise that could be enjoyed in the open air.

"The entity should keep close to all of those things that have to do with outdoor activities, for it is the best way to keep yourself young—to stay close to nature, close to those activities in every form of exercise that breathes in the . . . beauty of nature . . . breathe it into thine own soul, as you would a sunset or a morning sun rising. And see that sometimes—it's as pretty as the sunset!" (3374-1)

In the case of a patient (2533-6) suffering from hypertension, who asked the sleeping prophet to "give a simple method of reducing the blood pressure of this body to normal," the answer given was, "The simple method is to keep

---

A television interviewer once asked me, "Which are the best exercises?"

My reply was, "The ones you do."—**H.J.R.**

Edgar Cayce, again and again in his readings, emphasized the importance of consistency and regularity in all things, especially exercise. "Whenever something is begun and then left off, it becomes detrimental—[anything] that should have been kept up!" (457-12)—**H.J.R.**

Walking is the best exercise, but don't take this spasmodically. Have a regular time and do it, rain or shine. (1968-9)

Cayce, in fact, prescribed walking in 280 of the 1,469 cases in which exercise was part of the general therapy. He also frequently recommended swimming, bicycling, horseback riding, tennis, badminton, and any exercise that could be enjoyed in the open air.

—**H.J.R.**

The entity should keep close to all of those things that have to do with outdoor activities, for it is the best way to keep yourself young—to stay close to nature, close to those activities in every form of exercise that breathes in the . . . beauty of nature . . . breathe it into thine own soul, as you would a sunset or a morning sun rising. And see that sometimes—it's as pretty as the sunset! (3374-1)

away from fats, and this will keep it near to normal.

"Walk in the open early of mornings. This brings better activity of oxygen and ozone as to keep the balance in the blood flow through lungs, heart, liver, kidneys. These are the sources from which either the pressure or repression causes disturbance."

Many eminent doctors agree with Edgar Cayce's enthusiasm for walking, among them the noted heart specialist Dr. Paul Dudley White, who is quoted as saying, "A vigorous five-mile walk will do more good than all the medicine and psychology in the world."[4]

The American Medical Association's Committee on Exercise and Physical Fitness states, "Walking briskly, not just strolling, is the simplest and also one of the best forms of exercise."

Of course, we are not referring here to strolling or a window-shopping walk. Walking can be made extremely beneficial when performed vigorously.

There are a variety of ways of walking, but I recommend stride walking, which can be performed with short, medium, or long strides. I would suggest that perhaps the last fourth of a mile in your walk should be done in the fastest way possible, with long strides so that one can work up a good perspiration.

The benefits of brisk walking and striding are increased exercise for the heart, increased oxygen intake, and improved blood circulation.

Bristol-Myers has included in its advertising campaign the following message on the benefits of walking:

"The body has about 60,000 miles of blood vessels—mostly capillaries. These tiny vessels bring oxygen to the muscles. Only a few are open when a muscle is inactive, but 50 times as many open up when the muscle is being exercised. Another benefit is in returning blood to the heart. The body's muscles work like an extra blood pump. When a muscle is being actively used, it squeezes the blood out of the capillaries and back toward the heart.

"So next time you have a short errand, don't drive—walk briskly."

I have often been asked about the merits of jogging. If it's done carefully, especially after one has received a doctor's approval after a cardiovascular checkup, jogging can be a very beneficial exercise. However, it can also be detrimental, and there have been a number of unfortunate fatalities when undertaken without a proper buildup. I would say the best preparation for jogging is a series of walks, gradually increasing the length and speed of the walk. For the beginner, ordinarily after having done a few weeks of increased distance and speed walking, one of the best ways to start jogging would be to walk about 300 ordinary paces, then jog slowly with small steps about 100 paces, then 300 more walking paces, and 100 more jogging paces. One can do that for about half a mile, or about 1,600 paces.

Then after the second week, if you do this three times a week, you can decrease the walking by 100 paces and increase the jogging by 100 paces. After two more weeks you can decrease the walking again by 100 paces, so in about six weeks you would jog a little less than one-half mile.

I would suggest, if you go on to the second half of the mile, that you repeat the same formula: after jogging the half mile you increase the jogging as out-lined above. By building up slowly, there is almost no limit to your ultimate capacity and you can get the most benefit from it; it is also by far the safest method. This way you exercise to increase your endurance and vitality, not to use up what little you might have, so keep your ego under control.

In rainy or stormy weather one could practice jogging indoors by running in place. When you do that, you could lift your knees up high and just keep a running movement in the same place without covering any distance, legs up and down in a jogging rhythm.

In addition to walking and other outdoor sports, Cayce recommended a regular program of calisthenics and frequently used specific exercises as therapy:

> We find that the exercises such as the setting-up exercise when the body first arises of a morning would be well, for this will bring strength to the lungs, vitality to the blood supply, and a new life, as it were, to the muscular forces of the body. Take then, at least five to ten minutes of exercises of the arms and limbs when the body first arises each morning. (4462-1)

In general he advocated that breathing and vertical exercises should be done in the morning in order to force as much oxygen as possible into the body, for we breathe shallowly while sleeping.

He considered horizontal exercises to be the most beneficial in the evening. Since most people work sitting or standing during the day, the horizontal ex-ercises have a tendency to normalize circulation and take the strain off arterial capillaries and veins of the lower extremities.

In reading 1773–1, we find Cayce advising the following (see Fig. 1):

> Mornings upon arising take for two minutes an exercise in this manner—where the body, standing with the feet flat on the floor, gently rises to the toes at the same time bringing the arms high above the head. Then bring these as far back as possible or practical swinging both arms back. Then gradu-ally bring them towards the front, then let down. Breathe *in* as the body rises and *out* as the body brings the hands to the front, slowly. Do this three or four times each morning . . . This is an excellent exercise for posture and for aiding in keeping this balance which will be set up by the general manipula-tions as combined with the osteopathic corrective forces.

In reading 2454–2 he says this (see Fig. 2):

> Then in the morning before dressing, exercise the upper portion of the body; [by swinging] the arms up and down, straight up, straight down; then the turning motion as of swinging the arms around, for the movement . . . from the diaphragm upward . . . from the ninth dorsal upward—these exercises will take away the heaviness and the tendency to get tired easily.

Then in the morning before dressing, exercise the upper portion of the body; [by swinging] the arms up and down, straight up, straight down; then the turning motion as of swinging the arms around, for the movement . . . from the diaphragm upward . . . from the ninth dorsal upward—these exercises will take away the heaviness and the tendency to get tired easily. (2454-2)

In reading 470-37 Cayce remarks thus (see Fig. 3 series):

[Each morning before dressing] rise on tiptoe slowly and raise the arms easily at the same time [reaching] directly above the head, pointing straight up. At the same time, bend head back just as far as you can. When let down gentle from this, you see, we make for giving a better circulation through the whole area from the abdomen through the diaphragm, through the lungs, head and neck. Then let down, put the head forward just as far as it will come on the chest, then raise again at the top, bend the head to the right as far as it will go down. When rising again, bend the head to the left. Then standing erect, hands on hips, circle the head, roll around to the right two or three times. Then straighten self . . . will change all of those disturbances through the mouth, head and eyes, and the activity of the whole body will be improved.

My own breathing exercise, a Reilly variation of the Cayce classics, goes like this (see Figs. 4A and 4B): Rise on toes, at the same time raising your arms out to the side and then up over the head, inhaling through the nostrils. On the exhalation, bring arms down, lower heels, cross arms, and hug the body at the waist as you bend forward, forcing all the air out of the lungs. Finish with a "Ha, ha!" or a grunt to empty all the air from the lungs before beginning the next inhalation.

Cayce also occasionally recommended alternate nostril breathing—a standard yoga exercise that is supposed to be very energizing.

In the following reading, Cayce describes how this exercise can be performed:

Of morning, and upon arising especially (and don't sleep too late)—and before dressing so that the clothing is loose or the fewer the better—stand erect before an open window, breathe deeply, gradually raising hands *above* the head, and then with the circular motion of the body from the hips bend forward; breathing *in* (and through the nostrils) as the body rises on its toes—breathing very deep; *exhaling suddenly* through the *mouth,* not through the nasal passages. Take these [exercises] for 5 to 6 minutes. Then as these progress, gradually *close* one of the nostrils (even if it's necessary to use the hand—but if it is closed with the left hand, raise the right hand; and when closing the right nostril with the right hand, then raise the left hand) *as the breathing in* is accomplished. (1523-2)

The evening exercises are to be performed for the most part lying on the floor. Cayce's rationale is expressed in reading 288-11, when he says that to take blood away from the head, in exercising the lower body, lie prone and use circular or swinging motions of the legs.

Other Cayce classics are the cat crawl and rolling exercise and the buttocks walk:

No better exercises may be taken than . . . the cat-stretching exercises, which includes, of course, being able—(put very coarsely)—to do the split, be able to put the head on the feet, to put the feet behind the head, to make the head and neck exercises and *all* of those activities that may be said to be of the feline or cat exercise. To be sure, in the present period, present development, present conditions that exist, must be gone at gently; but be persistent morning and evening, working at it, still not letting it become *rote,* but *purposeful.* (681-2)

Be careful if you try this one:

The rolling exercise is to put the head between the knees and have someone roll you over two or three times. (308-8)

. . . let the exercise preferably be for the lower limbs [in the evening] . . . a movement as of sitting on the floor and walking across or swinging the limbs one in front of the other for 3 to 4 movements. (2454-2)

Now we come to the most popular exercises of all, the Cayce head–and–neck exercise and rolls. These are prescribed for both morning and evening, and are particularly valuable to relieve muscle tension for people engaged in desk work, typing, piano playing, and other activities that strain head, neck, eyes, shoulders, and arms.

Cayce, responding to a client asking, "How may my eyes be strengthened so as to eliminate the necessity of reading glasses?" replied, "By the head and neck exercise in the open as you walk for 20 or 30 minutes each morning." (2533-6) (See Fig. 3 series.)

In fact, Cayce recommended these exercises to 250 people suffering with various forms of eye and ear trouble and to fifty others for a wide variety of complaints. In addition to aiding vision and hearing, it is an excellent stimulant to the thyroid.

Cayce suggested that these be performed in the morning in a standing position and in the afternoon or evening in a sitting position.

I prefer my patients to start off with the sitting position so that they can press their shoulders and back into the back of a chair, keeping their posture erect and head straight and centered, and mentally reaching for the ceiling.

Cayce says (see Fig. 3 series):

When we remove the pressures of the toxic forces we will improve the vision. Also the head and neck exercise will be most helpful. Take this regularly, not taking it sometimes and leaving off sometimes, but each morning and each evening take this exercise regularly for 6 months and we will see a great deal of difference: sitting erect, bend the head forward three times, to the back three times, to the right side three times, to the left side three times, and then circle the head each way three times. Don't hurry through with it but take the time to do it. We will get results. (3549-1)

I would like to point out that while most people will find that performing the horizontals before going to bed is very relaxing and conducive to sound sleep, there is the exceptional person who may be overstimulated by them. If you are one of these exceptions, I suggest that these exercises be performed before dinner.—**H.J.R.**

An Exercise for Hemorrhoids

The Cayce exercises for hemorrhoids have been widely publicized in books and by the patients who have benefited from them.

In case 2823-2 Cayce had this to say:

But the best for the specific conditions of hemorrhoids is the exercise, and if this is taken regularly these will disappear—of themselves! Twice each day, of morning and evening—and this doesn't mean with many clothes on!—rise on the toes, at the same time raising the arms, then bend forward, letting the hands go toward the floor. Do this three times of morning, and three times of evening. But don't do it two or three times and then quit, *or* don't do it three or four times a week and then quit, but do it regularly! [See Fig. 1.]

I would like to point out that while most people will find that performing the horizontals before going to bed is very relaxing and conducive to sound sleep, there is the exceptional person who may be overstimulated by them. If you are one of these exceptions, I suggest that these exercises be performed before dinner. A side benefit is that they normalize the appetite of nervous people who tend to overeat or eat too fast at the evening meal. The exercise must be done slowly.

Horizontal exercises will have a tendency to normalize the circulation and take the strain off the arterial capillaries and veins of the lower extremities. Sometimes hard exercise will have a narcotic effect in which the fatigue of the body will relieve the mind of anxiety.

However, such exercises should not be attempted if one has a cardiovascular disorder of any kind, except under expert supervision. Then special exercise can be very good.

Cayce expressed it this way:

Exercises for the blood flow away from head . . . Swinging, circular motion then of lower portion of body in evenings, and the circular motion of hands and upper portion of body in mornings . . . (288-11)

By this he meant exercises of the type such as the leg circles and the leg raises described in the horizontal exercises in Chapter 7.

When Cayce was asked, "Should I *make* myself take the evening exercise of the lower limbs even when I am so tired and heavy that I can't put any pep into it?" he answered, "The best way to acquire the correct amount of pep is to take the exercise!" (288–38)

Cayce's advice to those who have sedentary occupations was: "Be mindful that there is sufficient of the exercises that use the areas through the lumbar and sacral [regions]: the bicycle riding, walking, horseback riding, rowing and the like." (1968–6)

This one was recommended for the evening. It is especially good for stimulating glandular activity also:

Then of an evening, just before retiring—[with the body prone, facing the floor and] with the feet braced against the wall, circle the torso by resting on the hands. Raise and lower the body not merely by the hands but more from the torso, and with more of a circular motion of the pelvic organs to strengthen the muscular forces of the abdomen. Not such an activity as to cause strain, but a gentle circular motion to the right two or three times, and then to the left. (1523-2) [See Figs. 5A and 5B. NOTE: Beginners may bend the arms at elbows as shown in Fig. 5B.]

To another sufferer he recommended this variation, which seems to be a form of early American acupressure:

Bending the body over—as over a table or chair—and pressing upon the nerves about the anus, where we would hold the ends of the ileum and scrotum plexus, will relieve easily. (555-7)

Then, each morning and each evening . . . Standing erect, raise the hands high above the head as possible, rising on the toes, then slowly bending forward until the hands will almost or quite touch the floor. Do this slowly, but do it at least three, four, five, six times, *very* slowly, stretching upward and forward and downward. (555-8)

For the feet Cayce gives the following: *strength arches*

(Q) What can be done to strengthen arches?
(A) The massage with the [specific] oils will be helpful. Also an exercise each day . . . would be well, of morning, before the shoes are put on—before the oil massage is given, of course (but do this daily); stand flat on the floor and spring on the toes, rising gently and springing. (3381-1)

(Q) Would you recommend special foot exercise?
(A) It would be well if there would be this exercise night and morning; night before retiring—but after the massage as indicated, see; and of morning just before putting on the hose—after the massage has been given:
    Stand erect (without anything on the feet, of course). Then raise the arms, gently, slowly, over the head—directly over the head. Then gradually rise on the toes. Then, as the body relaxes or lowers itself, lower the hands also—the hands extending in front of the body. Then rock back upon the heels, with the hands extended sufficiently to strain or to exercise the bursa of the heel, or those portions of the heel *and* the arch, you see, to aid in strengthening. Doing this, together *with* the massage of the properties indicated through heel and arch, and especially over the frontal portions of the foot, we will bring better conditions for same. (1771-3)

(Q) What is the most effective treatment to follow to stop the progression of structural destruction in my feet?
(A) Rising upon the toes twice a day, morning and evening—upon arising and before retiring. Before putting on shoes and stockings of morning. Raise the arms, rocking back and forth on the heel and toe. Gradually, as the body raises up, raise the arms high also. Such an exercise is most beneficial.
(1620-3)

> **An Exercise to Improve Assimilation**
> The better change should come within from the better assimilation of that eaten, which will be found to be more improved by the exercises of stretching arms above the head, or swinging on a pole would be well. This doesn't mean to run out and jump on a pole every time you eat, but have regular periods. When you have the activities, do have these exercises, for they will stimulate the gastric flow and let that eaten have something to float in . . . (2072-14)

As I have mentioned in earlier chapters, sometimes Cayce spelled out instructions in great detail when he referred men and women to me, and he often left the planning as well as the execution of the program entirely to me.

In any case, there was a striking similarity between Cayce and me, in our philosophy of exercise and even in the actual exercises themselves.

Over the years I have modified and adapted many of his ideas into the exercises and programs that I designed for individual clients both at the Health

Reducing Abdomen — roll on a barrel

Institute and in private practice and at the A.R.E. Clinic. You will find them listed in the following pages.

It was as though he had been reading my mind—perhaps that was exactly what he was doing—reading my mind, as well as the minds of all the masters of healing through the ages.

You will note similarities in the exercises in the following pages. Occasionally he even suggested something in a reading that already existed in the Reilly repertoire. For example, he told a thirty-five-year-old woman (540-11) who asked at the end of her reading, "Please give methods for reducing abdomen," that the answer was, "Roll on a barrel—this is the best!"

Many years ago one of the now-defunct New York dailies featured my exercises with a medicine ball, which can be a great beauty aid, and I had a model demonstrate the same principle of rolling—but on a medicine ball or hassock instead of on a barrel.

Before we get to the matter of the general exercises for conditioning and tone, I would like to say a few things about yoga. I am asked with increasing frequency about it, and its popularity in the modern culture has grown.

I have had a great deal of experience in evaluating the effect of yoga exercises through my association for many years with the world-famous yoga teacher, Blanche De Vries, who has private students at her magnificent estate on the Hudson River in Nyack, New York.

Frequently Blanche has me evaluate her students before they begin their lessons with her, and I have treated some of them with massage and manipulation to speed their progress. Unfortunately, not all yoga teachers are as careful with their students. Mrs. De Vries and I have often discussed a lack of certification by some yoga teachers, and as it has become more fashionable, more and more "instant experts" have arrived on the scene to waste the time, money, and even health of those who are interested in securing its benefits.

Men and women in their middle years, between forty and sixty-five, who have never exercised before, may suddenly become yoga-conscious. They may seek any kind of teacher without inquiring about background or credentials, and may, as a result, develop different kinds of disabilities caused by doing too much too soon. Deplorably, we are treating more and more cases of hiatus hernia (a rupture of the muscles of the diaphragm) caused by such exercises as extreme back bends performed incorrectly or prematurely before the muscles are sufficiently strengthened and stretched.

We are also getting many cases of torn or pulled tendons, especially in the region of the lower back, hips, and groin, and injuries of the neck and shoulder muscles that result from improper instruction. If you wish to take up yoga, be certain you have an experienced teacher with whom there would be very little danger of such mishaps. Some of the pupils of Blanche De Vries are in their sixties, seventies, and eighties, and they have found yoga exercises most beneficial in attaining and retaining the flexibility of youth far into what some call old age.

We find that Cayce's wisdom in regard to yoga, as in so many other ways, was prescient and just as relevant today as when he gave it. To a forty-four-year–old man who had been experimenting with yoga exercises and who was experiencing some physical and mental disturbances, Cayce gave this caution:

> These exercises are excellent, yet it is necessary that special preparation be made—or that a perfect understanding be had by the body as to what takes place when such exercises are used.
>
> For, *breath* is the basis of the living organism's activity. Thus, such exercises may be beneficial or detrimental in their effect upon a body.
>
> Hence it is necessary that an understanding be had as to how, as to when, or in what manner such may be used. (2475-1)

I know many of you will have to overcome an initial reluctance to the idea of exercise, a reluctance that will soon evaporate as you "come alive" in body, mind, and spirit as movement sends fresh blood and energy coursing through your veins. I can assure you that the time you spend maintaining health is going to be much more pleasant than the time spent in illness, struggling to repair the ravages of neglect, and to regain your health.

7

For Figure and Fitness—Exercises from Head to Toe

Many of us start a home physical-fitness program by purchasing a variety of expensive equipment. This is highly profitable for the equipment industry but hard on the home budget; and very often after the novelty has worn off the only exercise dividend the gadgets yield is that which you get crawling under the bed or reaching into a closet, where they have been stored, to dust them.

If you are serious about getting into shape and keeping fit, you can equip a Cayce–Reilly home-health institute with a bath towel, a striped beach towel, and resolution. The towel exercises in this chapter will give you a diversified workout for the least expense and expenditure of time. Performed every morning, the six vertical towel exercises will keep you limber, improve the muscle tone of the entire body, stimulate your circulation, and give you added pep and energy to meet the stresses of the day. They may also be performed before dinner to relieve fatigue.

The towel exercises incorporate many of the movements recommended in the general Cayce exercises, combined with the Reilly interpretation and basic principles. Some of the towel exercises will combine two to six or seven of the body movements suggested in the Cayce readings into one exercise. By using a towel we have tried to make the exercises easy to follow and more demanding. But they do limber most of the large joints of the body, and many of the small ones, too.

Preparation

1. Check with your doctor, preferably one who understands exercise, before undertaking any exercise or activity program. He or she will be able to diagnose your personal physical idiosyncrasies, such as hernias, your cardiovascular condition, etc., and is best qualified to prescribe the parameters of your individual abilities.

Check with your doctor, preferably one who understands exercise, before undertaking any exercise or activity program. He or she will be able to diagnose your personal physical idiosyncrasies, such as hernias, your cardiovascular condition, etc., and is best qualified to prescribe the parameters of your individual abilities.—**H.J.R.**

When I supervise exercises, I vary the order in which I call them and alternate the pointed heel and toe to keep the patient's mind from wandering. You might find this helpful in staying alert and concentrated. If you do your exercises with a partner, by all means spell each other in calling the order of the regimen.—**H.J.R.**

2. Prepare your equipment.

a. You will need a forty-inch bath towel that you will fold lengthwise into a four-to-six-inch width, and then bring the ends together until it is about twenty inches.

b. Place a large striped beach towel on the floor. Lie down so that the body is in a straight line from head to foot. Your feet should be about four inches apart. Have someone check you. Have your husband or wife or friend mark the outer and inner edges of your feet and then sew onto the towel two pieces of sponge rubber, felt, or other material that you can feel by touch. This is to ensure that you are always in the correct position when performing horizontal exercises.

NOTE: Frequently, even dedicated students worsen their condition by performing their exercises incorrectly in the wrong position, thus emphasizing their postural problems instead of correcting them. In the absence of supervision, the towel lines and the rubber or felt guides will help you monitor your own position to ensure that it is correct.

3. Wear an exercise suit, bathing suit, or any clothing that is light and permits freedom of movement.

4. Prepare your mind to concentrate and give full attention to what you are about to undertake. Exercises performed absentmindedly with your head full of postmortems or the upcoming problems of the day are not going to do you much good, either in mind or body. Visualize yourself as tall, slim, and flexible, and make a mental picture of the result you want to achieve. This will exercise your involuntary muscle system as well as your voluntary muscles. (This, by the way, is how I have taught paralytics and even paraplegics to regenerate some movement into their bodies, a matter that will be discussed in greater detail in a later chapter.)

When I supervise exercises, I vary the order in which I call them and alternate the pointed heel and toe to keep the patient's mind from wandering. You might find this helpful in staying alert and concentrated. If you do your exercises with a partner, by all means spell each other in calling the order of the regimen.

5. If you like to perform your exercises to music make sure the tempo is different from your natural rhythm. This is especially important if you are trying to reduce. I once had an instructor come to me at the institute to complain that he could not reduce the weight of a woman client no matter how hard she worked in the gym. She had exhausted the instructor, not herself. I observed her exercising and noticed that she worked with little effort. Questions disclosed that she was used to doing housework in a large house, cleaning it herself, and going up and down stairs, and she had developed a certain rhythm to her movements. She was exercising in the same natural rhythm and she was not expending enough energy to make a difference. We solved her weight problem by giving her first a fast exercise and then a slow one until we altered her natural rhythm. She then began to lose weight.

If you are doing hard physical work and are not overweight, this does not apply to you, as rhythm makes for economy of movement. But for maximum results it would be wise to have someone watch you or time yourself and vary your natural rhythm. Never break or change the rhythm too rapidly, though, as it bunches the muscles above the movement.

General Instructions

1. When you start your exercise program, do each exercise for six counts; then increase two counts per week until you are doing each one twelve times. You may work up to eighteen at the rate of two a week after a period of time.

2. Breathing: Inhale when straightening up or out, exhale on all forward or side bending movements. (Do not exhale on back bends.)

3. Keep feet parallel about twelve to eighteen inches apart. Knees should be slightly bent on all standing exercises. (Bending with stiff knees can cause back injury.)

4. Exercise slowly, steadily, and easily. Don't get overtired.

5. Always check posture before beginning exercise. Stand against a wall. Heels should be about two inches out, calves as close to the wall as possible, shoulders against the wall, and head against the wall. Pull the abdomen in and flatten the back against the wall. Raise arms slowly overhead and hold for a count of ten. Bring arms down to sides and walk away from the wall, keeping the position (Figs. 6A, 6B, 6C, and 6D).

Reilly Towel Verticals

These exercises incorporate most of the movements recommended by Cayce for morning verticals.

T1 Standing Kick

Stand high, heels twelve inches apart, feet parallel, hands straight above head, grasping towel firmly at ends.

Keeping arms and legs straight, kick right foot up to near shoulder level—lower towel to meet ankle at shoulder level. Return to position. Alternate first right, then left. Take no steps forward or backward. (See Fig. 7.)

T2 Pendulum

Without twisting the trunk, hold folded towel overhead full length, keeping the hands as high as possible. Bend the body to the left, keeping full tension on the towel, then straighten and bend to the right, making an inverted pendulum motion. Keep head and neck parallel with arms when bending to side. (See Fig. 8.)

T3 Wood Chopping

Holding towel overhead, and without moving feet, twist trunk to right, keeping tension on towel. Bend trunk, bringing left hand down between legs as far as possible, as in chopping wood. Return to position. Alternate first right, then

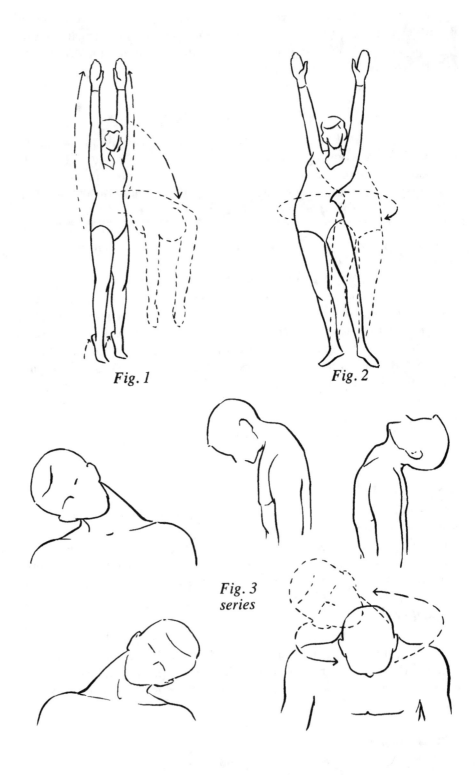

Fig. 1   Fig. 2

Fig. 3
series

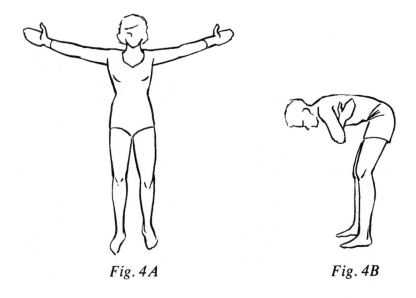

Fig. 4A   *Fig. 4B*

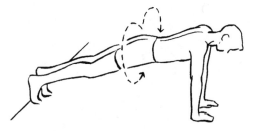

Fig. 5A

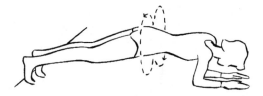

Fig. 5B

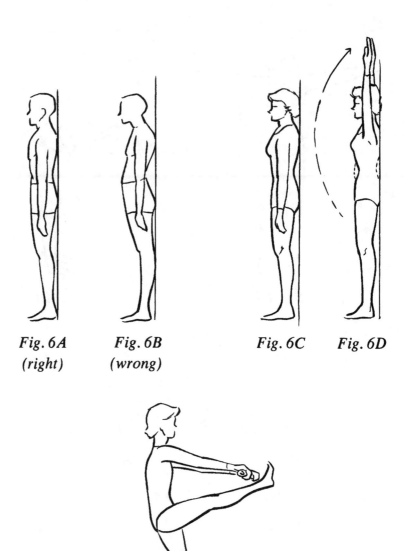

Fig. 6A   Fig. 6B   Fig. 6C   Fig. 6D
(right)   (wrong)

Fig. 7

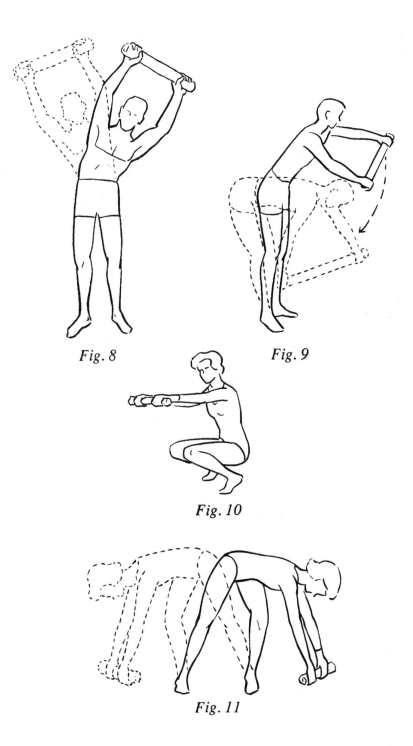

Fig. 8

Fig. 9

Fig. 10

Fig. 11

left. Feet should be parallel twelve to eighteen inches apart, and weight on toes. (See Fig. 9.)

T4 Knee Bend

Squat with the knees bent and the feet about twelve inches apart. Balance with towel held out in front at arm's length—at about height of shoulder. Return to standing position and repeat. Try squatting with knees front and parallel—then try with knees separated and out to the sides. (See Fig. 10.)

T5 Trunk Twist

Grasp the ends of a towel with hands high overhead. Twist the trunk sharply to the right. Bend at the waist and aim the center of the towel at the back of the right heel. Keep full tension on the towel. Straighten to position, turn sharply to the left and alternate, first right, then left. Keep right knee slightly bent. When turning to the right, bend right knee and keep left knee as stiff as possible. Reverse legs on left side—bend the left knee and keep the right knee as stiff as possible. (See Fig. 11.)

T6 All-Around

Start with hands high overhead. Grasp each end of the towel (full forty-inch length) and bend forward so the hands are about a foot from the floor. Then holding the ends of the towel taut, bring left hand to outside of left leg. At the same time, bring the right hand up and overhead (crossing the face with the towel), and then around the left side of the head. As the right hand goes down behind the shoulders and then backward to the right, the left hand comes up over and back of the head to the right, and then downward in front to the starting position. Let the elbows bend with the movement. After six counts reverse the exercise by bringing the left hand to the right side, etc. (See Figs. 12A–B, 12C, and 12D.)

Head-to-Toe Exercises

For scalp and face exercises, see Chapters 13 and 14, on beauty.

Eyes

All eye exercises are suitable for use any time of the day. They are especially beneficial to relieve eyestrain when working.

Eye Circles

Sit erect, eyes front. Do not move head during this exercise. If necessary to help you keep head still, hold it with opposite hand. Raise right arm to shoulder level—fully extended to right side. Keeping arm stiff and fully extended, describe an arc toward the middle of the head, wiggling the index finger as you draw the imaginary half-circle. Follow the movement of the finger with both eyes, rolling them to the extreme right, turning eyeballs up to the top of the socket, then to the extreme left and down to the bottom of the socket. Hold one second in each position. Begin with six times and work up to ten or twelve. Then repeat with left hand, having eyes travel in opposite direction. (See Fig. 13.)

Eye Focus

Sit erect. Extend right arm forward as far as it will go, holding index finger extended and raised upright. Bring arm and finger toward nose, following the movement with the eyes until they are nearly crossed as finger touches the nose. Be sure that head does not move. Then return arm and finger to starting position following with the eye. Begin with six times and work up gradually to ten or twelve times daily.

Palming

Squeeze eyes shut—tight, hold for count of eight, rest for count of eight, and repeat. Then slowly open wide, hold for eight seconds, and repeat three times. Close eyes. Hollow palms and cover eyes—be careful not to touch eyeball. Rest eyes by visualizing blackness. (Also use the Cayce head–and–neck exercises.)

A.M. Verticals

The following series V4 to V11 is excellent for correcting poor posture, round shoulders, kyphosis (dowager's hump), flabby arms, and lifting and firming bust.

Shoulders, Arms, and Bust

V4A Shoulder Shrug

A good shoulder exercise consists of raising the shoulders up and down as in a shrug.

V4B Shoulder Circles

A second move is to bring the shoulders forward, rotate them forward three to six times, then rotate them backward three to six times.

V5 Arm Circles

Bring the arms out to the side with the palms up, thumbs back, keeping shoulders level, rotating forward six to ten or twelve times. Then rotate backward six to ten or twelve times. This is a good exercise for the shoulders, upper arms, chest muscles, and bust. (See Fig. 14.)

V6 The Push-Pull

This is a coed chest developer for firming the bust for women and developing the chest muscles for men. Bring the arms forward eight to ten inches below the shoulder level, clasping the fingers of one hand into the fingers of the other, and push together, hold for about ten seconds, and then pull out and hold again for ten seconds. (See Figs. 15A and 15B.)

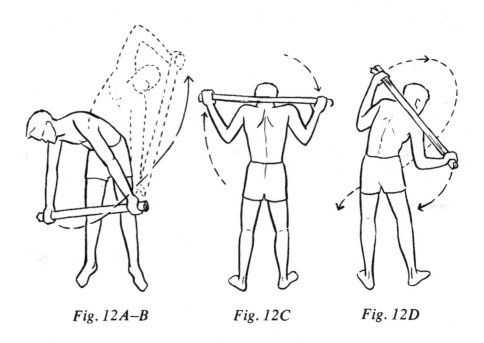

Fig. 12A–B   *Fig. 12C*   *Fig. 12D*

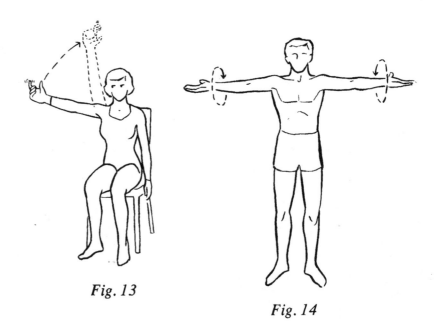

Fig. 13

Fig. 14

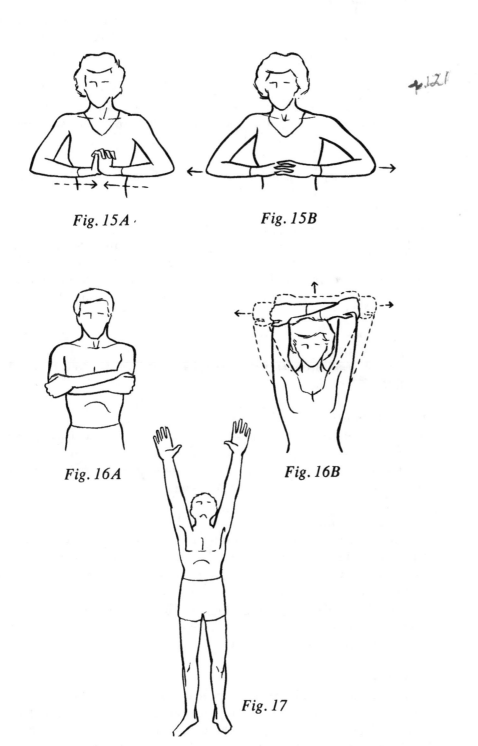

Fig. 15A

Fig. 15B

Fig. 16A

Fig. 16B

Fig. 17

V7A The Frame-Up

Clasp each elbow, holding the arms forward and bringing them above your head, back as far as you can, hold for about ten seconds. (See Figs. 16A and 16B.)

V7B The Second Move

Do the same thing as above, bring the arms over your head and then pull the elbows from side to side, up and sideways. Don't bend sideways at waist. This exercise is very good for upper arms, chest, bosom, and back. (See Figs. 16A and 16B.)

NOTE: See Chapter 13, on beauty, for other bust–firming and bust–developing exercises.

Arms, Shoulders, and Upper Back

These are excellent for shoulders, upper back, and arms. They are contraindicated in cases of neuritis, bursitis, or hiatus hernia. For strengthening your arms there are dozens of different exercises to be used with dumbbells and weights, depending on the individual and the degree of muscle buildup or toning desired.

V8 The "Hallelujah"

To reduce fat on upper arms bring hands up over your head and shake "Hallelujah." (See Fig. 17.)

V9 The Indian Rope Trick

Throw an imaginary rope up into the air and climb with one hand over the other until your hands reach as far as they can go. When you get to the top, don't hang on but climb down again. For slimming and firming arms, slimming waist, and improving posture. (See Fig. 18.)

V10 The Windmill

Sling the arms around—don't just turn them—using the body as a balancer, backward and forward six to twelve times. Then reverse the movement, coming forward and backward, slinging them around. First you do both movements with one arm, then with the other. When you get really good (contraindicated if one has pain in the shoulders), you can do the same movement with a dumbbell in your hand, beginning with a two–pound one and increasing to six pounds for women and ten pounds for men.

V11 Point Stretching

Stand against the wall, holding a pencil about two inches long in your right hand. Then reach up as high as you can, coming up on your toes, and make a little mark on the wall with the right hand. Switch the pencil to the left hand and repeat. Practice this every day and at the end of the month you will find that the pencil marks have moved up from one–half to two inches. This exercise is excellent to lift the rib cage, slimming the waist. It can actually pull the

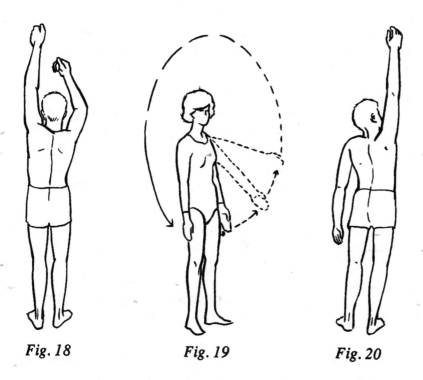

Fig. 18   Fig. 19   Fig. 20

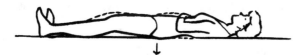

Fig. 21A

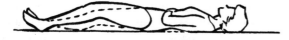

Fig. 21B

full height out of your body. (See Fig. 20.)

P.M. Horizontals

Lie flat on your back on the floor, preferably on a blanket or pad covered with a striped towel with foot markers. You must be on a hard surface. (Do not do these exercises in bed, even if you have a bed board.)

Abdominals

These exercises will influence the abdomen generally—help to reduce it, and also stimulate the liver, gallbladder, spleen, and all the glands and organs of the abdominal region. They also help to tighten the muscles, to control the forming of pockets or diverticulitis in the large colon, and to correct constipation.

H12A and H12B are corrective exercises for lordosis (excessive back arch).

H12A Pelvic Tilt

Lie flat on the floor, push down with your whole body so that your lower back is flat on the floor. (Make sure that there is no room for your hand to go between your lower back and the floor.) Then push down and make the lower back long. The force of that down–push usually brings the knees slightly off the floor and pulls up and tilts the pelvic girdle. Hold this for three seconds and work slowly up to a six–second hold. (See Fig. 21A.)

H12B

The second move in this exercise is, after you lie flat on the floor, to lift your knees up about six inches. Keep the back flat, breathe normally. Then bring the knees down slowly without raising your lower back. This is a very good exercise for straightening out a lordosis and keeping the lower part of the abdomen flat, because those muscles don't get exercised very often in ordinary exercise. (See Fig. 21B.)

H13A Elbow-Knee Kiss

Lie on your back clasping your hands in back of the head. Bring up the left knee, at the same time raising the right elbow, keeping the hands clasped, raising the body and bringing the right elbow to touch or go past the right knee. As you rise, exhale through the mouth and nose and then close your mouth. Hold this position for about three to six seconds, then release, and come back to starting position. Do the same on the alternate side, the right knee to the left elbow. Start with six of these, adding two a week, until you reach somewhere between twelve and sixteen. Do it slowly.

Be sure not to favor one side over the other or you may accentuate a lateral scoliosis (a lateral curve of lower back). You can help to correct this condition by checking to see that elbows and knees meet at the same points on both sides. If you have difficulty with this, try harder on the short side. It is a good correction for lateral scoliosis. (See Fig. 22.)

H13B Double Elbow-Knee Kiss

The next move is to bring both knees up to both elbows. Exhale, close mouth, and hold for three to six seconds. Do this four times to start, adding one a week till you reach about twelve. (See Fig. 23.)

H14A Knee-Over Twist ✓

Lie flat on the floor with your hands down at your side. Bring your left knee up at right angles to the body, then trying to keep the shoulders flat on the floor, twist at the waist, bringing the left knee over to the right side, trying to keep it at right angles. Hold for about three seconds, then come back to the starting position. Repeat the same exercise with the right knee to the left side. Do this alternate movement six times. If you have room it is preferable to extend arms, palms down, at shoulder level, adding two a week until you reach twelve to sixteen. Keep stretching a bit farther with each exercise until you can bring knee to floor. (See Fig. 24.)

H14B Double Knee-Over Twist ✓

Bring both knees up at right angles, twist them over to the right side, shoulders flat on the floor, then bring them back and down. Do the same movement on the left side four times to start, adding one a week until you are doing twelve. (See Fig. 25.)

H14C

A variation of the above exercise is to bring the leg up straight, without bending the knee, and repeat as above. In other words, left leg to the right side and right leg to the left side without bending the knee—the same movement with both legs. These are good waist whittlers and correction for upper–back spine. (See Fig. 26.)

H15 The Sit-Back

The next exercise starts from a sitting position. Hold your head forward and down, chin on chest. It is very important that the head remain forward and down. Sitting on the floor, legs stretched out, your hands at your side as a guide, lean back to a forty–five–degree angle, keeping the head forward, chin on chest. Hold it for the count of three to six and then come up. The head must always be kept down and forward even when coming up. If the head is not kept down, it makes the abdomen protrude. Keeping the head forward keeps a concave curve in the abdomen. This is an excellent exercise to flatten the abdomen. It tightens the muscles of the lower abdomen, and especially important for women, it helps keep the pressures off the lower pelvic girdle. It increases circulation and also gives movement to the organs, glands, and intestines. It will also help to pull up sagging organs into their proper position. (See Fig. 27.)

NOTE: The popular sit-up is potentially dangerous to weak backs and should be done only by experienced exercisers or under supervision.

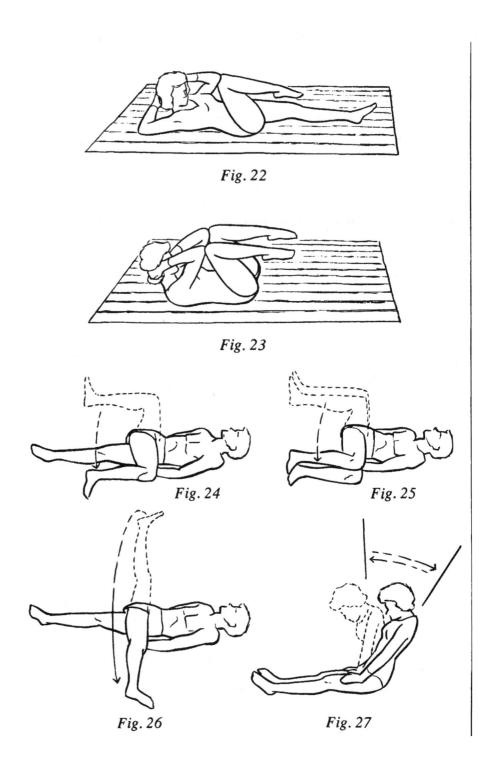

Fig. 22

Fig. 23

Fig. 24   *Fig. 25*

Fig. 26   *Fig. 27*

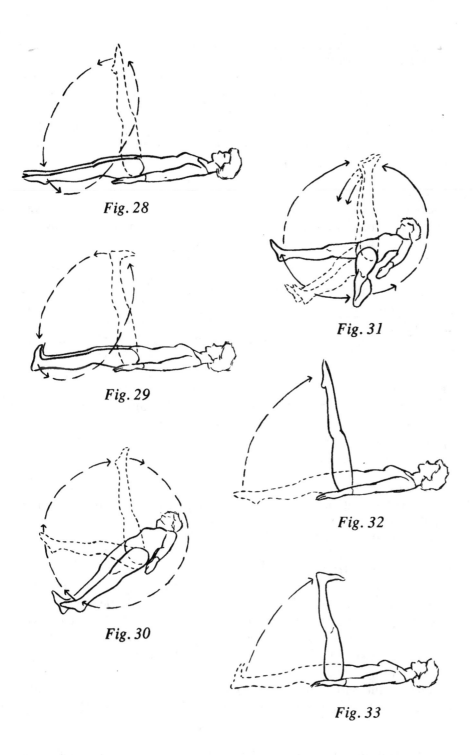

Fig. 28

Fig. 29

Fig. 30

Fig. 31

Fig. 32

Fig. 33

Hips and Legs

H16A Heel-Toe Leg Circles

Lie flat, point the left toe, circle it out and up and down, clockwise with the right, counterclockwise with the left. Rest. Then pull up the toe, stretching the heel, and circle the same way, out and up. Repeat with the right leg. Alternate about six times, increasing two a week until you reach from twelve to sixteen. (See Figs. 28 and 29.)

NOTE: The leg circles open the pelvic area, increasing circulation, and the up and down movement of the leg raises helps speed circulation to and from the legs and feet. *Keep entire back flat on the floor.*

H16B

Lie flat, point the left toe, circle left leg around up and out counterclockwise, and rest. Then bring the toe up, stretch and point heel, and repeat. Repeat the same with the right leg circling clockwise. (See Fig. 30.)

H16C

Circle with both legs out and in, clockwise and counterclockwise. Each leg goes away from the other. Do these first by pointing toes and then pull toes and point heels.

This exercise firms, tones, and shapes legs; flattens and tones abdomen. (See Fig. 31.)

H17A Leg Raise

Raise the left leg, point the toe, bring the leg up straight, keeping the knee as stiff as possible. Come down and rest. Pull the toe up and point the heel and repeat the same movement. Repeat on the right side. Perform at a moderate pace—not too fast. (See Figs. 32 and 33.)

H17 Double Leg Raise

Raise both legs at the same time, and lower. Be sure to keep the small of the back flat on the floor.

(See note following H18.)

H18 Double Leg Circles

Place both hands under the buttocks, keeping the knees stiff, and raise legs and rotate them in a circle from left to right, up to left, circle around to the right, then let them down. Do the same from right to left. Do it three times on each side. You may do it three times on one side and three on the other, or alternate it, working it up to six to twelve on each side.

The important thing to observe in this exercise is that the small of the back stays flat on the floor. If the small of the back is lifted so that you can put a hand under it, the exercise is not serving its purpose. (See Fig. 34.)

NOTE: Warning! If you cannot keep the back on the floor, don't do the exercise, because you may accentuate a lordosis (lower back curve).

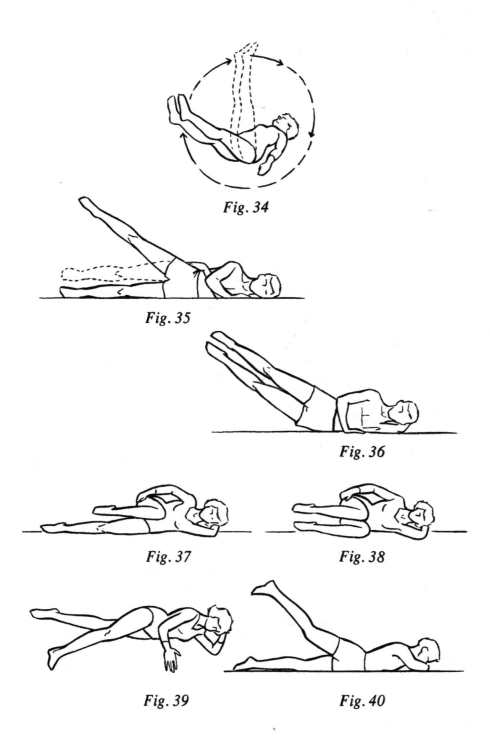

Fig. 34

Fig. 35

Fig. 36

Fig. 37   Fig. 38

Fig. 39   Fig. 40

H19 The Scissors

Raise legs about two feet from the floor. Point toes and scissors legs up and down. Then pull up toes and point heels and repeat scissors movement. Don't go too fast. The swing of the legs can be from six inches off the floor to a full right angle.

Keep the small of the back flat on the floor. This exercise is good for the legs and will tighten the muscles of the lower abdomen.

Lying–on–Side Position

The following series may be performed lying first on one side, then on the other. It is not necessary to change sides between exercises.

Check your position against towel lines.

Be sure your body is straight from head to foot.

H20A Side Leg Raise

Lie on the right side, lift the left leg up and put it down, keeping the knee stiff, first with pointed toe, and then pull up your toe, point the heel. Repeat on left side. (See Fig. 35.)

H20B Back Leg Raise

Keep knee stiff, stomach in, and raise leg backward as though taking a step back. Very good for the hips as well as legs and lower back.

H21 Double Leg Side Raise

Keeping the body in a straight line with the shoulders, keeping the ankles together, lift both legs up together. Be sure the ankles are together when you lift them up and try to keep the whole body in a straight line. You can do that three to six times. A good way to increase the efficiency of this exercise is to hold the legs for the count of three after lifting them up.

This exercise is good for side fat rolls and hips. (See Fig. 36.)

H22A Side Knee-Chin Kiss

Lying on your side, bend one knee and try to touch knee to chin. Then straighten the leg and rest. Repeat on alternate side. (See Fig. 37.)

H22B Double Side Knee-Chin Kiss

Lying on side, bend both knees and try to touch knees to chin. Then alternate the sides. (See Fig. 38.)

This stretches the muscles of the lower back and is good for buttocks, hips, and thighs.

H23A Side Leg Circles

Point the toe and rotate the leg in a circle first forward and then backward clockwise and then counterclockwise.

Then pull up the toe, point the heel, and perform the same circling movements. This is good for the waistline, abdomen, small of back, thighs, and legs.

H23B Double Side Leg Circles

Both legs straight, point the toes and then rotate both legs in a circle first forward, then backward. After that, you can rotate them backward and forward, also changing positions of the feet—toes pulled up and heels pointed, and vice versa.

CAUTION: Do not try the double side circle until you have been exercising for a month.

H24A Side Scissors

Lie on your right side, bring the legs up together, and then scissor back and forth. Swing back and forth, not too fast.

H24B: Turn over and repeat on the left side. (See Fig. 39.)

For the Back

These back exercises are very good for the average person, but anyone with hernia of any type or a lordosis (lower back curve) should avoid them.

H25 Back Leg Lift

In prone position on your abdomen, turn your head to the right, lift your left leg—knee stiff—reaching as far as you can to the right side, lift it high and over, and try to see your left foot. Then do it on the opposite side. Do this six to twelve times. (See Fig. 40.)

H26A Arm and Shoulder Lift

Still lying on your abdomen, arms at the side, raise your head, back, and shoulders from the floor. Hold for a count of four and increase to eight. Repeat with arms out in front. (See Fig. 41.)

H26B The Everything-Up Lift

Bring arms straight up over your head and lift head, shoulders, back, and legs up. Keep knees stiff. Hold for a count of four, and increase hold count to eight to twelve. (See Fig. 42.)

H27 Reverse Back Bend

Lie on abdomen, feet up in back. Bring arms backward and grasp ankles. Hold for a count of six. After some practice, try rocking on abdomen.

This stretches front thigh muscles, but be careful. (See Fig. 43.)

NOTE: Omit if any abdominal hernias are present.

Ankles and Feet

H28 Ankle Circles

Sit with your legs extended before you. Cross right foot and ankle over left leg midway between knee and ankle. Then rotate foot and ankle first right and then left. Then move the foot back and forth, alternate with left foot.

H29 Ankles Aweigh

Brace your weight on the outside edges of your feet. If standing, you can

A good follow-up to the ankle strengthening exercise is the tendon stretch. This can be very useful when high heels cause contraction of the Achilles tendon that might result in other disturbances of the legs and feet.—**H.J.R.**

steady yourself by holding on to a chair. If sitting, it will be easy to balance your weight. Then roll weight to inside and rest on full foot. Repeat.

H30 Ankle Stretch

To stretch and strengthen ankles, sit on a firm surface, preferably the floor, keep knees stiff, legs out straight in front. Fold towel lengthwise into a four-inch width. Place the middle of the towel on the sole of the foot, under the toes. Grasp both ends of the towel and pull toward you and back. Then push the toes and the front of the foot forward. Resist this movement by holding back on the towel so that considerable force must be exerted by the foot in its forward movement. *Be sure* to keep the ankles in a *straight line*, and keep pressure on the towel so that the foot and ankle have a real workout. At the start, give six of these resistive movements to each foot. (See Fig. 44.)

H31 Tendon Stretch

A good follow-up to the ankle strengthening exercise is the tendon stretch. This can be very useful when high heels cause contraction of the Achilles tendon that might result in other disturbances of the legs and feet. Combining both of these exercises will give best results.

In the same position as the previous exercise, keeping the folded towel under the toes with knees stiff, pull the front of the foot back toward you, and pull back very hard, and using the weight of the body, S—T—R—E—T—C—H. This will stretch and lengthen the contracted tendon at the back of the heel. When starting, stretch each foot about six times with full weight and strength. Hold each stretch about ten seconds, and rest five seconds. (See Fig. 45.)

H32A "Charlie Chaplin" Walk

The "ten-minutes-to-two walk": Put your toes at an angle that would approximate ten minutes to two on the clock (à la Charlie Chaplin). Walk about twelve to sixteen steps forward. Try a few backward, even sideways, when you are really adept. (See Fig. 46.)

H32B Pigeon-Toed Walk

Turn your feet inward, pigeon-toed, toes together and heels pointing on the clock to twenty minutes to four. Take twelve steps forward and some backward. (See Fig. 47.)

H32C

Pull up your toes and walk on your heels twelve to sixteen times. You can do all of these movements forward, backward, and sideways.

Feet

H33 Foot Roll

Take a milk or coke bottle. Sitting on a chair, roll your foot back and forth over the bottle. Place a hand on a knee and lean your weight on it while you roll the foot back and forth. This gives a little more pressure.

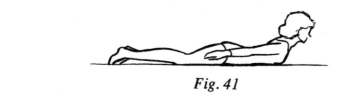

Fig. 41

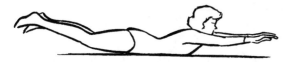

Fig. 42

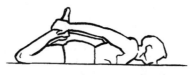

Fig. 43

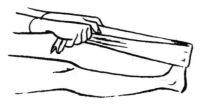

Fig. 44

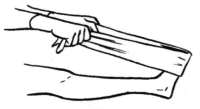

Fig. 45

One of the advantages that women enjoy in chairless societies is the custom of squatting, which facilitates childbirth. The old-fashioned birthing stool and methods used in developing nations—whose natural wisdom we might do well to emulate—enable women to bear many children with less fuss and pain than their unfortunate sisters in industrialized countries.—**H.J.R.**

H34 Pick-Up
Take a small Ping-Pong ball or marble and try to lift it with your toes.

H35 Toe Wiggle
Hold your foot. Stretch and wiggle each toe separately with your hand.

Buttocks and Hips

H36 Fanny Walk
Sit down on the floor, roll your arms in front of you, swing the body to the right, push the left leg forward, walk on the hip, swing the right leg forward, and swing the body to the left. Keep walking across the floor about ten feet. Then try doing it backward for the same distance.

H37 Fanny Bounce
Lie flat on the floor, bring your knees up, lift the buttocks to one side and let them hit the floor, then the other side. This is just a moderate contact, not a blockbuster.

Sexercises

During her childbearing years, it is important to a woman to keep her pelvis, abdomen, back, and thighs strong and flexible for easy delivery. One of the advantages that women enjoy in chairless societies is the custom of squatting, which facilitates childbirth. The old-fashioned birthing stool and methods used in developing nations—whose natural wisdom we might do well to emulate—enable women to bear many children with less fuss and pain than their unfortunate sisters in industrialized countries. The modern delivery table must have been invented by a sadist or one ignorant of elementary biological processes. The conscientious performance of exercises from childhood on will greatly enhance a woman's life—in coitus, in childbearing, in easing menstrual and menopausal discomfort, and in maintaining a youthful figure throughout the years.

Here are three special exercises to add to the preceding ones in this chapter.

S38
Practice squatting whenever possible—not just deep knee bends but squatting—knees spread apart as wide as possible; buttocks suspended as close to the floor as possible, hands and arms resting on knees. If at first it is difficult for you to maintain balance, you can support your weight by holding on to a chair.

S39 The Chinese Kow-Tow
Assume a knee-chest position as shown in Fig. 48. You may use a pad or thin pillow to protect your knees until you get used to kneeling. Sink back on your heels and cough as hard as you can three times. You should feel the cough vibrate in your pelvis and throughout the lower abdomen. Then stretch

your body and arms forward along the floor as far as you can reach in the Chinese kow-tow or "Praise Allah" position. (See Fig. 49.)

Return to the knee-chest position and repeat this exercise three times.

This exercise can help to normalize a tilted-womb position and other gynecological problems.

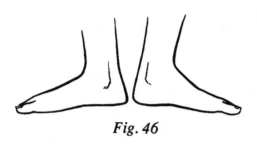

Fig. 46

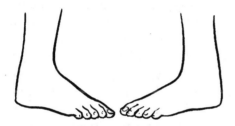

Fig. 47

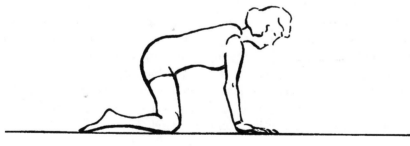

Fig. 48

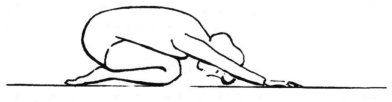

Fig. 49

An important part of the chief muscle of the female pelvic diaphragm is known as the pubococcygeus, or PC. It is like a thick, wide rubber band, which acts as a sling to support the organs of the pelvis. When this muscle becomes lax or stretched through poor muscle tone, childbirth, or pelvic disorders, it often results in urinary incontinence and unsatisfactory coitus.—**H.J.R.**

S40 For Men and Women

The Cayce pelvic-circles exercise described in Chapter 6 is excellent for stimulating glands and sending rejuvenating blood to the sex organs.

Men should increase the circumference of the circles they describe with their hips. Also practice jackknifing the torso up and down in a V position as far and high as the legs and back permit. However, start very slowly and gradually, increasing the up-and-down movements very gradually to avoid back injury.

No one with any kind of back pain should try the latter movement—stick to the circles.

S41 To Improve Feminine Response in Marriage[1]

An important part of the chief muscle of the female pelvic diaphragm is known as the pubococcygeus, or PC. It is like a thick, wide rubber band, which acts as a sling to support the organs of the pelvis. When this muscle becomes lax or stretched through poor muscle tone, childbirth, or pelvic disorders, it often results in urinary incontinence and unsatisfactory coitus.

Dr. Arnold Kegel, a professor at the University of Southern California School of Medicine in the early 1940s and who now has a clinic at Los Angeles County General Hospital, was studying the problem of urinary incontinence when he found that "when the PC was a firm, straight platform, giving good support to the internal organs, urinary stress incontinence was almost unknown."[2] In developing treatment, he found that in correcting the urinary problem, he was also correcting long-standing unresponsiveness and frigidity in many of his female patients. A simple exercise corrects both the coital and urinary problem and has brought more satisfying sexual relationships to many couples.

The PC Exercise

Since the PC controls the flow of urine, if the flow is interrupted by contraction of the PC, the muscle is exercised and tightened, and in time it regains its elasticity. Dr. Kegel recommends that the patient begin with five or ten contractions and increase the exercise gradually until one is doing ten or more contractions each waking hour. Mrs. Brod, who has interviewed many women on this subject and practiced it herself, reports that the effectiveness of the exercise is enhanced if the contraction is held longer—beginning with a count of four and working up to a "hold" of ten or twelve.

S42 Urinary Control

Many older men as well as women suffer from urinary incontinence, which we have found is cured by bicycle riding. Dr. William McGarey of the A.R.E. Clinic reports that he has had similar success with older patients, and reports from other doctors have confirmed this simple remedy.

Preparation for Sports

A steady program of physical conditioning is important if you wish to pursue and enjoy any recreative or competitive sport. This is of paramount importance if you are a weekend athlete and don't want to become one of the millions of Monday-morning casualties in orthopedists' offices.

The preceding exercises should get and keep you in good condition. The following special exercises will give you better coordination, flexibility, and muscle tone for different sports. If you are a beginner, they will improve your performance; if a veteran, they will aid you to stay flexible, especially when weather or lack of time makes outdoor sports impossible.

Many of our sports are hazards to good posture. Bowling, golf, and tennis are one-sided and tend to develop a lateral, or side, curvature of the body. While the crawl stroke in swimming is a wonderful exercise, too much of it has a tendency to accentuate a round-shouldered posture.

These sport hazards to posture can be overcome by reversing the practice movements and doing them from the left side as often as from the right.

Do not neglect the general exercises given earlier in Chapters 6 and 7.

H37A Dry Swimming—Breast Stroke

Use a stool, hassock, or chair without arms. Balance on the abdomen and go through the motions of the breast stroke. Use a frog kick for the legs. (See Fig. 50.)

H37B Dry Swimming—Crawl Stroke

Bring the hands back and forth as in crawling. At the same time, kick the feet up and down, keeping the knees as stiff as possible.

H38 Indoor Golf

Take a golfing stance. Use a book of about the same weight as a golf club. Swing up and back, then down and around to the left side. Start on the left side and do the same to balance posture.

H39 Book Tennis

With right hand, swing book high to the right side. Hold another book in the left hand at the right side of the abdomen. Then swing downward and to the left with the right hand, and up and to the left with the left hand, to give the effect of forehand and backhand strokes. Alternate this movement, starting with the left hand up, right down.

40A Chair-Ski

Place the right foot on the seat of a chair. Support yourself by holding on to the back of the chair. Bend forward, flexing your knee, until weight is on the front of the right foot. (See Fig. 51.)

40B

Push and raise your body on a chair by pushing with the right arm and straightening the right leg as much as possible. This will lift the left leg off the floor. Then let the body down to the first position. Alternate with the left arm and leg. With practice, this exercise should result in more work for the leg and less for the arm. (See Fig 52.)

A steady program of physical conditioning is important if you wish to pursue and enjoy any recreative or competitive sport. This is of paramount importance if you are a weekend athlete and don't want to become one of the millions of Monday-morning casualties in orthopedists' offices.—**H.J.R.**

41 Heeling

For skaters and walkers, exercises 32A and 32B (as shown in Figs. 46 and 47) will strengthen the ankles and relieve fatigue of the feet.

Bend over and take hold of the toes. Try to walk forward and then backward. (See Fig. 53.)

Posture

The story of the evolution of the human race can be told in terms of posture. It can be said that when an anthropoid stood on its hind legs and reached for the stars it became a human being.

Posture expresses the life span of the human being in a ninety-degree angle. We start off horizontally and then we rise as babies and start walking bent over like an ape, because we have not yet developed a back curve. About the age of two or three the curve starts to develop and as children we stand straight. At the height of our vitality, most of us stand as straight as possible, and then as we grow older we begin to stoop, unless we have kept fit, and then we are horizontal again.

Posture does, to a large extent, mirror your reaction to life. The expression "facing the world with your chin up" is psychologically descriptive and significant.

Just having good posture, of course, will not ward off all the unpleasant aspects of life, but the state of physical fitness necessary to maintain good posture will surely help to minimize them. To some extent our spirit, our courage, in fact our whole reaction to life can be related to good posture. Although some intelligent people have poor posture, it is a fact that good posture usually ties up with a good mind. It has been brought out in testing college students that, as a group, persons with good posture score *better* in psychological tests than those with poor posture.

As we grow older, especially when physical fitness has been neglected, we develop a "sad sack" droop that advertises our defeats to the world. But good posture is also important for your health as well as your looks and psychological well-being.

From an anatomical viewpoint, good posture in the upright position is just not really natural. In human beings, however, the forces of evolution are upward—in ideas, ideals, and posture. In the use of our brains and the many facets of our intellect, humans are favored above all living creatures, and we have developed skills of the hands and fingers that are beyond compare. This was brought about by the change from the natural horizontal position, which favored the positions of the organs of the body and the circulation to the legs, to an upright one, which favored both circulation and increased stimulus to the brain. It also freed the arms and hands. While there are some animals that can stand on their hind legs for short periods of time, ability to completely function in an upright position is ours alone.

Let us consider the advantages of our upright position. In the erect position, the return flow of the toxin-laden blood from the head is speeded up. In this way the brain receives more rapidly the fresh blood with its rich load of oxygen and blood sugar for nourishment and better brain function. The upright position releases the hands and arms from use as supporting devices. Together with the increased coordination of the eyes, the hands can be used in many skilled occupations. With use they continue to develop coordination, flexibility, and great skill. It is interesting to note that centers of speech in the brain are located in the same section that controls the movements of the hands. We can speculate that when our ancestors stood up and communicated with their neighbors in sign language, a stimulation of the speech centers occurred. Then sounds and finally words were used to express ideas.

One of the most important developments of our upright stance was the stimulation of the brain through the nerve reflexes. While standing and walking seem easy and natural to most of us, great coordination is necessary for balance and movement in an upright position. There are three important adjustments that the nerves must make in order to achieve good balance. Those that:

- respond to stimulation from the muscles,
- regulate the adjustments of the eyes, and
- affect the regulation of balance from the semicircular canals of the inner ear.

Stimulation of the reflex–nerve centers by a continual change of balance, the stimulus that comes from learning new skills with the hands, the attempt to express ideas by the sign language, and rudimentary speech were important factors in the development of the brain.

Another development that came with the upright position was a change in muscular and bone development. When two legs do the work of four, they must be strong, both for balance and weight carrying. Consequently, there is a greater development in certain muscles of the legs and also in the lower back. There is also more strength in the human leg bone. Even from a physiological standpoint, an upright human being must have more backbone for proper erect carriage. *It was important that the upright postural muscles of the leg, back, and neck be exercised to maintain better this upright position.*

In an erect position it is very necessary to have good muscular tone in the upper part of the body for proper breathing. In the horizontal position the rib frame is below the spine and the chest frame hangs loose. In that position very little muscular effort is necessary for breathing. Therefore, when we stand upright, the weight of the chest wall must be lifted with each breath.

"Bad posture can lead to physical problems as you grow older," says Dr. Gerald Finerman, a prominent Los Angeles orthopedist and assistant professor of orthopedic surgery at the University of California at Los Angeles (UCLA) School of Medicine. Dr. Finerman points out that bad posture can lead to "lung, heart, and circulatory problems, arthritis and neuralgia in the neck and back, indigestion and poor eating habits, aging—causing you to look older before your time."

"Round shoulders and back can lead to heart failure at an early age—as early as your forties and fifties," said Dr. Finerman. "It could cause a malposition of the heart and increase lung resistance to pumping blood, which can result in pulmonary hypertension."

One of the most important developments of our upright stance was the stimulation of the brain through the nerve reflexes. While standing and walking seem easy and natural to most of us, great coordination is necessary for balance and movement in an upright position.—**H.J.R.**

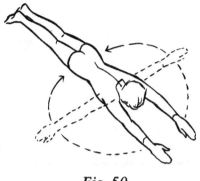

Fig. 50

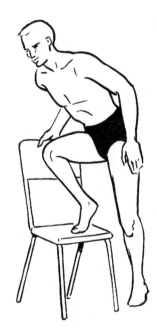

Fig. 51

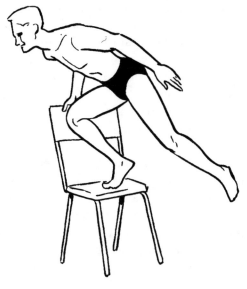

Fig. 52

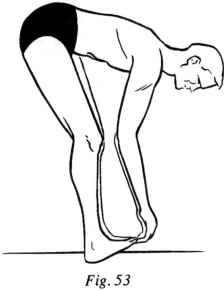

Fig. 53

Round shoulders and back can lead to heart failure at an early age—as early as your forties and fifties. It could cause a malposition of the heart and increase lung resistance to pumping blood, which can result in pulmonary hypertension.
—Dr. Gerald Finerman

Nothing is worse for the lungs than round shoulders. They limit the amount of space in which the lungs can expand to take in more air. Air able to reach deep into the lungs flushes out stagnant air, and the blood, liver, brain, arteries, and kidneys all benefit. It is essential, for instance, that the brain receive plenty of fresh oxygen if one expects to be fresh and bright, Dr. Finerman said.

"Round shoulders also cause the chest to press down on the stomach and the stomach hasn't the room it needs to work properly. And round back will also make you look old before your time," he added. "You look much better and much younger if you stand straight."

Downward pressure on the organs is another disadvantage that can come from our upright position if we are careless in posture and neglect to keep the abdominal muscles in good condition. When we are young and active, the muscles of the abdomen are usually firm and have good tone, but as we grow older they become weak and gravity pulls the upper body forward and downward. As time goes on, the burdens and negative factors of life seem to sit on our shoulders and press us down; the chest sags, the ribs sink in, and the abdomen settles lower and lower. But even more important than appearance is the amount of damage all this downward sag can cause.

When the organs of the abdomen sag downward and press upon each other, you may be heading for trouble, for the downward drag on the nerves and blood vessels interferes with normal circulation and causes considerable nerve irritation. Sometimes the intestines are pushed down five inches or more. This continued downward pressure on the vital glands and organs of the pelvic region can, in time, cause pathological changes and functional degeneration. With all this pressure and interference, it is logical to suspect that many abnormal and diseased conditions of the glands and organs are influenced by bad posture and lack of good muscular support for the abdomen. The abdominal fat, both internal as well as external, is often influenced by poor posture as well as lack of exercise and overeating.

I have drawn a rather dreary picture of the effect that poor posture and weak abdominal muscles can have on our general health and appearance, but it is amazing what a little understanding, perseverance, and exercise can do in the way of both correction and prevention.

To realize how important posture and muscle tone are for good function of the vital organs and glands, let us consider the anatomy of the abdominal cavity. The organs are attached to the back of the inside wall of the body by weak elastic tissue. This tissue carries the arteries, veins, and nerves to the organs. Actually, without muscular support it can hold the organs properly in place only when the body is in a horizontal position. To secure the organs when standing erect, it is necessary to bring into use four pairs of large abdominal muscles. These muscles contain and hold in proper position the stomach, the liver, the small and large intestines, and other glands and organs contained in the abdominal and pelvic cavity. The four main muscles of the abdominal wall come in pairs—for internal and external support. The so-called "washboard" development of the abdomen of the athlete shows the pattern of these muscles. In front we have two sets of muscles—one set on each side. For best function of the glands and organs it is necessary to keep these muscles toughened and exercised. By keeping these muscles *up*, your body won't let you *down*.

The more we learn of the importance of building up and maintaining the necessary muscles for good posture, the more we realize how important it is to give time and effort to proper exercise. When we are truly aware of the great harm that can be caused by a poor posture and a flabby abdomen, I am sure that we will always find those ten to thirty minutes a day for proper exercise to develop and maintain a real corset of muscle to hold the body in good position.

For those who have been accustomed to artificial abdominal support for some time, here is a word of caution: *don't discard the support too suddenly*. The muscles have become weak and must be trained slowly. A good procedure is to start on some light abdominal exercises, for three minutes twice a day. Then slowly increase by adding each week one to two minutes to each exercise period. It is surprising how soon the muscles tighten up and give us a secure feeling of firmness. If you are really interested in doing a good job on your abdominal muscles, you can increase the exercise period to ten to fifteen minutes, twice a day. Be sure to add a few postural and limbering movements for all-around development. (Use Horizontal Exercises 12A–14C on pages 126–127.)

In discarding an abdominal support, begin by leaving it off one hour, then two hours, and so on. With a developing exercise program it is surprising how soon you will find artificial support unnecessary. If for some medical reason you must continue to wear a support, it is still advisable to try in some manner to give movement to unused muscles, otherwise it will be difficult for them to regain their necessary tone and strength. If, on the other hand, it is impossible for you to exercise, your physician might advise exercise equivalents to prevent atrophy of the nerves and muscles.

> *To realize how important posture and muscle tone are for good function of the vital organs and glands, let us consider the anatomy of the abdominal cavity. The organs are attached to the back of the inside wall of the body by weak elastic tissue. This tissue carries the arteries, veins, and nerves to the organs. Actually, without muscular support it can hold the organs properly in place only when the body is in a horizontal position.*
>
> **—H.J.R.**

> *The more we learn of the importance of building up and maintaining the necessary muscles for good posture, the more we realize how important it is to give time and effort to proper exercise.*
>
> **—H.J.R.**

Correcting Lordosis (postural defect)

Some people have great difficulty in keeping the abdomen in good position although the muscle tone is excellent. Even with firm musculature and much physical activity, many dancers have a deep curve in the lower back and a protruding lower abdomen. One also sees protruding abdomens in people who are otherwise quite thin. This is often a result of a postural defect known as lordosis, or hollow back, an exaggerated curve of the lower back, with the back above the buttocks curving deeply inward. Lordosis increases the normal lumbar curve by many inches.

In very severe cases, expert advice and assistance are necessary to correct the position of the back and the pelvis. However, there are many methods of correction through exercise, exercise equivalents, and habits of daily living. For instance, you may practice standing up with the back of the head held as high as possible and pressing the buttocks in and downward. You may also try sitting high in a straight-backed chair and pushing the small of the back against the back of the chair with pressure downward on the hips. Be sure to hold the

People with a hollow back usually find it difficult to keep the small of the back on the floor when exercising. Putting the hands under the buttocks sometimes helps. Try stretching out before you exercise, pushing the buttocks down and under while pressing the lower back against the floor. —**H.J.R.**

head high and the shoulders back. Try pressing the lower back against the chair for twenty seconds to start. Repeat about six times. After a bit of practice you can work the holding time up to two or three minutes.

When you are doing the chair–posture work fairly well, try changing to the floor. Keep the knees *stiff* while in a sitting position with the back against the wall. Make sure all parts of the back, including the shoulders and back of the head, are pressed against the wall. Also use Horizontal Exercises 12A and 12B.

People with a hollow back usually find it difficult to keep the small of the back on the floor when exercising. Putting the hands under the buttocks sometimes helps. Try stretching out before you exercise, pushing the buttocks down and under while pressing the lower back against the floor. It is not easy, but quite necessary; otherwise the abdominal exercise might increase the inward curvature. Another precaution might be necessary. If you find it impossible to keep the small of the back on the floor, use a single limb in all leg exercises. Until proper position of the lower back against the floor is firmly established, lifting of both legs at the same time might bring up the small of the back. You can test this by trying to put the hands, palms down, under the small of the back while exercising. There should be no space for the hand.

If your grip is good, try hanging from a horizontal bar, bringing the knees up in front. This will help to lengthen, stretch, and strengthen the back. Also, doing the horizontal bicycle exercise, bending from the hips as far toward the head as possible, will tend to straighten the lower back. All exercises that stretch the back from the hips up are beneficial. Remember to stand and sit tall with the hips pressed downward and back. If you have a tendency to a hollow back, *never carry heavy loads with the arms extended in front.*

If you have a tendency to lordosis, try to avoid any activity or exercise that makes the lower abdomen protrude. Even if you like to amaze your friends, don't show off by doing back bends.

Some of us imitate the posture of the chimpanzee, whose lower back is in direct contrast to the hollow back that we have described previously. The ape posture is observed when the pelvis is held flat and the buttocks pressed far forward, so that in a sitting position the buttocks are too far forward and the lower back, or lumbar curve, is completely eliminated. This has a tendency to round the shoulders and bring them forward. Many of us assume this position when fatigued, and it is quite restful, especially when we have been holding our body stiff and tight because of too much tension. If, however, the natural lumbar curve is flattened for too long a period, the shoulders droop forward and we start to look as sloppy as Brother Chimp. When this flat–back condition is too fixed or severe, professional advice and direction are necessary. Unless you require a physician's treatment, there are many ways of self–correction.

Lower–Back Exercises

When the lower back is too flat, we need exercise that will flex and bend it backward; we also need exercise that will stretch the contracted muscles of the back of the legs and hamstring that pull the pelvis forward. Here are a few everyday exercises that can be of help:

1. Stand about a foot from a wall, then with the arms full length over the head, bend backward until you touch the wall. As you progress, increase the distance from the wall. This will help to limber and increase the arch of the lower back.

2. Another good exercise is the Towel Exercise 1, the Standing Kick. Be sure to stand high with shoulders held well back.

3. A good way to loosen the spine and improve the lumbar curve is to lie on the floor with a medicine ball or narrow hassock under the small of the back. Gently, at first, roll the lower back over the ball—roll about a foot, backward and forward. Do this about six times, adding three a week until reaching eighteen or better. After loosening the back with this exercise, remove the ball and, still lying on the floor, draw up the knees and keep the feet flat on the floor. Then arch the small of the back by supporting the weight on the buttocks and shoulders. At first it might be necessary to have some fairly firm support to raise the small of the back. Rolled-up newspapers or several thicknesses of tightly folded blanket will do A rolling pin also could be used for a back support. Increase the thickness by wrapping with newspapers and blankets—one inch a week—until it is about four inches in diameter.

These exercises, if continued faithfully, should help take the "ape" out of your back and give you a nice lumbar curve.

Correcting Round Shoulders

The word "droopy" describes a posture of round shoulders and flat chest and a forward droop of the head and neck. This position can result from fatigue and negative emotional impacts, and can be influenced by occupation and play habits. Lack of muscle tone in the back, shoulders, and neck, and neglect of posture correction are the main contributing factors to permanent round shoulders. In some occupations and in general daily living, there are many positions that favor round shoulders—it is common with those who do much reading, writing, and studying. There are also occupational round shoulders afflicting surgeons, dentists, podiatrists, laboratory workers, designers, and architects, to name a few. Machine workers who do fine precision work or even the busy homemaker who does too much sewing, in fact all men and women who are engaged in tasks that keep them bending forward and downward are candidates for the "round-shoulder club."

When, in modern living, we are exposed to round-shoulder occupations, it is necessary to compensate by exercise that will keep the chest and head up and the shoulders back. This will also help in better breathing. Even in such a healthful sport as golf, we have to watch our posture, for golf tends to pull the shoulders too far forward. Television viewing has also influenced the tendency to sag and have round shoulders. If you are looking at television for any length of time, get up occasionally and stretch high with the hands over the head as far as possible—a good seventh-inning stretch, as in Fig. 17, the "Hallelujah" exercise, on page 124. Another good idea is to straddle a hard straight-backed

The word "droopy" describes a posture of round shoulders and flat chest and a forward droop of the head and neck. This position can result from fatigue and negative emotional impacts, and can be influenced by occupation and play habits. Lack of muscle tone in the back, shoulders, and neck, and neglect of posture correction are the main contributing factors to permanent round shoulders.

—H.J.R.

I believe that most of us are aware that positive thinking and constructive action have a most beneficial effect on posture. On the other hand, negative thought and adverse circumstances can not only depress the mind and spirit, but also show their effects on body posture.—**H.J.R.**

A physical fitness program that keeps us standing and sitting tall and erect and develops the necessary musculature to hold the organs and glands in good position will give us a more vital and cheerful outlook on life.—**H.J.R.**

chair, fold the elbows on the back of the chair, and sit high.

If you are in good physical condition, the effect of a round-shouldered position would be only temporary, for then you have the muscle elasticity and flexibility that are yours when you are fit. A few extra minutes of posture exercise will offset the effects of a round-shouldered position.

I invented a correction for neck and round-shoulder strain during World War II for the workers at the Curtiss-Wright airplane plants. The women suffered from pains and fatigue from bending over, with heads down and shoulders hunched, concentrating on the fine precision instruments they were assembling. The following exercise relieved them.

I taught them to place a large paper cup filled with bolts on their heads and hold it there for three minutes. This forces the head back into correct position and rests the cervical spine, relieving neck pain. If you prefer, you may use any weighted object on the head for this purpose.

Also use exercises V4A, V4B, and V5 to correct round shoulders and relieve strain.

I believe that most of us are aware that positive thinking and constructive action have a most beneficial effect on posture. On the other hand, negative thought and adverse circumstances can not only depress the mind and spirit, but also show their effects on body posture. The relationship of postural changes to insecurity and lack of spirit is well known to psychiatrists and psychologists. When we hear some good news or have some business, professional, or social success, we "pick up," as the saying goes. We walk straight and hold our heads higher. The man or woman returning from church worship seems to walk straighter and with more buoyancy.

For many years psychiatrists, psychologists, and physiotherapists have studied the effect that negative thinking, emotional shock, and reaction to negative environment can have on posture. Such descriptions as "sagging," "droopy," "pressing down," "collapsed," "slumped," and "sad sack" all describe a weak-muscled posture stance. Besides the poor posture caused by occupational positions and careless habits of daily living, we must also take into consideration those caused by unfavorable reaction to environment—frustration, distress, or negative thinking with a so-called poker face. But your walking, standing, and sitting position will give you away. Fortunately, we usually counteract most of the negative impacts and then straighten up again. (As straight, that is, as we have been accustomed to.) But some negative impacts are more lasting and can cause definite changes in posture. One defense posture I refer to is "turtle neck." The shoulders are rounded and the neck and head pressed down; the

position is that of a person warding off a blow. Another is that of the defeated-looking individual who shuffles along, body bent inward, and head hanging down.

I do not say that good posture will completely change an introvert or a confirmed pessimist, but a fitness program that improves the posture will help. You can't be in good physical condition, standing straight and high, and at the same time harbor negative thoughts for too long!

A physical fitness program that keeps us standing and sitting tall and erect and develops the necessary musculature to hold the organs and glands in good position will give us a more vital and cheerful outlook on life. We are then better equipped to tolerate or throw off negative impacts. As earth people we must continually fight the downward pull of gravity by knowledge, physical fitness, and positive thinking. Standing up to life takes a vibrant spirit, an active mind, and a straight, well-conditioned body.

Posture Pointers

Alterations in the spine and posture from disease or injury are in many instances difficult to correct and require orthopedic supervision and perhaps surgery. Although the corrective exercises given in the preceding pages can be helpful, here are a few tips on prevention:

1. Standing too much on one leg, or sitting too much on one buttock, or crossing the legs in a manner that puts more weight on one side or the other may cause lateral curvature of the spine. Shift weight frequently from one side to the other and try to stand or sit squarely.

2. Avoid carrying heavy books, briefcases, or other weights, if possible. A knapsack is preferable, especially for schoolchildren carrying books. If you are a busy executive carrying a briefcase, shift the case from one hand to another frequently. If a housewife, try bringing packages home in a cart if you are not driving.

3. You might look odd carrying your groceries home from the market on your head, but in the countries where this method is used for transportation, the women and men have beautiful carriage and posture. Practice carrying objects around on your head at home.

4. Curling up in a fat armchair or on a soft couch can play havoc with posture. To read a book, paper, magazine, or any reading matter, it is best to keep your reading material at chest level, held at a forty-five-to-sixty-degree vertical reading angle. If you maintain a good upright sitting position with the head high, there is very little, if any, pressure on nerves and blood vessels in the neck. The spine is held in good position and the organs are not compressed.

5. For long hours of study, sit at a fairly high table, for then the reading matter will be in position. In an easy chair, a narrow piece of plywood, eight to twelve inches in width, on which to rest the book, placed across the arms of the chair, can help.

6. If you read in bed, be sure to change position continually from side to side and from back to abdomen; don't read in the back position too long. Try sitting up in bed with the back braced on backrest and reading matter on knees.

7. When much time is spent at a typewriter, try sitting as tall as possible. Occasionally stretch the head and shoulders as far up and back as possible.

Exercise your eyes as described on pages 120-121. Try the Cayce head-and-neck exercises and shoulder shrugging. A good posture chair is very helpful.

8. If you do have occasion to write, use a straight-backed chair that is drawn up fairly close to the table. If your abdomen is in the way, take the abdominal-reducing exercises and do the push-aways from the dining, not the writing, table. The height of the table is best when it is two to three inches higher than the elbows. Sit in close with the back straight. Slightly shifting the position helps to avoid the round shoulders and forward bending of the neck and spine.

In any case, whether typing, writing, or reading, it is best to stop every once in a while and stretch to snap back to good posture and relieve fatigue.

9. Be sure that when bending over to pick up something from the floor, you bend your knees, not your back. Keep the back straight, squat, and pick up. Keep heels together and you will have to bend knees.

10. For lifting—keep heels together and bend the knees. Use the leg muscles to do the lifting, not the back. Never lift heavy weights without help.

11. Sleep on a firm mattress and/or use a bed board. Avoid sleeping on your stomach.

The best position is to sleep on either side with one knee bent, with a small pillow under your head to keep head and shoulders on an even level.

If you sleep on your back, you may use a small, downy pillow or sleep without one. However, be sure to place a pillow under your knees.

8
Massage and Manipulation: Rubbing People the Right Way

*For the hydrotherapy and massage
are preventive as well as curative
measures. For the cleansing of the
system allows the body-forces
themselves to function normally,
and thus eliminate poisons, congestions and conditions that would
become acute through the body.*
(257-254)

*Take not just a few minutes, but
set a period and make of it an occasion when the massage is given.
Take from thirty minutes to an
hour or hour and a half to do it!*
(1688-7)

*About twice each week, almost
bathe in olive oil or peanut oil;
especially peanut oil.* (1688-7)

The scrawled pages in my hand literally screamed an anguished cry for help. The handwriting, at times almost illegible, proclaimed the pain and effort it had cost the writer to commit his despair to paper. He was completely paralyzed.

"I am writing to you in the hope that maybe you can help me," the letter, dated June 13, 1969, began. "My name is Lenny Contino. I am twenty–nine years old and an artist. In '59 I had an accident while swimming. I broke my neck, dislocated the fourth vertebra, fractured the fifth, dislocated the sixth vertebra."

The letter went on to describe the surgical and medical procedures used on him through the years, including traction, multiple surgery, drugs, and other conventional therapies. He was still completely paralyzed and deteriorating steadily.

"I am very afraid of doctors," Lenny went on, "but not of you, and if you were willing to take the chance with me, I sure would be willing to do the same with you . . . I have written to so many people, but they never even bother to write back and I am in a chair and there is only my mother who cares . . . All I ask is, if you think maybe you can help me, 'great' . . . but if you think you can't help, please could you just send me a line saying 'no'? That would be more than anyone else I've written to has done . . . Please excuse my handwriting . . . I have to use a hand brace to write."

It was a difficult dilemma for me. We are so besieged with requests for help that it has been a strict rule not to accept new patients. Yet how could I withhold whatever help he could receive from massage and manipulation from this brave boy, who kept hoping and trying in the face of such discouragement?

I wrote back giving him an appointment three months later. That was five years ago [1969]. I taught his mother how to give him a massage for at least an hour each day, and she has been faithful in her ministrations. Today that young

I have treated many so-called "hopeless" cases similar to Lenny's and have witnessed many patients improve in varying degrees. In nearly all of these cases, the necessary ingredient, besides the person's will and determination, has been the daily massage and manipulation given by a devoted person.—**H.J.R.**

man has a new hold on life. He can sit up in his wheelchair without slumping over like a rag doll and can paint "pictures that are taller than myself." He is readying a collection of paintings for a one-man show. His arms are useful once more. He can stand up on all fours, and many muscles that were dying from disuse are restored and steadily growing in strength and tone.

"All the boys who were my friends in the hospitals that I was in are now dead," Lenny told Mrs. Brod when she interviewed him. "I couldn't lift my neck without a lot of pain when I came here. Now . . . I get up on my hands and knees and I jog my body up and down, and it has the same effect as if I ran—it exercises my body and I think up exercises that I can do in addition to the ones Dr. Reilly gives me. And, of course, my mother massages me every day like Dr. Reilly taught her to do. It's been slow but steady and the improvement is a real miracle."

The boy's spirit and perseverance cannot be underestimated in the salvaging operation that we have undertaken, but the role of the daily massage and manipulation given by his devoted mother between his monthly visits to me cannot be overestimated.

I have treated many so-called "hopeless" cases similar to Lenny's and have witnessed many patients improve in varying degrees. In nearly all of these cases, the necessary ingredient, besides the person's will and determination, has been the daily massage and manipulation given by a devoted person.

This is dramatically illustrated in the story of Mr. and Mrs. B.M. A successful lawyer and businessman, Mr. B.M. found himself at the prime of life and productivity virtually cut down by an ailment diagnosed as Charcot–Marie–Tooth disease. He was told at a rehabilitation center that he would be confined to a wheelchair for life.

In a letter dated January 2, 1970, his wife graphically described what happened to her husband:

"In the early months of 1967, I noted that Ben [not his real name] had difficulty in handling steps. I found that on occasion he was falling—or tripping; while walking he would bump into a door—or a wall. I noted a general weakness and other indications. Going up steps got progressively difficult until it was necessary for me to drive him back and forth to business. He had difficulty in getting up from a chair and sitting down . . . It got to a point that he could not get in or out of a chair without help.

"He walked with difficulty, dragging his feet . . . He couldn't raise himself up on his hands when he was on his stomach. The nerve running along the side of his legs [peripheral nerve] protruded very noticeably. Atrophy of the buttocks was present. He was not able to work and when he did—he had difficulty in concentrating. His memory was affected. His coordination was affected. He couldn't drive. The outlook was bleak . . .

"He was getting Vitamins E, C, and B$_{12}$—the latter, B$_{12}$, by injection daily and then we proceeded to taper off gradually to twice a week—1,000cc.

"We tried a chiropractor who gave some measure of help—but with the diagnosis of Charcot–Marie–Tooth and with his general condition so bad—I, of course, was desperate for help for my husband. One evening while listening to the radio I heard of Dr. Reilly and Edgar Cayce. I went out the next morning and purchased the book *The Sleeping Prophet* and immediately thought I must find the answer here. I started with massaging with Vitamin E oil . . . As you know, it took a while for me . . . to locate you and ask your help for my husband who was a 'medical reject', a verdict which I couldn't accept . . .

"On New Year's Day 1967, we made our pilgrimage to you with the files I had gotten from the A.R.E. and my reports, and you read them and took Ben on as a patient. From that day on, God and you have been on my side. I have been fortunate enough . . . to have you teach me to massage Ben and this is my faithful job which I do daily. I have seen Ben come back to good health—he pursues a normal existence. He puts in a day as good as any man in good health. We are both eternally grateful. Dr. X of the rehabilitation center says his case is 'one in a million' . . .

"May I also add . . . what you have done for me. I broke my wrist in . . . 1968; it was set and I developed a frozen shoulder, the pain was excruciating—I had complications with my blood condition—as I developed secondary hemorrhage (I am a pseudohemophiliac and suffer with fragility of the capillaries also)—so I had complications. I had another mishap while I was still in the cast—I ended up with the advice that I would lose 60 percent of the use. Due to your untiring help, the shoulder was relieved—and I don't think I lost 3 percent of the use. I massaged Ben even with the cast on—the hand and the wrist are as good as new. I never had or have any pain or discomfort due to weather, etc.

"I could go on indefinitely about how wonderful you are—and how wonderful you have been to both Ben and me and to the many people who come to you for help, many of whom I have seen regain their health through your treatments . . . I only hope that you and your good work can be spread to the four corners of the earth to benefit people like my husband and the doctor you treated last summer, who came as a vegetable and left a whole human being, able to live a full life.

"Bless you and Betty, whose untiring efforts have made it possible for the 'medical rejects' to be able to again live full lives."

Another dramatic example of the role that increased circulation plays in healing is the story of one of the great ladies and horsewomen of Westchester County in New York State. Some years ago, she slipped on ice and fractured her hip. When she entered the hospital, the doctor offered her the choice of having a pin in her hip for quicker results or taking her chance with traction and slow, natural healing. They predicted that without the pin she might, if she were lucky, get off with six weeks for good behavior.

I advised her to take the traction instead of the pin and then instructed her husband how to massage her; in addition I gave her a Cayce remedy—a concentrated but easily digested calcium preparation called Calcios. Her husband had to bootleg both the Calcios and the massage into the hospital; one night he was so concentrated on massaging his wife that he did not notice it was late, and a nurse making her rounds caught him at it. She called the security officer to put him out, and said, "My God, that woman is going to die of a thrombosis; he's rubbing her!"

About a year later, that same young lady walked into my office and said that she had an offer to make a television commercial that involved parachuting from a plane. She wanted to learn some more exercises to strengthen her ankles and legs. I was absolutely stunned at her spirit and courage—from crutches to parachuting in one year—**H.J.R.**.

I had been taking care of the woman for years and was quite sure she was not going to have a thrombosis. In fact, she was up and in a walker in eleven days; out of the hospital and walking on her own two feet with crutches in seventeen; and riding a horse a few months later. The improved circulation expedited the healing of the bones.

I shall never forget the beautiful young girl who hobbled into my office in the Capitol Theatre Building on crutches. She said, "My name is Jane Benson. I am a dancer and ice skater, and the doctors say I will never dance again. I would as soon be dead. Sidney Kingsley told me that there is only one person who can help me and that is you." She was referring to the famous writer and theater producer whom I had never met.

"I knew the minute I walked into his office that everything was going to be all right," Jane confided to Mrs. Brod. "I was modeling and dancing at the School of American Ballet with George Balanchine. I received a call from Dick Button to join his Ice Show at the World's Fair . . . One day [at rehearsal] I slipped on the ice. I grabbed a railing as I felt a shooting pain radiating from my ankle up my leg. My ankle started to swell, and Dick had me rushed off to a doctor who takes care of a lot of ballet dancers. Dr. B. shook his head and said I would have been better off had I broken my leg—he said my injury would take a long time to heal. He gave me a shot of cortisone and I went back to the rehearsal. I kept taking shots of cortisone and rehearsing and I got worse and worse. First it was my right leg that I had injured and then both legs. Finally I went to an orthopedic specialist who put me on crutches and wanted me to wear orthopedic shoes. He said he doubted that I would be doing any dancing or skating for a while, maybe never. I did not want to wear those horrible old orthopedic shoes, and he said if I didn't I would be crippled for life. I had been doing some work with Lee Strasberg and Sidney Kingsley and they told me about Dr. Reilly. I went to him three or four times a week. He worked with those blessed hands—deep, deep massage . . . and I started to get better—not later, but immediately.

"Dr. Reilly also had me doing the ankle exercises with a towel and my whole leg got stronger. I was able to go back to everything, modeling, dancing, and skating."

This story has an amusing sequel. About a year later, that same young lady walked into my office and said that she had an offer to make a television commercial that involved parachuting from a plane. She wanted to learn some more exercises to strengthen her ankles and legs. I was absolutely stunned at her spirit and courage—from crutches to parachuting in one year.

Yes, she made it with the exercises and renewed massage treatments. She not only made the commercial, but she took up sky diving as a hobby and that is how she met her husband, Maj. James Rowe, Vietnam hero and POW, the first American prisoner to escape from the North Vietnamese. He wrote a book about his adventure, *Five Years to Freedom*, that enjoyed considerable success.

Professor Robert J. Jeffries, an engineer by profession, retired from a very successful career in business to teach at the University of Bridgeport and to pursue his interest in Edgar Cayce's work and other paranormal healing. In the following letter, Professor Jeffries reports dramatic improvement in an eye condition brought about by massage and manipulation as recommended in the Edgar Cayce readings:

> Prior to my visit to Virginia Beach during July 1967, I had great difficulty with vision in my one good (left) eye. (My right eye has been essentially blind since birth.) The symptoms included "double-vision," "halos" around point-sources of light, and "floating blind spots." I could not see sufficiently well to drive or to read normally. Various local ophthalmologists at the Retina Institute in Boston and Columbia-Presbyterian Medical Center in New York diagnosed the difficulties as due to optical refractions resulting from "corrugations" or "roughness" of the surface of the cornea—cause unknown.
>
> Anna, my wife, drove me to the Beach, where her reading of the Cayce files suggested that in several cases bearing a similarity to my symptoms, Cayce had recommended manipulations of the spine and/or massage, and had in some instances referred specifically to you as the desirable therapist . . .
>
> I mentioned Anna's findings to Lucille Kahn, who happened to be at the Beach that day, along with her husband, David . . . He introduced me to you . . . You very kindly gave me a "treatment" and instructed the resident masseur with respect to a continuing type of "massage," which I followed daily for the ensuing five days.
>
> By the end of the third day I could see well enough to read normally. By the end of the fifth day I could drive. On the seventh day I drove home to Connecticut. Ophthalmological examination on my return confirmed "no apparent" corrugations or roughness of the cornea. I have had no recurrence of the symptoms mentioned above to this date (September 30, 1968).
>
> The above are facts. Was it coincidence? Would the problems have disappeared by themselves? Was the massage responsible for the change? There is no way of proving anything. The facts are, however, as I have stated them.

I treated Professor Jeffries for a back injury in 1973 and can report that he still has had no reoccurrence of the symptoms and is still enjoying the improved vision of his massage–manipulation therapy.

I could go on and on citing case after case of the healing power of massage but that would make another book.

Manipulation (which includes massage) is probably the oldest and most instinctive of all healing methods. One naturally reacts to a hurt or an injury by stroking or rubbing the affected parts; a mother soothes a crying baby by stroking its head or back. Psychologists confirm that this stroking is not only soothing to the baby but plays an important role in its mental and emotional development.

Even among animals a primitive form of manipulation is used. Many animals will lick their wounds to cleanse them. Licking with the mouth and tongue hastens healing by increasing the flow of blood. Deer, horses, dogs, cats, and many other animals will rub their heads, sides, and backs on the bark of a tree

Manipulation (which includes massage) is probably the oldest and most instinctive of all healing methods. One naturally reacts to a hurt or an injury by stroking or rubbing the affected parts; a mother soothes a crying baby by stroking its head or back.

—H.J.R.

The use of manipulation has been noted in the oldest records of history. There are written records of massage being used in China as far back as 3000 B.C. In those early days the Chinese had seven classes of physicians who used some form of manipulative therapy.

—H.J.R.

or rough surface to give themselves a massage, sometimes for cleansing or healing, but other times for the sheer delight of it. How quiet and appreciative a horse, cow, or even a fierce bull will become when massaged with a curry-comb or when the human hand is run over the head, back, or limbs. Most animal trainers use some form of stroking in their work.

In humans, quiet stroking of different parts of the body brings about a relaxing semi-hypnotic feeling that has a more favorable effect on the nervous system than tranquilizers and sleeping pills—with none of the detrimental aftereffects.

At this point, let us ask, "What is manipulation?" Manipulation is a skillful or dexterous treatment by hand or mechanical apparatus. It includes massage, and active and passive movements of the joints, muscles, connective tissue, tendons, and ligaments. Pressure and stretching are also used in this therapy.

Massage, an important part of manipulation, is defined as systemic therapeutical friction, stroking, and kneading of the body.

Mechanotherapy, another part of manipulation, is treatment by mechanical means, such as vibrators, Zander machines, etc.

The use of manipulation has been noted in the oldest records of history. There are written records of massage being used in China as far back as 3000 B.C. In those early days the Chinese had seven classes of physicians who used some form of manipulative therapy.

Massage is usually given with the hands, but among some peoples the elbow or forearm is also used. This technique is quite frequently used by the Japanese. Among the Burmese and some tribes of India, massage is given with the operator using his or her feet and legs while sitting down or reclining on one side. Among the ancient Polynesians, massage was given by walking up and down on the patient while he or she was lying on the ground or with a mat underneath. As late as 1939, while visiting the Hawaiian Islands, I found that a few of the native Hawaiians could still do the "walking massage." They supported their weight by using heavy sticks or rods. Also they often used a device similar to a parallel bar to support their weight. By these means they could control the amount of weight pressure and deliver a pressure movement from that of a featherlike stroke to the full weight of the operator. The sensation was very pleasant, especially the steady, deep pressure.

Another form of both massage and manipulation was used by employing an animal as the masseur. In the past, at the numerous post-harvest fairs held in the rural parts of Russia, they had a practice known as "walking the bear." For this purpose, a small honey bear weighing 100 to 300 pounds was trained to walk up and down the patient's back. This gave the effect of a kneading massage and was a substitute for a crude form of osteopathic and chiropractic manipulation. For the farmer who had been bending over and working in other distorted positions for weeks, this straightening out of skeletal structure, muscles, tendons, joints, and connecting tissues really made him feel he was on holiday. (It was not recorded what type of license the bear was required to have!)

While manipulation is basically massage, much more knowledge and skill have been added in modern times. When special forms and techniques were utilized in treating a specific ailment or deformity, osteopathy and chiropractic were born.

The ancient Hindus have recorded the use of manipulation in the Ayur-Veda, or "Art of Life." The Persians and Egyptians were familiar with and used many types of manual therapy. The "anointing of oil" was an expression used over and over again in the Old Testament. The ancient Greeks mention anointing, rubbing, friction, and active and passive movements almost as long ago as 1000 B.C. Hippocrates used and recommended many types of manipulation.

Perhaps one of the oldest records of an attempt in the Western world to use manipulation as a definite therapy in the treatment of disease was a description of the technique of Asclepiades, who lived about 140 B.C. He practiced in both Greece and Rome, and founded a very successful school in Rome in which he expounded his theory of the use of diet, water, massage, and active and passive exercise. He taught that movement of the body was necessary to health. What we are now learning about the importance of the lymph glands and their circulation, Asclepiades sensed over 2,000 years ago. While he did not know the dependent nature of the lymph circulation, he did attempt to restore the free movement of nutritive fluids by means of rubbing and other forms of manipulation.

In the records of the ancient Greeks of about 1000 B.C. and in reading Homer's *Odyssey* we learn that the weary returning warriors were massaged and anointed with oil by beautiful handmaidens to refresh and restore them. The ancient Greeks and Romans had many forms of manipulation for many different purposes—pinching, rubbing, massage, active and passive exercise, and a form of shampooing. These procedures were used both as a luxury and with the baths; for therapeutic purposes in disease and deformities; for preparing athletes for competitions or exhibitions; and for repair after battle. Massage was also used to put old decrepit slaves into good condition so that they would bring higher prices on the auction block—a kind of "body simonizing" job.

Manipulation was used and recorded by the Romans from the first century B.C. The Roman physician Celsus, who lived in the first century, mentioned the rubbing of different parts of the body for different diseases and the many different types of manual therapy that were employed. A century before him, Julius Caesar had himself pinched all over for the relief of neuralgia. The emperor Hadrian, the famous Pliny, and the learned physician Galen used and advocated manipulation in the treatment of disease and in the general maintenance of health.

Paracelsus, in the sixteenth century, extolled the benefits of massage. Massage and other forms of manipulative therapy were also mentioned in the sixteenth century by Mercurialis, the Italian physician, and Gabriel Tallopius, the famous surgeon of Padua. In the fifteenth century, the Japanese were also using all types of manipulative therapy. At that time they published a book called *San-Tsai-Tou-Hoei*, with many drawings of the anatomy, of active and passive exercise, and of all types of massage and passive movement. This therapy

Perhaps one of the oldest records of an attempt in the Western world to use manipulation as a definite therapy in the treatment of disease was a description of the technique of Asclepiades, who lived about 140 B.C. He practiced in both Greece and Rome, and founded a very successful school in Rome in which he expounded his theory of the use of diet, water, massage, and active and passive exercise.

—H.J.R.

Manipulation was used and recorded by the Romans from the first century B.C. The Roman physician Celsus, who lived in the first century, mentioned the rubbing of different parts of the body for different diseases and the many different types of manual therapy that were employed.—**H.J.R.**

In the fifteenth century, the Japanese were also using all types of manipulative therapy. At that time they published a book called San-Tsai-Tou-Hoei, with many drawings of the anatomy, of active and passive exercise, and of all types of massage and passive movement. This therapy was used in disease, postfractures, muscular contractions and cramps, and the relief of fatigue.—H.J.R.

was used in disease, postfractures, muscular contractions and cramps, and the relief of fatigue.

At the beginning of the seventeenth century the physician Sydenham turned to manipulative therapy to effect many of his cures. In the same century, Hoffman, the Prussian physician, made use of all types of mechanotherapy, both active and passive. In the eighteenth century there was considerable agitation for the use of manual therapy in disease and deformity. This movement was headed by Siton André Tisset of France, who wrote several books on the curative values of massage and manipulation.

The nineteenth century brought a great revival of all types of active and passive manipulation in the Western world. The famous Swedish fencing master, physiologist, and poet, Peter Henrik Ling, founder of the Swedish–massage system, brought the knowledge and some of the practices of the ancients up to date. He tried, as far as possible, to put the art of manipulation, as known up to his time, on a scientific basis. Most of the basis of our work in manipulation and medical gymnastics has stemmed from Ling's efforts to coordinate and rationalize this field.

About the middle of the nineteenth century the famous Douglas Graham of Boston wrote the first comprehensive book on manipulation. The work of D.A. Sargent in the field of mechanotherapy and physical education has had its influence in this field right up to the present. The nineteenth century also introduced the field of mechanotherapy and the many machines of Zander. These machines were used to exercise different parts of the body and to imitate the movements of exercising, such as horseback and camel riding and bicycling. In 1874 Dr. Andrew Taylor Still brought osteopathic medicine into the healing arts. Twenty years later Daniel David Palmer founded chiropractic. In the early part of the twentieth century there were the works of Drs. R. Tait McKenzie and John Harvey Kellogg in the field of manipulative therapy.

Although for many years the medical profession was reluctant to utilize the full therapeutic range of manipulation and massage, thus losing many of their patients to osteopathic physicians and chiropractors, the two world wars greatly stimulated the science of rehabilitation in the treatment of veterans. This gave great impetus to the acceptance by the medical establishment of the healing role of massage and manipulation in physical medicine. In fact, my first institute was called the Reilly Physicians' Service, and at the Rockefeller Center Institute we treated patients referred by over 3,000 doctors.

In paranormal healing the hand is the agent used by the healer. Can human hands heal? An affirmative answer seems to be emerging from laboratory experiments conducted by a nun, Sister Justa Smith, a distinguished and talented biochemist and enzymologist working at Rosary Hill College and the Human Dimensions Institute in Buffalo, New York, with healer Oskar Estebany.

When the retired Hungarian army colonel, Oskar Estebany, who had notable success in healing through the "laying on of hands," held test tubes containing enzyme solutions, Sister Justa Smith was able to observe a significant change in increased activity of the "treated" enzymes when compared with "untreated" controls.

It is interesting to note that Sister Justa reports that when the colonel was indisposed or emotionally upset, the enzymes did not respond in the same way.

Sister Justa Smith's experiment seems to indicate that massage, when administered by someone with a healing attitude and ability, can influence the enzyme activity of the body as well as the circulation.

Incidentally, this same healer, Colonel Estebany, had already demonstrated in other carefully controlled experiments conducted by Dr. Bernard Grad of McGill University at Montreal that he could hasten the healing process in plants and mice by the "laying on of hands."

With this kind of scientific evidence confirming the intuitive wisdom of thousands of years of experience, it should be easy to understand why massage administered by the human hand can never be satisfactorily supplanted by any sort of machine or vibrator, although the latter have their uses when nothing better is available.

Massage can be both stimulating and relaxing. It affects every part of the body—nerves, organs, glands, circulation, and muscular tone—helping to rid the body of toxins and fatigue poisons. Years ago I observed some experiments performed by Dr. John Harvey Kellogg at the Kellogg Institute in Battle Creek, Michigan, as well as the work of Dr. Douglas Graham, which led us to the conclusion that a good massage with the proper drainages was the equivalent of about four hours of sleep.

In some experiments, a man had to lift a kilo (about 2.1 pounds) until his fingers were completely fatigued. On the first go-round he lifted the kilo 840 times. He was then massaged for five minutes—first his palm, then his fingers were worked on—and he was then able to lift the kilo 1,100 times, an increase of almost over a third of his capability before the massage. As fatigue took over, without the massage his performance dropped to 500 times on the next try and decreased again to 200 times on the last try.

Years later, I wrote an article about the role of massage in overcoming fatigue and it attracted the attention of the noted Tibetan scholar Theos Bernard, later known as the "White Lama." He was undertaking a crash course in Sanskrit at Columbia University, trying to complete his doctorate in three years and nine months before leaving for Tibet, and he wanted to be able to do it with only four hours of sleep, so he could devote the additional hours to study.

I arranged for my brother, Dr. Pat Reilly, an expert physiotherapist, to go to Bernard's home every morning for almost nine months to give him a massage. At the end of the time, Bernard passed his exam, completed his doctoral thesis on yoga exercises, received his doctorate in Oriental languages, majoring in Sanskrit, and proved the claim that forty-five minutes of massage was equal to four hours of sleep. The warmly autographed copy of his doctoral thesis, expressing his appreciation to my brother, is a cherished memento of this experiment.

Manipulation and massage were an integral part of Edgar Cayce's drugless therapy. I don't believe we ever had a comprehensive count of the number of cases in which he prescribed massage because of the varied terminology he

Massage can be both stimulating and relaxing. It affects every part of the body—nerves, organs, glands, circulation, and muscular tone—helping to rid the body of toxins and fatigue poisons.

—H.J.R.

With this kind of scientific evidence confirming the intuitive wisdom of thousands of years of experience, it should be easy to understand why massage administered by the human hand can never be satisfactorily supplanted by any sort of machine or vibrator, although the latter have their uses when nothing better is available.—**H.J.R.**

Manipulation and massage were an integral part of Edgar Cayce's drugless therapy. I don't believe we ever had a comprehensive count of the number of cases in which he prescribed massage because of the varied terminology he used— sometimes he called for rubs, sometimes for osteopathic massage, sometimes just massage.—**H.J.R.**

used—sometimes he called for rubs, sometimes for osteopathic massage, sometimes just massage. Certainly nearly all the cases he sent to me called for massage and/or manipulation, often in combination with diet, hydrotherapy, electric therapy, exercise, and other treatment. This was characteristic of the Cayce work, in which each human being received an individually orchestrated composition of therapies designed to restore the person's harmony of body, mind, and spirit.

Cayce advised a New York businessman as follows:

> For the hydrotherapy and massage are preventive as well as curative measures. For the cleansing of the system allows the body-forces themselves to function normally, and thus eliminate poisons, congestions and conditions that would become acute throughout the body. (257–254)

> (Q) Shall I resume peanut oil rubs?
> (A) There is nothing better . . . they do supply energies to the body. And, just as indicated in other suggestions—those who would eat 2 to 3 almonds each day need never fear cancer. Those who would take a peanut oil rub each week need never fear arthritis. (1158-31)

Cayce's understanding of how massage benefits the system was graphically illustrated in the following case which describes one of its many functions. It occurred in a patient who had acute leukemia, an eighteen-year-old boy:

> The massage is very well, but we would do this the more often, see? As long as there is an opportunity of it producing the effect to all areas of the better activity to the organs of the body. The "why" of the massage should be considered: Inactivity causes many of those portions along the spine from which impulses are received to the various organs to be lax, or taut, or to allow some to receive greater impulse than others. The massage aids the ganglia to receive impulse from nerve forces as it aids circulation through the various portions of the organism. (2456-4)

Cayce gave this advice to a forty-five-year-old man suffering from incoordination of the nervous system (5467-1):

> In the *mornings,* thoroughly massage the whole of the cerebrospinal, rubbing into same—*after* the massaging thoroughly with that of cold applications, see, following the massage—massaging into the centers along the spine, equal parts Tincture of Myrrh and Olive Oil. *Heat* the oil, not to boiling, but nearly so, and add the Myrrh. About a tablespoonful of each should be used. This, the quantity to be used at each application . . .

I want to underscore two interesting aspects of this reading. When asked, "Who should give the massage?" Cayce replied, "One that is in attune with that [which] is being attempted."

Attunement is the key in healing—and particularly in massage. I have learned over the years that with a few lessons you can teach any average person to give elementary massage. But the difference in the result comes from the practitioner's attitude.

In the cases I have cited earlier in this chapter, the devotion of a mother and a wife were key elements in their loved ones' recovery and progress.

In a very recent case, a son has been the instrument of healing for his father. When Mr. R., an attorney, came to me, I knew immediately that it would require daily treatment to help him. He had been pretty badly crippled in an explosion—his left leg had been broken and had terrible rips in it; his kneecap had also been broken. He had been told by his doctor that he might always limp and have to use a cane or crutch.

I told Mr. R. I could try to help him, but if he could arrange to have a daily massage at home, he might be able to walk properly again. I suggested that I teach his son how to give him the treatments, and father and son agreed to try. They came for eight to ten visits; I would give the father a treatment, at the same time teaching his son what to do at home.

Mr. R. has recovered 95 percent movement in his leg and has discarded both the crutches and the cane. On his most recent visit he told me:

"You know, Doc, my son and I have never been such good friends or so close, because he feels he has done so much for me. You have been the means not only of making it possible for me to walk normally again, but also of promoting and enhancing my relationship with my son."

Some relatives who learn massage to help a member of the family become good enough at it to become professionals. This is what happened to Mrs. K.F., who brought her daughter to me for treatment. The daughter was developing what doctors had told her was multiple sclerosis and was losing her coordination. In such cases we can never guarantee results, but we find that the steady application of manipulation and massage keeps the patient from getting worse and often keeps them ambulatory. Sometimes if you can build up their general health and condition, they enjoy a remission from the disease. Then if the muscle tone and circulation have been maintained, the patient can begin to function normally, whereas if muscles are left to atrophy for too long, even with remission, they will not be functional.

I taught the mother how to work on the daughter and then the daughter returned to her husband and home in another city. One day, the mother went to visit a friend who was hospitalized with paralysis of one side. Mrs. K.F. started to rub her friend's arm and hand which were totally numb; then she rubbed the leg. The patient's son came in—he was a doctor in that very hospital. He watched Mrs. K.F. work and asked her if she would come in every day and give his mother a massage. (He, of course, offered to pay her.) The mother had a 60 to 70 percent recovery from the paralysis and her physician–son has now recommended Mrs. K.F. to other patients and doctors. She has a full-time profession now—working for doctors.

Another point I would like to call to the reader's attention is the precise directions given in the readings for the mixing of the massage solution. Cayce used a wide variety of lubricants and he has willed us a legacy of combina-

The Edgar Cayce Handbook for Health Through Drugless Therapy

Edgar Cayce on Peanut Oil

Cayce recommended peanut oil, alone or in combination with other oils, more often than any other, particularly in cases of arthritis. As previously mentioned, in reading 1158-1 he said: "Those who would take a peanut oil rub each week need never fear arthritis"; in reading 1206-13, "[Using] the [peanut] oil rubs once a week, ye will never have rheumatism nor those concurrent conditions from stalemate in liver and kidney activities."

tions, which we have used with great effectiveness for over forty years. For example, peanut oil, alone or in combination, is repeatedly found in the preparations used for the prevention and treatment of arthritis and rheumatic aches and pains; mixtures with a kerosene or gasoline base appear in his formula for a popular strain lotion, and for treating patients who have had infantile paralysis, cerebral palsy, and paralysis. Cocoa butter, alternated with olive oil or olive oil combinations, was recommended for children suffering various illnesses from whooping cough to cerebral palsy. For example, Cayce reading 5568-6 is for a six-year-old boy with cerebral palsy:

> Well that the body, each evening, be rubbed *thoroughly* with those forces as may be found in an ointment—which acts as a lubricant for the whole system. These may be alternated between cocoa butter and olive oil, or olive oil and myrrh and then cocoa butter. These will make for bettered condition for the body's rest and for the activities of the extremities—as well as centers along the cerebro-spinal system . . . this would also be helpful for this body, were the spine rubbed very thoroughly, not in the ordinary treatment as of manipulation, but a more coarseness, so that we will stimulate the nerve ends as they function through the muscular portion of the body.

Cayce recommended peanut oil, alone or in combination with other oils, more often than any other, particularly in cases of arthritis. As previously mentioned, in reading 1158-1 he said: "Those who would take a peanut oil rub each week need never fear arthritis"; in reading 1206-13, "[Using] the [peanut] oil rubs once a week, ye will never have rheumatism nor those concurrent conditions from stalemate in liver and kidney activities."

Cayce did not always explain his selection of a particular oil or mixture, but where we do find explanations there always seemed to be a therapeutic rationale, rather than caprice or custom. Certainly we know from his wide use of fume baths (to be explained in Chapter 10) and his attention to lubricants that he understood the important role of the skin in assimilation as well as elimination.

For example, in reading 440-3 he says, "Olive oil—properly prepared (hence pure olive oil should always be used)—is one of the most effective agents for stimulating muscular activity or mucous-membrane activity that may be applied to a body."

In the case of a woman with impaired locomotion who was also suffering from asthenia (weakness) and toxemia, he did explain the purpose of the massage lubricant:

> Twice each day massage the body, especially along the spine. In the evening massage same with olive oil, *pure* olive oil in each segment, each vertebra, along the spine, massage this well into the body; massaging along the limbs, especially that of the sciatic nerves and along those of the arm that come from the brachial plexus, or along the portion of the arm in the forearm on the exterior, inside on the upper portion, see? Bathe off, after this has been

thoroughly massaged into the body, taking at least twenty to twenty-five minutes of such massaging, see? Of a *morning,* see, massage the body with Tincture of Myrrh, weakened, see? This to toughen, the other to relax and strengthen and feed the muscular conditions, and to bring about the better locomotion from the effects of the poisons as are being eliminated from the system, and to strengthen the body throughout. Do that for at least fifteen days, see? (5421-6)

In reading 618-4 Cayce stated that myrrh was good for the muscles and would stimulate the superficial circulation.

In another reading, 440-3, he said, "Tincture of Myrrh acts with the pores of the skin [in] such a manner as to strike in, causing the circulation to be carried to affected parts . . . "

In my many years of experience both at the institute and in my current practice I have found five or six mixtures to be the most useful; you will find the formulas for them at the end of the next chapter.

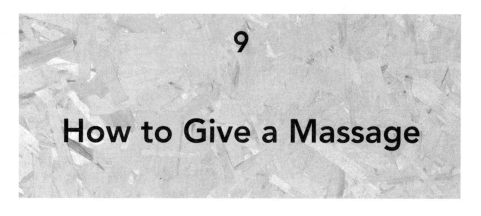

9

How to Give a Massage

And [using] the [peanut] oil rubs once a week, ye will never have rheumatism nor those concurrent conditions from stalemate in liver and kidney activities. (1206-13)

Those who would eat two to three almonds each day need never fear cancer. Those who would take a peanut oil rub each week need never fear arthritis." (1158-31)

The peanut oil rubs [massages] supply energies to the body . . .
(1158-31)

. . . and olive oil is one of the most effective agents for stimulating muscular activity or mucous-membrane activity that may be applied to the body. (440-3)

Instructions for Home Massage

While I would not attempt to compare the benefit of home massage to that given by a competent operator, you will be surprised at how much benefit you can derive from mastering some simple techniques. The benefits to your body, mind, and spirit are inestimable and the benefits to your pocketbook obvious. We will begin with how to massage one's self.

Auto Massage

1. Take an ordinary bath towel, about forty inches long (the twin of the towel from your exercises), and fold it to a width of about six inches. With this simple aid you can give yourself a good friction rub and get some exercise, too, as an added dividend. A towel rub will improve your circulation, help to condition you, and definitely firm up the arms, chest, and shoulders:

Let the towel hang over the right shoulder, then grasp the end on the chest side with the right hand, bring the left hand up and around the back, and grasp the other end of the towel. Then work the towel back and forth across the back, producing a nice friction glow. Then reverse, with the towel on the left shoulder, left hand in front and right hand in back. Putting a twist in the towel will make for variety.

2. Another method of massaging the back of the neck and back with a towel is as follows:

Put the folded towel flat against the back of the neck, hold the ends of the towel fairly tight at about shoulder level. Have the towel firm against the flesh, then pull slowly back and forth about two to four inches. Try to move the underlying flesh and muscles rather than the surface. Then, holding on to the towel, let the hands drop so they are against the chest. Then, with maximum pressure on the towel give a short back and forward pull. This will massage the base of the neck and the large trapezial muscles of the shoulders. Dropping the towel to the level of the armpits, you can give yourself a toweling massage of the back at that section. Then drop the towel lower until the entire back has been covered. The hips can be massaged in the same way. In working the hips you can wiggle against the towel movements so you can double the action—a sort of Hula counterpoint.

In using the towel in this way you can give yourself both a friction and a compression massage. For friction the towel is held less taut and the movement is freer and longer. Be sure not to continue after the skin becomes very warm, as a friction burn can result. For compression massage the movement of pulling the towel back and forth is much shorter, but a great deal of pressure must be applied to the ends of the towel. This is necessary to move the underlying flesh and muscle.

3.   A method of massaging the feet and legs with a towel is as follows:

Fold the forty-inch towel as described previously. Then, while sitting on a kitchen chair, loop it around the foot—one loop. Work the towel back and forth, then zigzag it. Use the same technique with the calf and upper leg.

You can also give yourself a rudimentary percussion massage by hitting a wall with your hips and buttocks—not so hard as to injure either yourself or the wall. This is very useful in breaking down fat. You can also get the benefits of percussion massage by hitting your buttocks with the inside of your fists, a procedure highly beneficial in breaking up congestion in cases of prostatitis.

Preparation

The most important thing to remember in giving a massage is that to get effective results you must have a desire to help the person you are going to be working on.

1.   Ideally, massage should be given on a table. Professional tables are between 27 and 30 inches high, 28 to 30 inches wide, 72 inches long—about the right height for the average man or woman. If the table is too high, you will not have good leverage, and if too low, you will wind up with a backache and needing the services of a professional yourself.

A massage can be given in bed if the operator sits on a chair. Directions will be given later in this chapter.

Although some contemporary massage advocates recommend putting the subject on the floor, I personally have found that this is more suitable for people from those cultures where they are used to squatting or kneeling. So if you are going to include massage in your new lifestyle, it is wise to invest in a table or make one at home.

You can make a table at home by using two carpenter's sawhorses to support a plywood top. This should be at least 3/4 inch thick, 30 inches wide, and 72 inches long.

You can improvise a homemade massage table by using a backless and headless studio couch or other daybed and setting it inside wooden blocks to raise it to the correct height. (These blocks were frequently used in our A.R.E.

clinic to accommodate the various heights of our operators.)

2.   If you are not using a padded table, cover with several layers of blankets or foam pads (beach pads are inexpensive, and waterproof and stain proof, too). Cover with a sheet.

3.   For general tonic massage we prefer to use as a lubricant the Cayce mixture given near the end of this chapter. Variations of the mixture are also given in the same place.

4.   Have the lubricant ready. It is best to place it in a plastic squeeze bottle, which is easier to handle and more hygienic than an open container. I find for beginners it is also handier, because it can be kept close so that tactile contact with the patient is not broken off when reaching for more oil and it will not spill if it tips over.

5.   Prepare a pillow that will be placed under the ankles of the massagee when he or she is prone (lying face down) and under the knees when supine (face up). This helps to relax the body.

6.   Remember to wash your hands thoroughly before touching the patient.

Before learning the various strokes (or movements and techniques), my students have to learn something about the body mechanics, for massage is not something done only with the hands and arms, but with the whole body.

In the great classic, *A Treatise on Massage*, Dr. Douglas Graham, a fellow of the Massachusetts Medical Society and alumnus of the Jefferson Medical College, wrote as follows:

> No matter how precisely and carefully worded the description may be, it is not likely to be comprehended, unless one sees, feels and attempts to do massage himself and compares his efforts with others; for massage, though it may be studied as a science, has like everything else in medicine and surgery, to be practiced as an art . . . there is much that cannot be systematized, that cannot be conveyed from mind to mind in books and articles.
>
>   The definition and manner of doing massage is not rendered any clearer by calling slow and gentle stroking in a centripetal direction, effleurage, or by speaking of deep-rubbing as massage à friction; or by using the term petrissage for deep manipulation without friction, or by calling percussion "tapotment" . . . The multiform subdivisions under which the various procedures of massage have been described can all be grouped under four heads, namely friction, percussion, pressure and movement.[1]

Starting with this disclaimer from so eminent an authority as Dr. Graham, I will urge the amateur masseur and masseuse not to get discouraged by the technical terminology they are likely to encounter in massage manuals and books. For practical purposes the beginner can use just a few basics, and as Dr. Graham also said, "The advantages of ordinary rubbing are not to be despised," as long as you rub them the right way. You will be surprised once you start, to discover how many movements will come to you instinctively and naturally, for as a great nineteenth–century doctor said, "A careful study of the structure of the human body, its contours and conformations together with the most

I will urge the amateur masseur and masseuse not to get discouraged by the technical terminology they are likely to encounter in massage manuals and books. For practical purposes the beginner can use just a few basics . . . —**H.J.R.**

agreeable and efficacious manner of applying massage to it, results in proving, either that the Creator made the body to be manipulated, or else that He put it into the heart of man to devise massage as a means of arousing under-action of nerve, muscle and circulation."

Body Mechanics

Before attempting a massage, it is necessary to learn how to move your own body with rhythm and balance. The bottoms of the feet, the calves of the legs, and the small of the back are all involved, as well as the shoulders, arms, and hands.

Loosen your shoulders with some of the shoulder-shrugging and shoulder-rotating exercises in Chapter 7. Loosen the legs, particularly the knees. Take a modified fencer's stance and flex knees, bouncing up and down with a springing motion—one leg should be forward and one leg back. Then swing the shoulders and hips back and forth in a coordinated movement—not unlike those of the dancers who enjoy rock music. Rhythm is everything. That is why I can manipulate as many as eighteen people a day without suffering undue fatigue.

Strokes (Movement)

Touching

This is used to make contact with the subject as an introduction to help both of you to relax. Place hands around the left arm or shoulder, your thumb on the upper arm, with fingers molding the contour of the arm. There is no movement — just a gentle reassuring pressure. Touching can be used on the shoulder, upper arm, or forearm. (See Fig. 1.)

Stroking (Effleurage)

This is the most commonly used movement. It is used to apply the lubricant, and for most of the traveling your hands must do to cover the length of the body and limbs. The entire hand is used in stroking with fingers close together and the entire surface of the hand in use and molded to the contour of the part of body which is engaged at the time. Stroking can be done in long or short or interrupted movements (explained in the following instructions) and can be applied with light, medium, or heavier pressure.

Stroking can also be done with fingertips, thumb, and knuckles, but for novices we will stick to the most common usage. Stroking is a most valuable movement; it increases circulation of blood and lymph, improves the return of the venous circulation back toward the heart, improves the tissues, and is soothing and relaxing, inducing sleep. (See Fig. 2.)

Kneading (Petrissage)

This is the most important movement, therapeutically, as it affects the nerves, the blood vessels, the glands, improves cellular change, normalizes the blood flow and the lymphs, and helps to remove toxins. Kneading is done by making small circles with the right hand moving clockwise and the left hand counter-

---

The Basic Massage Strokes
- Touching
- Stroking (Effleurage)
- Kneading (Petrissage)
- Friction
- Rolling
- Wringing
- Nerve Compression
- Percussion
- Manipulation

Effleurage is the most commonly used movement. It is used to apply the lubricant, and for most of the traveling your hands must do to cover the length of the body and limbs.—**H.J.R.**

clockwise, always in an upward and outward direction even when you are massaging the limb downward. Pressure is exerted by the thumb with the kneading being performed by the four fingers close together. The hands roll rhythmically as does your whole body swinging from the shoulders, hips, and legs. (See Fig. 3.)

Friction

This is a stroking movement, which is applied to the surface of the skin (frequently without a lubricant), not working the underlying muscles. It is usually performed more rapidly than stroking and is more superficial, stimulating the surface skin. The position of the hands is the same as in stroking. (See Fig. 2.)

Rolling

Holding the hands flat, fingers straight and pointed outward, roll the leg or thigh back and forth as you would a piece of dough or clay that you are rolling into a rope strip. While the left hand moves forward, the right hand moves back and vice versa. This is a movement that is good to use for athletes, skaters, or anyone who is muscle–bound or suffering from muscle fatigue. (See Fig. 4.)

Wringing

This movement is often used on the sides, where there is an accumulation of fat over the girdle. Place open hands with fingertips pointing away from you on your subject's waist or limb. Squeeze the fat or flesh with both hands, then pull toward you with the right hand and away with the left, using the same motion you would employ in wringing out a towel. This drives the blood from the muscles, stimulates the nerve cells and breaks down fat cells. (See Fig. 5.)

Nerve Compression

Place both hands on subject's arm as in *touching*, with thumbs on top of the arm, fingers molded around the sides and underside of arm, and squeeze upward and outward, applying pressure with body weight behind the squeeze. This is very useful for normalizing circulation and is relaxing. (See Fig. 6.)

Percussion

This has a number of variants known as *cupping, beating, hacking,* and *slapping.* Percussion has specific therapeutic uses in breaking up cold congestions and in treating prostatitis and other problems. Many masseurs and masseuses like to finish up a general massage with hacking on the back, a feature popularized in so many Hollywood movies. *Cupping* is usually performed in short staccato movements, usually on back or chest with the hand held in a cupped or hollow position. (See Fig. 7.)

Slapping is done with the flat of the hand (see Fig. 8), *beating* with doubled–up fists; and *hacking* is done with the sides of the hands, the fingers held loose (see Fig. 9).

*Petrissage is the most important movement, therapeutically, as it affects the nerves, the blood vessels, the glands, improves cellular change, normalizes the blood flow and the lymphs and helps to remove toxins.—*__H.J.R.__

for
cold
congestion

prostatitis –
infection of
the prostate

cupping – fig. 7

There are many other strokes: draining, fulling, raking, chopping, etc., with as many different names; but those given above should serve most needs for home massage.

Manipulation

These are simple passive movements of the person's limbs performed by the masseur or masseuse (rotary and hinge joints). Do not permit the subject to help. See that he or she remains relaxed.

Reilly Method of Home Massage

General Principles

1. All general massage movements should be *upward* and *toward* the heart, except for the neck and head.

2. It is best to massage the upper part of a limb first, beginning at the distal end and proceeding up: elbow to shoulder, hand to elbow, etc.

3. In general, strokes are begun lightly, and with each succeeding repetition the pressure increases and then diminishes until the last stroke is soothing, slow, and light. Movements are applied with more pressure ascending and are lighter descending.

4. Slow tempo is used for relaxation—let us say 60–90 movements per minute; rapid movement is used for stimulation—from 120–180 strokes per minute.

5. Remember, try to maintain constant touch with the subject even when changing your position. If you must move to the other side or from the head to the feet, try to keep one hand in touch.

6. Try to become alert to possible "danger signals": spots that are too hot or too cold, stiffness, pain, acute tenderness, etc. If they persist, be sure to call these to the attention of your subject's doctor—they may be early warning signals of some disorder.

7. The following order, which I use and teach, has been found to be effective if the recipient is at all nervous and apprehensive. Massage the arms first because this warms the operator's hands and the arms are the least sensitive part of the body. Do the abdomen before the head and shoulders, because if you loosen any gas or toxins in the colon it can produce a slight headache, which the head massage will clear. I have found it easier and more efficient to work on the feet when the patient is prone and the legs are flexed at the knee, giving good access to the feet.

Remember to apply enough oil to the limb so that the skin is smooth and your hands do not drag along the patient's skin. Keep the strokes long and firm. Take it slowly—a tender, loving-care approach. If you apply too much oil, you will not be able to go as deep, so wipe excess off with a towel or tissue. For rapid stimulation, use "friction" without a lubricant.

The Routine

1. To begin, place your subject in a supine position (lying on back) with a pillow under the knees. Use two towels to protect the bosom and pubic area of a woman, or a sheet and towel. Men may wear shorts, towels, or sheet. This is to prevent chilling as well as to protect modesty.

2. Your first approach to the subject will be through TOUCH. Place one or both hands on the arm or shoulder before beginning massage therapy. This is an important way to establish rapport and make contact.

3. Put a lubricant on your own hands.

4. Apply the lubricant, stroking the entire arm.

5. Begin with the left arm at the elbow and massage up to the shoulder.

6. Starting at the wrist, massage up to the elbow.

7. Then do the hand.

8. Manipulate the hands and arms as directed.

COMPLETE ONE ARM BEFORE STARTING THE OTHER.

Repeat this procedure on the right arm.

9. Nerve compression.

10. Finish by *stroking* the whole arm upward from the hand and fingers up to the shoulder and down.

11. Do the abdomen carefully, following cautionary directions, and stimulate the liver.

12. Do the sides and waist.

13. Starting with the left leg at the left knee, massage to the buttocks.

14. Massage around the knee.

15. Starting at the left ankle, massage the lower leg up to the knee.

16. Manipulate the knee and hip.

17. Nerve compression.

18. Finish with stroking of the entire leg—feet to buttocks.

19. Do the face.

20. Do the neck and shoulders.

21. Turn your subject over to a prone position (face down).

22. (a) Do the back of the legs, knee to thigh; (b) do the ankles to the knees.

23. Massage the feet and toes.

24. Manipulate the feet and legs as directed.

25. Nerve compression and optional strokes to the entire leg.

26. Finish with long stroking.

27. Work the back, buttocks, neck, and shoulders as directed in the following pages.

28. Finish with long stroking from the neck down the back to the buttocks, and up again.

NOTE: When using optional back, leg, or shoulder strokes, do them before the final stroking.

Technique Instructions

The following instructions are based on a 30- to 45-minute general tonic massage. As you develop experience and enthusiasm, you can expand to 60 minutes by increasing the number of times each movement is applied and adding more strokes.

Arms

1.   Your subject is now lying on the table or bed, face up, with a pillow under the knees, suitably draped. You should be standing on his/her left side with your right leg forward, left leg balanced comfortably, facing the subject. You will begin with the left arm.

If you are giving the massage on a bed, consult instructions later in this chapter. (See Fig. 10.)

2.   TOUCH the subject on shoulder and arms.

3.   Put a lubricant on your own hands.

4.   Apply the lubricant to the subject with long STROKES upward on the entire arm—gently STROKING it two or three times, from hands to shoulder. Use the entire hand, keeping the fingers together and molded to the contour of the arm.

5.   Beginning high at the shoulder, use a KNEADING MOVEMENT on the arm, working your hands alternately, keeping your hands close together. Work up, but move downward. The circular motion of the hands is always *upward*. When you reach the elbow you start to work back to the shoulder. Do this two or three times, in a continuous, smooth flow, always draining up, following the venous blood flow to the heart.

To keep your subject more relaxed you can support the arm under your own "wing"—tucking it under your armhole when you are using your two hands as in kneading.

Try to remember your "knee action," rocking your body back and forth while working on the subject. Increase the pressure so that you are molding the flesh like a piece of dough or clay. (See Fig. 11.)

6.   To do the forearm (from wrist to elbow), bend the arm at the elbow, resting it and the upper arm on the table, or tuck it under your "wing" as described above.

STROKE the forearm from wrist to elbow two or three times. Be careful that there is no pressure on the inner artery of the arm; keep the pressure on the outside of the arms. Knead the forearm one or two times. You may add rolling if you are giving a longer massage or if there is muscle strain, as after tennis or golf.

7.   Next we do the hand. Spread the hand open to relax it. If your subject is a nervous person he/she may have a tendency to clench hands and feet, so proceed slowly and gently. Massage the fingers, beginning with the little finger, with spiral motions on each finger, from tips to knuckles, as if you are turning a screw. This drains the blood and changes the circulation. Another technique is to hold the subject's finger between two of your own and wiggle

it as if you were screwing it into a socket. Be gentle. Then rotate each finger in each direction. Work the hinge and rotary joints of the hand and fingers back and forth. Pull the fingers and stretch the hand as wide as possible without strain.

Massage the palm of the hand with your thumbs, using both of your hands and moving in small circles, in opposite directions. Then massage the outer hand by holding your thumb firmly in the subject's palm and moving your other fingers in a circular movement on his/her outer hand.

Rotate the thumb clockwise; rotate the hand, using your own two hands to make the movement. Flex the hand at the wrist back and forth.

DO NOT LET THE SUBJECT ASSIST YOU. KEEP HIM/HER RELAXED. THE OPERATOR PERFORMS ALL THE MOVEMENTS.

(This leads into the manipulation of the arm.)

8.   For joint manipulation, flex the elbow. Place your own hand under the arm of the subject just above the elbow and the other hand at his/her wrist. Bend the subject's arm back and forth gently at the elbow as if it were on a hinge, bringing the hand as close to the shoulder as possible. (See Fig. 12.)

ROTATE the shoulder. Put your hand over the triceps on the back of the arm and clasp the subject's wrist or forearm. Rotate the arm and shoulder in both directions. (See Fig. 13.)

9.   NERVE COMPRESSION is used next to the finishing movement, which is STROKING. Position your hands on the subject's arm as in TOUCHING; your fingers are molded around the sides and underside of the arm. Starting at the top of the shoulder, press upward and move hands down the arm. The motion is an outward, upward squeeze. You can put your body weight behind this. Work all the way down to the wrist and then go up the same way (one or two times).

BE CAREFUL NOT TO PRESS THE ARTERIES ON INSIDE OF THE ARM.

(This movement is good for circulation and relaxation) (See Fig. 6.)

10. FINAL STROKING consists of STROKING from hand to shoulder two or three times. The first STROKE can be medium pressure and slow; the second, lighter going up, and TRAIL your hands very lightly back to subject's hands. End by going up arm very lightly, then back down very lightly.

Place the subject's hand quietly and gently on the table and do the right arm.

Abdomen

11.   TOUCH the abdomen with the whole hand, and STROKE the oil on lightly, establishing contact with this very sensitive area of your subject's body. Stand at the left side of your subject, with your own feet parallel, instead of one in back of the other, and balanced comfortably.

Have your subject bend the knees, placing the feet flat on the table or bed. It is more comfortable if the knees are supported with one or more pillows. With your fingers flat, begin to knead at the lower left side of abdomen, rotating your fingers and hand clockwise, moving backward to about an inch or two under the left ribs, across the abdomen to a couple of inches below the right ribs, and then continuing down in little circles to just above the right hip. Remember, the small movement is up and out. After you have finished this, complete circles of the torso. Repeat the same motion from the right side to the left side, following the movement of the large bowel. Do this three times in each direction.

To stimulate the peristaltic action of the intestines, place the entire right hand on your left hand (or vice versa if you are more comfortable), and starting at the lower left, work backward to the right in a big circle of the abdomen, with light kneading from right to left, shaking and vibrating the hand that is in contact with the subject's body. Do not press on the bladder.

Following the abdominal massage, bring your hands to the front of the lower ribs on the right side, and placing one hand in back and above the rib and the other in front, shake the liver—just shake up and down and this will stimulate it. (See Figs. 14A, 14B, and 14C.)

Sides

12. While your subject is still supine, and after you finish the abdomen, you may want to work on the sides, using kneading and wringing movements, if the subject (particularly a woman) has fat deposits there. (Many women would like to get rid of this unsightly girdle roll, which I often call their "hanging garden.")

Standing on the right side, reach across the left side of your subject's waist and squeeze loose flesh at the waistline between your thumb and fingers. Lift as much flesh as you can, grasp and squeeze and knead it. Then with a "pulling and pushing" (wringing) motion, pull the sides up and in toward the navel, defining the waistline—back-and-forth kneading and wringing, pushing and pulling up. Do this at least six to eight times.

KEEPING your hand on your subject's body, walk to the other side of the table and repeat on other side.

Legs

13. Upper leg: Begin with the left leg. You are standing at the side of, and facing, your subject, with your right leg forward and your left leg back. (See Fig. 15—the subject has a pillow under the knees.)

The movements and routine will be the same as for the arms—first LUBRICATING, then STROKING, and then KNEADING from the knee to the hips, and up to the top of the thigh. Throw your whole body weight on the leg for this movement, three times.

BE CAREFUL TO AVOID PRESSING ON THE FEMORAL ARTERY (inside of leg). (See Fig. 16.)

Deep-knead the upper leg, especially on people who are getting a little flabby there—this drains out edema and promotes muscle tone. If you want to get more circulation and muscle tone, use shorter strokes. REMEMBER, WHEN YOU ARE MOVING DOWN THE LIMB, YOUR SMALL HAND MOVEMENTS WILL STILL BE UPWARD AND OUTWARD.

14. Knees: Next, massage the knee in a circular motion, using your thumb

and fingers. Work around the side of the knee, loosening muscles and flesh. Use pressure on your thumbs when you want to go deeper.

15. Lower leg: STROKE, KNEAD, and ROLL the front of the leg from the ankle to the knee. Then bend the leg slightly and work on the inside of the lower leg (especially the calf). Knead up along both sides of the bone, using the fingers and thumbs with small circular movements. This upward pressure will increase circulation and drain edema.

16.   Manipulation: Flex knee and then rotate the hip socket by holding the bottom of foot or ankle with one hand and holding the knee with the other hand. Rotate first up and out clockwise and then counterclockwise. Then bend the knee toward the body, up and down, working the hinge joint of the knee. (Do each of these three to six times.)

Full Leg

17. Nerve compression: Use this movement starting at the top of the thigh and moving down to the ankle as directed in the arm massage.

18. Stroking. Finish with long STROKING movements FROM ANKLE TO UPPER THIGH, using medium pressure going up and lighter coming down (three times). Each time get lighter. Repeat this procedure on the right leg.

Head and Face

19. (a) Standing in back of the subject, we begin first with the sinus areas on the forehead. Place your fingers over your subject's forehead in between and just above the eyebrows. Tap the fingers of the hand lightly with the fingers of your other hand (eight to ten times). (See Fig. 17.)

(b) Using a circular motion, gently massage both sides of the nose with your fingers, beginning at the sides of the nose and working outward on the cheeks to the ears (six to eight times). (See Fig. 18.)

(c) Massage the gland below (and slightly behind the ear) with light to medium circular motion, then work up behind the ears with the same circular motion (five times on each side). (See Fig. 19.)

For this part of the massage it is very relaxing to the subject to hold his/her head in your free hand. Don't pull or stretch the skin of the face.

Neck and Shoulders

20. (a) Standing or sitting behind subject's head with your feet parallel and balanced, start at the base of the neck and work fingertips along both sides of the spinal cord, rotating up and outward in small circles. Work from the base of the skull down to and including the shoulders (six to eight times). (See Figs. 20A and 20B.)

(b) Standing at the side of the table, tilt the patient's head to one side and hold the forehead lightly with one hand. Use the fingertips of the other hand (keep fingertips flat) and massage the back of the neck, pulling lightly forward on the neck. Work on the shoulder and back as far down as possible. Switch head position to the opposite hand and do the other side of the neck, shoulder, and back. (Do six times on each side.)

(c) Push downward against both shoulders at one time, then alternating one at a time. Go slowly, easily, and hold for a few seconds. Do not push in a jerky manner. (See Fig. 21.)

Other neck and shoulder massage movements are given when the subject is prone.

The Prone Position

21. Turn your subject over and place a pillow under the ankles. Place a rolled-up towel under the forehead to keep him/her more comfortable. (See Fig. 22.)

Back of the Legs

22. (a) STROKING:

Apply lubrication with STROKING movements starting high near the buttocks and working down toward the ankle and then back up again.

(b) KNEADING:

Using the same kneading upward and outward circular movement that you have been using on the arms and the front of legs, start high near the buttocks and work to the feet. Increase pressure and go deeply into the leg. Apply the weight of your body when moving your hands down the leg. Then starting at the ankles, KNEAD upward to the buttocks. The ankles can be thinned and drained of edema in this way (two or three times in each direction). Increase to six times if there is much edema.

23. Do the feet. Apply lubrication with long strokes to the bottom of the foot and then knead them with your thumbs in small circles, clockwise and counterclockwise. (See Fig. 23.)

Work the toes with the same spiraling movement you used on the fingers of the hands.

Massage the side of the foot using both of your hands—one on each side of the foot, and then do the heels.

Apply pressure with the heel of your palm to the front and back of toes and the ball of the foot. A circular movement, using the heel of your hand on the ball of your subject's foot, is very effective for foot fatigue.

When doing the instep, apply more pressure in long strokes with your thumbs.

Spread and stretch the ball of the foot with your two hands.

24. Do manipulation of feet and leg. Rotate the ankles as you did the wrist—clockwise and counterclockwise. (See Fig. 24.)

Then pull foot up and down, slowly and carefully. (See Fig. 25.)

Finish by folding the legs back, bringing the heel to touch the buttocks if possible, or as far back as your subject can bend leg comfortably.

FINISH THE ENTIRE LEG WITH THE NERVE COMPRESSION AND STROKING AS DESCRIBED IN THE FOLLOWING DIRECTIONS.

25. Nerve compression: Starting at the buttocks, perform the movement with both hands, sliding lightly down the leg, about an inch at a time, until the foot is reached. Repeat going from foot to buttocks.

26. Stroking: Start at the ankles and STROKE up to buttocks with a slow, deep motion. Come back with a lighter pressure. Repeat two or three times very slowly and lighter each time.

NOTE: If you are trying for stimulation, all forms of percussion can be used on the back of the legs (like hacking) and on the buttocks (slapping and beating).

Back

27. (a) As usual, lightly stroke the oil onto the skin. Work from the neck to the buttocks, standing over the patient's head, if possible. Use long strokes from the neck all the way down to the buttocks, leaning on the patient with your whole body weight. This won't hurt the patient; it will feel good. Lean into the stroke going down and ease up coming up. Work *very, very slowly* to relax the autonomic nervous system. You can tell the patient is relaxed when the body comes up to meet the hands.

(b) Working on the side portion of the back, from the side toward the spine and back to the side—where some of the fat is sometimes accumulated—use a rolling, wringing, kneading motion. Use both hands—one alternating movement with the other—and establish a pleasant but constant rhythm. Push with the whole hand, pull with the other hand, curl the fingers under the ribs, lifting them slightly, and work down the back, starting at the shoulders down to the buttocks. (See Fig. 26.)

(c) Next, knead the upper part of the back (the shoulder area), site of the trapezius and deltoid muscles (shoulder muscles). Roll the muscles under your hand, between the thumb and base of thumb and the index finger and the four fingers of your hand, lifting and squeezing them. (See Fig. 27.)

(d) Massage the back and sides of the neck with your fingers and then with your thumb. People who do a lot of mental and desk work are usually very tight there. (This is done better when sitting behind the subject's head.)

(e) Next flatten the fingers of one hand and place your other hand on top of it. Starting at the top of the spine, start loosening the muscles alongside the vertebrae with an upward and outward half-circle. Starting at the top at the base of the head, work down the entire side of the spine and then go up again. Repeat on the other side of the vertebrae. Always push up and outward from the spine with your body weight behind the hands as you descend. (See Fig. 28.)

(f) Next, move to the buttocks, where you will work on four different points. Standing on the right side of the body, a little below the buttocks, put one hand on top of the other to increase pressure, and with a rocking movement of the knees and feet start rotating the upper part of the buttock on the inside toward the spine. Rotate it up and out. Then drop to the lower part of the buttock and rotate it the same way—up and out. Do each three to six times. (See Fig. 29.)

Then you take the upper outside part of the buttocks above the hip socket and rotate it up and out—also the same movement to the lower outside of buttocks (over hip socket). Repeat on the other side. Then put both hands on first one, then the other buttock, and rotate up and outward with the full weight of your body—six to twelve times.

(g) Interrupted stroking: Put your thumbs on the spinal column with hands outspread over the side of the back. The four fingers of the hand should be close together—the thumb spread away as far as you can hold it comfortably. Leaning the weight of your body on your hands, go down the spine for about 8 inches and then pull up underneath the ribs; as you pull up, exert a little force, almost lifting the ribs up. Then go down another 6 inches, and when you come to the end of the ribs, shift your pressure downward to the thumb so you don't press on the kidneys—and then you go down another 6 inches and pull up again—then another 6 inches until you have reached the upper part of the buttocks. (See Fig. 30.)

The benefit of this movement comes not only from STROKING down but the pulling up and raising of the rib cage.

28. Start at the base of the neck and slowly STROKE down, with pressure, to the end of the spine at the sacrum. The hands are held in the same position as for the interrupted stroking—thumbs on spine, fingers together and spread out to the full size of the hand. (See Fig. 31.)

Go down with medium pressure and return, trailing fingers lightly. Repeat a second time, throwing more body weight on the arms going down, very, very slowly with total body weight behind it—all the way down to the end of the spine.

Then finish with lighter stroking two to six times according to the degree of relaxation you wish to impart to your subject. (See Fig. 31.)

Optional Back Strokes

For advanced work you may add these movements to your back massage:

29. (a) Mass kneading: Begin at the top of back, press down and lift the muscles back up. This is sort of a squeezing action. (See Fig. 32.)

(b) Mild springing action: Press down with both hands a few times, working down to just above kidney area—do just the spinal column at the kidney area, then the whole area again below the kidney, and then work back up the same way. (See Figs. 33A and 33B.)

(c) Separation traction: The hand at the base of the spine remains stationary with pressure down and toward the feet, while other hand is working down along the spine with pressure down and toward the head. Count to six or seven at each position. (See Fig. 34.)

EXTRA massage is additional work at the base of the skull down the neck and into the shoulders at the base of the neck (for people who do lots of mental work).

Massage Therapy for Cold Congestion

"Cupping" is very effective in loosening cold congestion. It can be administered both on the chest and back. Hollow the hand so that a suction effect is created when the hand strikes the chest or back. Keep the wrist flexible so that there is a staccato and slapping action at the same time.

"Hacking" also can be used for this purpose. Follow earlier instructions.

For a Head Cold

Use the sinus massage on the face, then massage the back of the neck first. Loosen tension muscles behind the ears carefully—for this is a very sensitive, tender area—following earlier instructions.

For Neck and Shoulder Strain

(This is performed in a supine position, before turning the subject over to the prone position.)

Here are two ways of loosening the trapezius muscles. Good for fatigue, cold congestion, and general muscular and postural discomfort:

1. With the subject supine, stand behind his/her head and with thumbs on the back of the shoulder, and your fingers outstretched toward the chest, rotate the muscle putting your own body weight behind the movement.

2. Standing on the right side, place your own left hand on your subject's forehead, turning the head toward you. Balance the head, but don't lean on it. Then with fingers of the right hand, start at the base of the neck, rotating upward and outward. Move up to base of the skull, then down the neck and outward to the shoulder. Do this four to eight times. Don't slide fingers over skin (avoid friction). Lift the muscles and loosen them from the bones.

Special Instructions for Bed Massage

If you are using a single bed, which permits you to go around to both sides, you will sit on the side of the bed facing your subject. The subject may lie with his/her head at the head of the bed or at the foot—it doesn't matter, except when the neck is being done. Then the patient must lie with the head at the foot of the bed so that you can sit behind it.

For massage in a double bed, first do one side—for example, the left arm and left leg. Then move your subject to the other side of the bed and do the right arm and right leg. Sit facing the subject. The back of the legs can be done at the same time by turning the subject over. But when you do the head, the patient must lie with his/her head at foot of the bed.

It is better to stand when doing the back. You may remain seated for the face, neck, and shoulders, sitting behind the head.

Floor Massage

You may do the back of the legs and the back of your subject while using the floor instead of a massage table or bed, but I do not recommend the floor for massaging the abdomen, the front of the arms, and legs. It takes a bit of practice to squat or kneel while performing massage movements without shutting off your own circulation and possibly incurring some back trouble of your own.

Cayce Massage Mixtures

In reading 1968–7, Cayce said of the following formula that it is "For making or keeping a good complexion—this for the skin, the hands, arms and body as well . . . " It is not surprising, therefore, that it is the one I use for general tonic massage.

General Tonic Massage
Peanut oil .... 6 ounces
Olive oil .... 2 ounces
Rosewater .... 2 ounces
Lanolin, dissolved .... 1 tablespoon

Shake well each time before using.

Peanut Oil and Olive Oil Mixture
For arthritis, rheumatism, Parkinson's disease, multiple sclerosis, the aftereffects of anesthesia, kidney disorders, toxemia, injuries from accidents, menopausal complaints, etc.:

Peanut oil .... 2 ounces
Olive oil .... 2 ounces
Lanolin (liquified) .... 1 teaspoon

Shake this solution and massage thoroughly into the lumbar and sacral areas, and especially along limbs . . . under the knee, in the foot, especially in the bursa of the heel and the front under the toes or in the instep. (3232-1)

For prostatitis:
After the massage, each time, we find it would be well to massage the affected area—that is, of course, across the small of the back and extending all the way over the prostate area, you see, and on either side of the limbs—with an equal combination of Olive Oil and Peanut Oil. Massage in all the body will absorb. Do this after the manipulations are given, each time. (1539-4)

Peanut Oil Alone
For multiple sclerosis, paralysis, apoplexy, palsy, Parkinson's disease, polio, menopause, cholecystitis, low vitality, fatigue, poor circulation, coronary occlusion, ulcerated stomach, glandular disturbance, etc.:

About twice each week, almost bathe in olive oil or peanut oil; especially peanut oil—in the joints, the neck, across the clavicle, across all the areas of the spine, the rib and the frontal area to the pit of the stomach, across the stomach and especially in the diaphragm area; then across the hips and the lower portion of the back and across the sacral area and then the limbs themselves. (1688-7)

Praise for Peanut Oil

From Pittsburgh, Pennsylvania, came this testimonial on the use of pure peanut oil: "As a rheumatoid arthritic, I have found it to be of great benefit to my condition. After using peanut oil as a massaging oil for several years, I have to agree with Cayce's belief that it not only lubricates but heals as well. I am sure that had I known about the oil in this use I would have been spared much misery."

Another glowing report from Mrs. H. regarding the use of peanut oil in a case of paralytic stroke: "The massage for limbs with the peanut oil relieves cramping. Relief [comes] in five or ten minutes—Massage of both legs and feet with peanut oil—results good. I appreciate the information very much as it gives quick relief in a chronic case."

March 13, 1954, report from Mrs. G.L.: "Yes, the peanut oil rubbed on arthritic joints certainly works! By constant use of it, I can continue to wear my wedding ring without having it enlarged."

March 27, 1951, report from Dr. W.O.R., Washington, D. C.: "My arthritic patient's first reaction [from the peanut oil massage] was an increase in vitality and elimination."

Castor Oil Alone

For arthritis, back pain, muscular and joint pain, contractions, and spasms:

The REILLY VARIATION is to use castor oil for any arthritic, rheumatic, or muscular and joint pain as an unction.

Using an infrared lamp (metal, if possible), place it about 12–18 inches above the part to be massaged.

Apply the castor oil to the painful area and let the lamp warm it and help it to penetrate into the skin for about 5–10 minutes. Then keep rubbing with the fingers and hand until the oil is well worked in. As the skin absorbs the oil, keep replacing it with new oil. Repeat the process of heating and rubbing. This can be continued 10–60 minutes.

CAUTION: Put oil on the back of your own hand for protection from the lamp when giving the treatment.

Praise for Castor Oil

From California, this report: "Mother had arthritis so bad she was committed to the hospital . . . The arthritis was centered in her fingers which were doubled back in her palms—she didn't think she would ever be able to open up her fingers again. Father brought her home and started a treatment of hot castor oil—rubbing her hands, arms, shoulders, and legs three times a day. Within a period of three or four months her condition improved to the extent that she could walk, use her arms, and her fingers straightened out, and today she is completely cured. She was seventy-six years old when she was at her worst and is now eighty-one."

Other Cayce Mixtures

To speed the healing of injured ligaments and for use after stroke and in paralysis:

Massage the body with the following combination of oils, adding in the order named:

Nujol, as the base	6 ounces
Peanut oil	2 ounces
Pine needle oil	1 ounce
Sassafras root oil	1/2 ounce
Lanolin (liquified)	1/2 ounce

This formula (3118–1) was used successfully in several cases of skiing accidents.

For leg and foot pain:

To 4 ounces of Russian white oil add:

Witch hazel	2 ounces
Rub alcohol (not wood, but *rub* alcohol compound)	1 ounce
Oil of sassafras	3 to 5 minims (drops)

Shake this together. Only use a small portion of same at the time. Begin with the hips and rub down [with upward pressure of the hands].

This would be good for anyone that stands on the feet much, or whose feet pain . . . (555–5)

For muscular sprains, strains, backache, and bruises (formula given in Cayce reading 326–5):

To 1 ounce of olive oil, add:

Russian white oil	2 ounces
Witch hazel	1/2 ounce
Tincture of benzoin	1/2 ounce
Oil of sassafras	20 minims
Coal oil	6 ounces

Rub small amount well into affected portions once or twice daily and apply heat if desired.

For varicose veins, tendinitis, strains, and fracture—especially good for the lower limbs:

> Do use an equal combination of Olive Oil (heated) and Tincture of Myrrh to massage in knees, limbs and feet, right after these have been bathed in hot water. Massage these oils well into them. (3523-1)

Massage Myrrh and Olive Oil—opposite from what is usually given but specifically indicates *heating* (not boiling) Myrrh and oil, mixing together to achieve an ointment rather than a solution; massage daily; especially for lower limbs:

> The activities of the massage, especially on the lower limb, should be once each day. Heat the Myrrh and add the oil (Yes, this is opposite from what has usually been given) but *heat* the *myrrh* and stir in. This doesn't mean boiling, but heat and mix together; for this will make for more of an ointment (while the other would remain in a different solution entirely). (4873-1)

> The next day we would use the Salt (plain sodium chloride; not that carrying other properties, but this well powdered) and *pure* Apple Vinegar.
>
> Use one one day, the other the next. Continue in this manner, and we find that these ingredients will supply calcium, acids and oils that will prevent accumulations of water . . . or prevent the tendons becoming so taut as not to allow movement in the knee and the kneecap. (438-5)

A Mixture for Arthritis ✗

Add these in the order named:

Usoline or Nujol as the base	4 ounces
Olive oil	2 ounces
Peanut oil	2 ounces
Oil of pine needles	1/2 ounce
Oil of sassafras root	1/2 ounce
Lanolin (liquified)	1 ounce

[Shake before applying.] (3363-1)

To prevent the recurrence in the muscular forces about the knee and the limb of the stiffening, so as to pull the ligaments loose again, we would massage the whole of the limb each day, as follows:

One day we would use equal parts of Olive Oil and Tincture of Myrrh for the massaging.

The next day we would use the salt (plain sodium chloride . . .) and *pure* Apple Vinegar. (438-5)

For incoordination of nervous system, facial tic, prostatitis:

. . . gently stimulate the ganglia, particularly in the 3rd cervical, 4th & 5th dorsal, 9th dorsal, and through the cervical area, stimulating also the limbs *and* the arms and shoulders and neck. Not too severely, but very firmly, gently; using the combination of Camphor Oil and Peanut Oil—equal proportions . . . (2952-1)

For constipation and tumors:

. . . two parts Russian white oil, or Usolene, or Nujol, to one part Pine oil. And use the regular Pine Oil, not pitch, not pine needles, but Pine Wood Oil, see? (2966-1)

For central nervous disorder (cough; also for children's whooping cough):

Then, before ready for retiring . . . gentle massage over the cerebro-spinal system . . . Cocoa butter, or any good cream (cold cream) may be used to massage in same . . . (143-7)

To remove scars:

To relieve much of the scar tissue on the left limb we would use sweet oil [peanut oil] combined with camphorated oil [in] equal parts. Massage this each day for 3 to 6 months and we would reduce the most of this. (487-15)

Scarmassage Skin Lotion

For burns and externally caused scars (from reading 2015–10):

Camphorated oil .... 2 ounces
Lanolin, dissolved .... 1/2 teaspoonful
Peanut oil .... 1 ounce

Once daily, massage into the scarred areas, using an amount the skin will completely absorb. Avoid contact with the eyes and mucous membranes.

NOTE: Some of these formulas can be obtained already made up. See the source of supply listed at the back of this book.

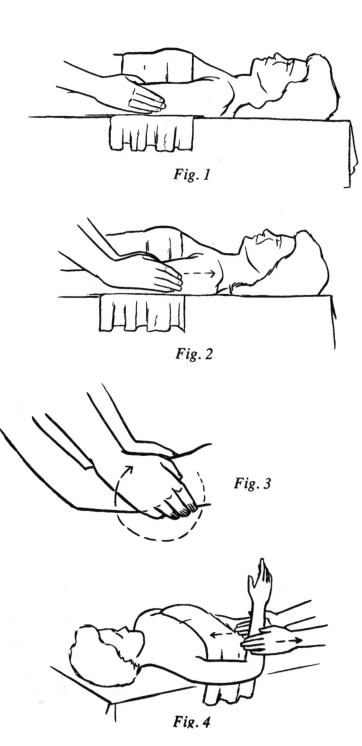

Fig. 1

Fig. 2

Fig. 3

Fig. 4

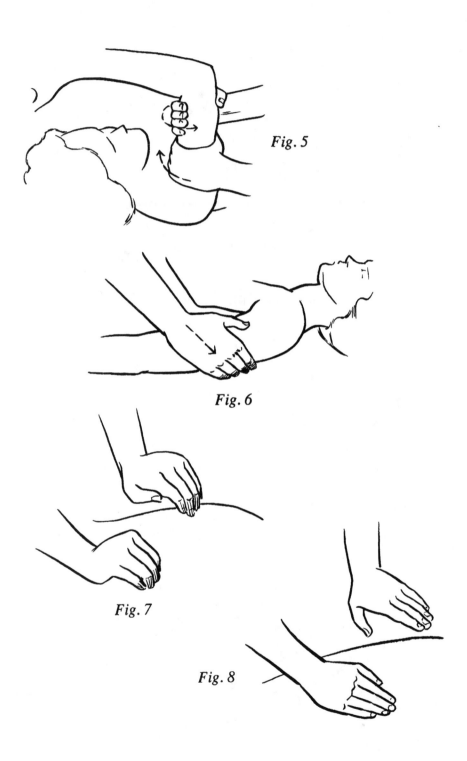

Fig. 5

Fig. 6

Fig. 7

Fig. 8

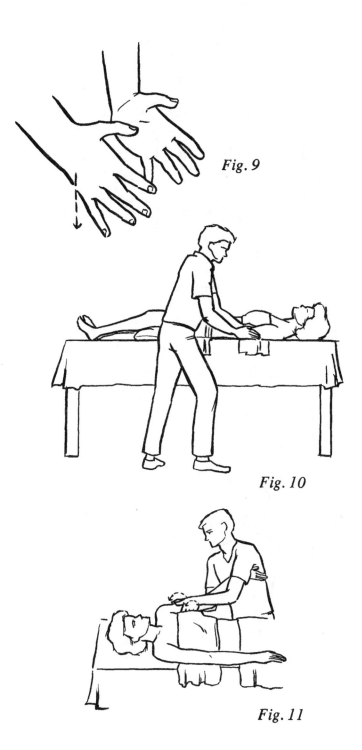

Fig. 9

Fig. 10

Fig. 11

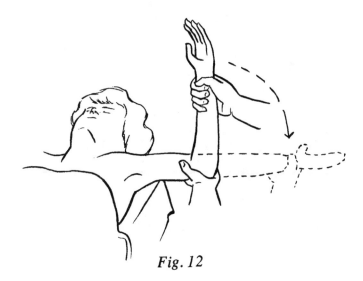

Fig. 12

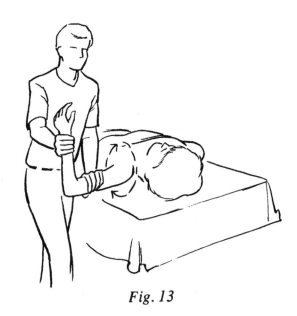

Fig. 13

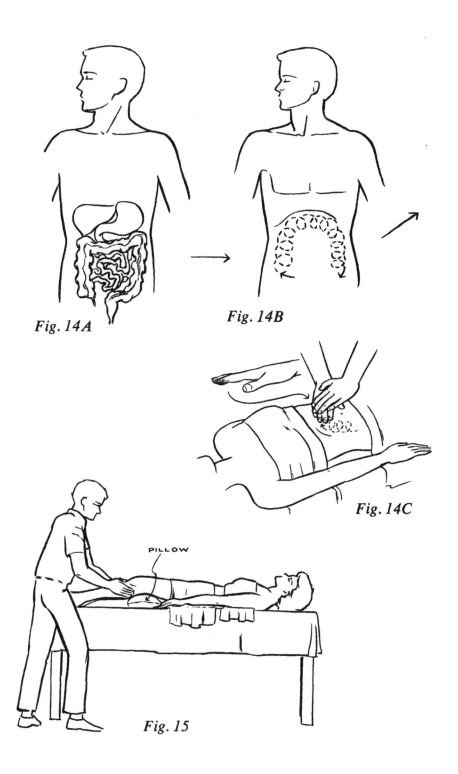

Fig. 14A

Fig. 14B

Fig. 14C

Fig. 15

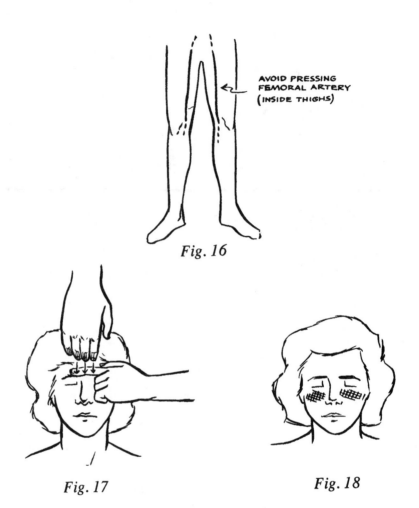

AVOID PRESSING
FEMORAL ARTERY
(INSIDE THIGHS)

Fig. 16

Fig. 17

Fig. 18

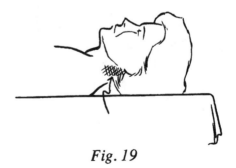

Fig. 19

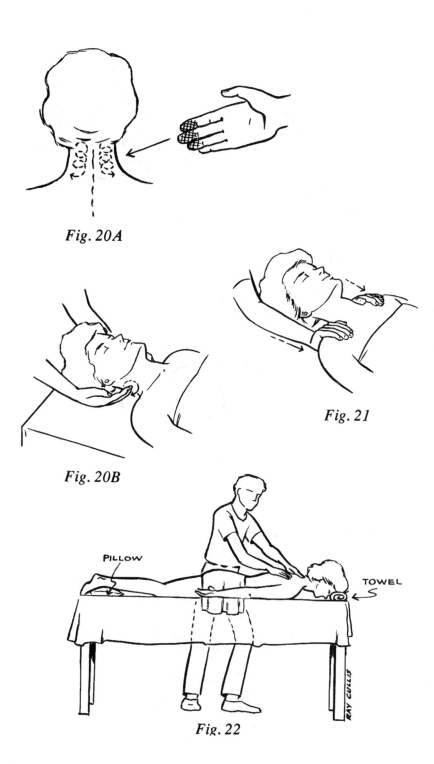

Fig. 20A

Fig. 21

Fig. 20B

Fig. 22

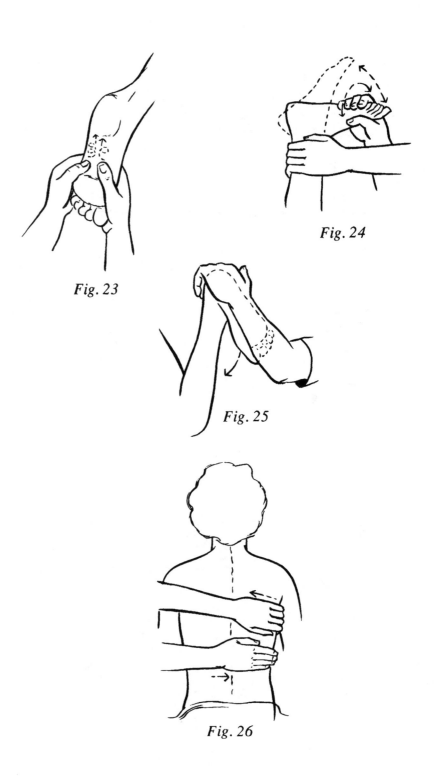

Fig. 23

Fig. 24

Fig. 25

Fig. 26

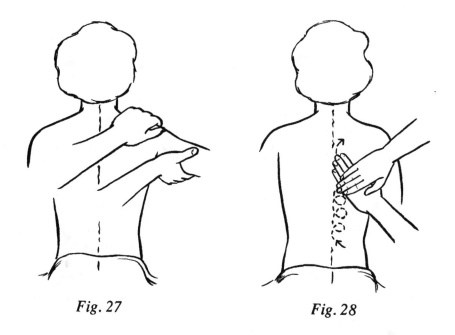

Fig. 27

Fig. 28

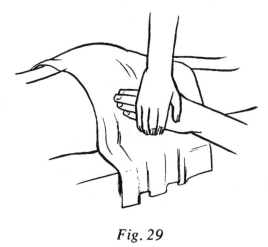

Fig. 29

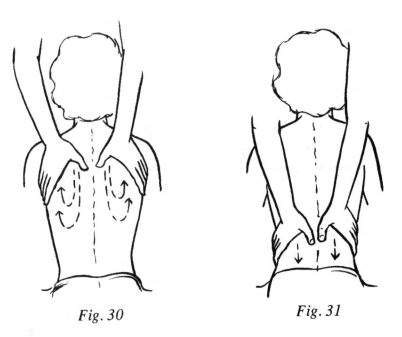

Fig. 30   Fig. 31

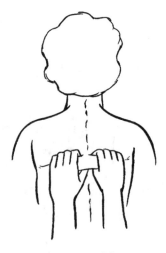

Fig. 32

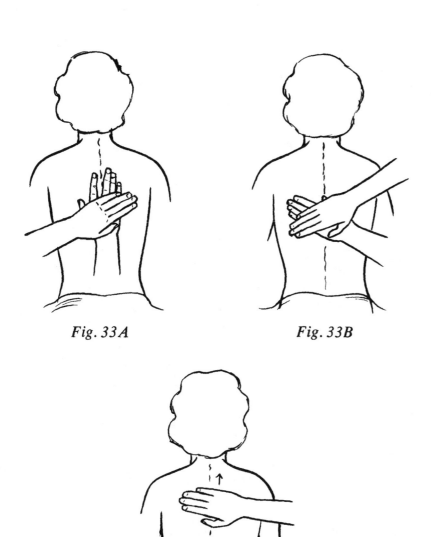

Fig. 33A   Fig. 33B

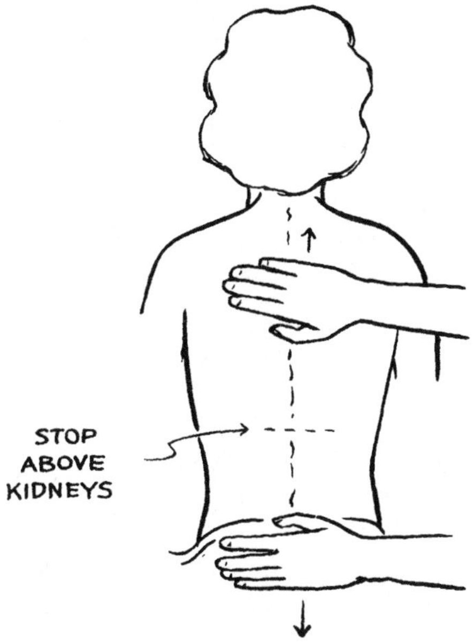

STOP
ABOVE
KIDNEYS

Fig. 34

10
Hydrotherapy: Healing with Water

(Q) How often should the hydrotherapy be given?
(A) Dependent upon the general conditions. Whenever there is a sluggishness, the feeling of heaviness, oversleepiness, the tendency for an achy, draggy feeling, then have the treatments . . . It'll pick the body up. (257-254)

*In my own career, hydrotherapy—which is the science of the application of water in all its forms for healing and health—is associated with some of my most memorable experiences.—*H.J.R.

Through the ages, water has been identified with magic, miracles, humanity's loftiest spiritual aspirations, and healing. Humankind, yearning to defeat aging and death, continually searches for a "Fountain of Youth." The healing miracles of a Lourdes come from a divinely blessed spring of water; the Bible is soaked with miracles associated with water. Babies are welcomed into the world by a baptism of water, and the dead are prepared for their entry into another world by being washed with water. Most religions use water to cleanse, sanctify, and purify. It has become an important symbol and carrier of culture from the Roman baths, the Japanese communal baths, to that American miracle of plumbing—the modern bathroom.

Water and life are synonymous. Life cannot be sustained without water. We can live for five weeks without food, but for only one week without water; hence, we have had to build our homes, farms, cities, and industries near water. The use of water for healing, as well as for drinking, cleansing, and luxury, has existed for thousands of years.

In my own career, hydrotherapy—which is the science of the application of water in all its forms for healing and health—is associated with some of my most memorable experiences.

During the 1940s, my wife and I had a vacation home in Key West, Florida, where we had become close friends of Jessie Porter (Mrs. E.L.) Newton, the grande dame of the Florida resort founded and developed by her ancestors. Mrs. Newton's home was a center for visiting artists, writers, musicians, and intellectuals from every field—the creative elite of the country.

One day she called me to hurry over to "fix the back" of one of her guests. The man was in his later years with a shock of thick, graying hair. He was very quiet and reserved during the treatment, and I did not know until it was over that I had been treating the famous poet, Robert Frost. I treated him three or four times until his back was well again. He was a very good patient—a shy, modest man. On another occasion, I treated John Dewey at Jessie's home.

197

The boy began to make splendid progress, but there was still one great handicap to overcome. Like all paraplegics, he could not control his eliminative functions. This is the most demoralizing aspect of most handicapped men and women.—**H.J.R.**

In another instance, Jessie summoned me on a sunny winter's day shortly after I had arrived from New York. She had taken an interest in a fourteen-year-old boy paralyzed from birth by spina bifida (a birth defect in which there is incomplete fusion of the spinal cord). In addition, this boy had been born with his feet bent backward, and the doctors had had to cut the tendons at birth to bring his legs down. He was doomed never to walk. He lived in virtual isolation, shut away from life in his rooms, cared for by attendants. Jessie, stirred by his plight, determined to do something about the boy's tragedy. Her first maneuver was to persuade his family to bring the boy to vacation in Key West.

The boy (let's call him David, though it's not his real name) was little short of a vegetable; his wasted body belied his age. Worst of all, the lackluster eyes announced that he had long since abandoned the will to live. This was more than a medical case, and I am sure it was only the stubborn spirit of Jessie Porter Newton that kept me from shaking my head hopelessly as other doctors before me had done and leaving the bright, sunny room in her home to which she had had the boy transported from Kentucky.

"Now, Harold, I just know you can do something for this boy." Jessie's voice was honey-sweet, but there was iron will in the tone. I don't know whether it was my desire to please her or guidance from the Greater Intelligence that moves us to the creative inspiration that produces works of art, music, literature, and new discoveries in science. In any case, I had an inspiration right then and there—and I scooped the boy up in my arms, walked down to the beach, and straight into the water with him. The waters of the Gulf and the area surrounding Key West are gentle, warm, and healing. Later, I recalled that Cayce had advised Tom Sugrue to settle in Clearwater and bathe in the Gulf—this, after Tom was paralyzed.

"It was a miracle, a real miracle like out of the Bible," Jessie told Mrs. Brod when she was interviewed. "Harold picked that boy up in his arms and literally carried him to the ocean and into life.

"What he did was motivate the boy—gave him a reason to want to live," Mrs. Newton recalled. "He told him, 'Son, everyone has limitations—sort of handicaps. Now the only thing you can't be is a professional athlete. But you can be a doctor, a lawyer, judge, senator—anything you want to be. And you're going to go to college.'

"Well, Doctor Harold taught the boy to swim and to exercise, to develop his upper body first in the ocean and then out of it. He taught David's male attendant how to massage, manipulate, and exercise him, too."

The boy began to make splendid progress, but there was still one great handicap to overcome. Like all paraplegics, he could not control his eliminative functions. This is the most demoralizing aspect of most handicapped men and women.

Then another inspiration hit me. I would use ice-water packs on David's groin and lower abdomen to shock the autonomic nervous system, which controls involuntary muscles, to contract with shock—and perhaps in time, like Pavlov's dogs, they would react. I told David's kindly attendant, who had become very interested in all the new therapy techniques, to watch the boy virtually twenty-four hours a day. Whenever any involuntary action of the bladder or bowels took place, he was to slap an ice-cold pack on the boy's groin and lower abdomen. For that purpose, we kept beside the bed a basin filled with ice water and ice cubes, with a pack cloth soaking in it.

It took months of devotion and training, but the method worked. David was still paralyzed from the waist down, but the muscles receiving signals from the autonomic nervous system contracted as they would in a normal person. Eventually David was able to go on to college. He learned to use braces and canes, drive a car, move about, and lead a near-normal life.

I have since used this system of ice-water packs on a number of paraplegic patients with equal success. All that is required is the devotion of some member of the family who is willing to work with the handicapped person. I used it recently on a Vietnamese veteran whose spine had been severed and on a young man paralyzed by an automobile accident who is now studying law; on Lenny Contino, whose story I related in an earlier chapter; and on others.

When I carried David into the sea, I was unconsciously emulating Hippocrates, the Greek father of modern medicine, who back in the fifth century B.C., it is said, made much use of the salubrious waters of the sea surrounding his island in the treatment of his patients. We do know that he advised boiling water before drinking it, putting him well in advance of the rest of the world by many centuries, and that he wrote extensively on the use of water, internally and externally, in the treatment of disease.

Archimedes, the Greek mathematician who lived around 212 B.C., discovered the important principle now bearing his name—that a body wholly or partly immersed in a fluid is buoyed up by a force equal to the weight of the fluid displaced.

This principle would one day, centuries later, lead an American president (Franklin D. Roosevelt), crippled with polio, to found a rehabilitation center in Warm Springs, Georgia. The Archimedean principle has had an important bearing on the future development of hydrotherapy treatment for physically handicapped patients.

Galen, a Roman physician of the second century A.D., also advised that water be boiled, then cooled before drinking. He was a firm advocate of the baths so popular in Rome, and used them with friction, or massage, and exercise to effect his famous cures.

Emperor Augustus of Rome is said to have been one of the first and most famous of the patients who recovered through a water cure when all other therapies failed, further popularizing the Roman baths, of which at one time there were 850 in Rome alone.

During the Middle Ages, bathing and water fell into great disrepute, for reasons it would take a historian to chronicle, although the plagues may have been partly responsible. On the other side of the still-uncrossed Atlantic, the American Indians were using baths to cure many diseases and had developed into a high art vapor baths similar to Cayce's fume baths, usually followed by plunging into a cold stream. In the fifteenth century, the Turks in

---

Water Therapy in Ancient History

The use of water as therapy for healing has existed for thousands of years. Baths and remedies are mentioned in Sanskrit as early as 4000 B.C. The White Lama told me that he found a description of water therapy in old Tibetan writings. The Babylonians, Egyptians, Cretans, and the Persians all used baths and water therapy extensively, long before the Romans inscribed their history on the architecture of their luxurious baths, which they left all over Europe and Africa. In Crete, one may see in the restoration of the ancient ruins of Knossos indoor bathrooms and the equivalent of modern plumbing systems with intricate drains for bringing in fresh water and flushing out the used water. The Spartans of Greece immersed newborn babies in ice-cold water to immunize them against disease and to toughen them.—H.J.R.

Galen, a Roman physician of the second century A.D., also advised that water be boiled, then cooled before drinking. He was a firm advocate of the baths so popular in Rome, and used them with friction, or massage, and exercise to effect his famous cures. —H.J.R.

Emperor Augustus of Rome is said to have been one of the first and most famous of the patients who recovered through a water cure when all other therapies failed, further popularizing the Roman baths, of which at one time there were 850 in Rome alone.

—H.J.R.

John Wesley on Good Health

Observe all the time the greatest exactness in your regimen or manner of living. Abstain from all mixed drinks, from all highly seasoned food. Use plain diet, easy of digestion; and this as sparingly as you can consistent with ease and strength. Drink water only if it agrees with your stomach. Sup at six or seven, on the lightest food. Go to bed early and rise betimes [early]. To persevere with steadfastness in this course is often more than half the cure. Above all add to the rest, for it is not labor lost, that old-fashioned medicine, Prayer, and have faith in God.

—John Wesley

Father Sebastian Kneipp cured Archduke Joseph of Austria of Bright's disease in 1892 with his water cure.—**H.J.R.**

Constantinople constructed marvelous baths and popularized the hot-air bath, which is still popularly called the "Turkish bath."

In 1776, John Wesley, the famous evangelist and founder of the Methodist Church, published his famous *Primitive Physick Easy and Natural Method of Curing Most Diseases.* Wesley used cold-water bathing for curing over seventy diseases and used it as part of therapy in 200 diseases. He wrote, "Cold bathing is of great advantage to health. It prevents abundance of diseases. It promotes perspiration, helps the circulation of the blood, and prevents the danger of catching cold."

Father Sebastian Kneipp cured Archduke Joseph of Austria of Bright's disease in 1892 with his water cure.

At the dawn of the nineteenth century Vincent Priesnitz, an uneducated farmer's son in Austria, was crippled in a bad accident when he was only seventeen years old. He cured himself with water treatments. His own success, later practiced on neighboring farmers and their animals, led him, at the age of thirty, to establish a "water cure." His fame spread, and when royalty and government and national leaders came to him for help, the "water cure" became the "in" thing in Europe, and similar cures sprang up wherever there was a "spring" whose magical properties could be used to cure or at least comfort the sick. Priesnitz's effort won the backing of the Austrian government.

In the United States, hydrotherapy attained great popularity through the efforts of Dr. Simon Baruch, father of the famous financier and presidential adviser, Bernard Baruch. Dr. Baruch wrote and published *The Principles and Practice of Hydrotherapy* in 1899 and the *Epitome of Hydrotherapy* in 1920. Equally important was the work of Dr. John Harvey Kellogg, who opened the Battle Creek Sanitarium in 1876 to pioneer in dietetic and hygienic drugless treatment. Dr. Kellogg did a great deal to establish hydrotherapy as a scientific system in this country, along with diet, exercise, and electrotherapy. In 1900 Dr. Kellogg published *Rational Hydrotherapy,* a comprehensive 1,100-page work. He invented the cabinet heated with electric-light bulbs, and today I am still using one of the first models to give the Cayce fume baths.

Water, in its multitudinous uses, variations, and effects, is unparalleled as a therapeutic agent. It is as fluid in application as its own nature. It can relax, stimulate, relieve pain, heal, and purify the body internally and externally. It functions in a manner that cannot be duplicated by any other modality, with maximum stimulation of the body's own healing powers and a minimum of aftereffects. Its very naturalness and flexibility make it possible to adapt this therapy to any degree of delicacy or strength of application dictated by the patient's condition. It is readily available (or was until we polluted it) and it is cheap.

Hydrotherapy is the science of the application of waters to the human body for the cure or prevention of disease, correction of physical and mental disorders, and maintenance and improvement of general health. Water can be used in three different forms: as a liquid; as a solid, or ice; or as a gas, that is, steam or vapor.

The application of water may be external or internal. It can be used for simple cleansing; for internal cleansing, orally or rectally; for stimulation of the circulation by alternate hot and cold water; for relaxation in a tepid bath; for massage by pressure or percussion; for healing action by various combinations of the various hydrotherapeutic modalities; and to relieve pain with heat or extreme cold (as ice).

Water can by conduction carry either heat or cold to the body: warm baths for relaxation; hot baths to relieve the pains of arthritis and rheumatism, neuritis, and gout; short cold baths for stimulation and to conquer fatigue; sitz baths to stimulate and prolong sexual activity. The effect of these baths, especially the hot baths, can be increased by adding salts and chemicals such as sulphur, pine, Epsom and other salts, etc. Water for internal cleansing introduced into the body by drinking, colonics, enemas, and douches is one of the most powerful therapeutic tools in nature's armamentarium. Vapor and steam baths given to stimulate elimination directly through the skin, lungs, and kidneys can be made more effective by the addition of chemicals to the vapor.

While ice is not used as commonly as liquid water and vapor, it has a definite therapeutic place. We apply it in short applications for stimulation, to increase circulation or to increase muscular tone. It is used in fever to cool the head and neck; to relieve headache or head pressure; as first–aid for burns and injuries; to control inflammation; and sometimes, in severe infection, to slow the circulation, thus inhibiting the action of pathogenic bacteria.

While my idea of using ice–water packs as I did on David and other paraplegics may have been original, at least so far as I have been able to discover, the use of cold compresses and packs, hot fomentations, or cloths soaked in herbal, oil, or chemical or mineral substances is as old as drugless therapy and has always had an important place in healing.

In *Water for Health and Healing*, Dr. Frederick M. Rossiter states, "The skin on a human being is the largest, heaviest organ of the body. It takes about 17 square feet of skin to cover the average man or woman . . . the entire skin is one great sentient membrane of closely knit nervous and vascular tissues. Thus, water therapy can aid the entire system.

"It has been estimated that in one square inch of true skin there are several millions of cells of various tissues, several feet of minute blood tubes, a dozen feet of nerve fibres, one hundred sweat glands, and a score of oil glands."[1]

Thus it is easy to understand why applications to the skin of water at varying temperatures and in its various forms can affect many parts of the body.

Edgar Cayce was a strong believer in the virtues of hydrotherapy and frequently prescribed it in some form or combination, as you have read in previous chapters. In fact, a survey carried out by the Cayce headquarters of 670 persons treated over a two–year period revealed that Cayce had advised one or more forms of hydrotherapy 109 times—the third most frequently prescribed therapy.

This is what he told David Kahn about the need for hydrotherapy:

(Q) How often should the hydrotherapy be given?
(A) Dependent upon the general conditions. Whenever there is a sluggishness, the feeling of heaviness, oversleepiness, the tendency for an achy, draggy feeling, then have the treatments. This does not mean that merely because

What Is Hydrotherapy?
Hydrotherapy is the science of the application of waters to the human body for the cure or prevention of disease, correction of physical and mental disorders, and maintenance and improvement of general health. Water can be used in three different forms: as a liquid; as a solid, or ice; or as a gas, that is, steam or vapor.—**H.J.R.**

While ice is not used as commonly as liquid water and vapor, it has a definite therapeutic place. We apply it in short applications for stimulation, to increase circulation or to increase muscular tone.

—**H.J.R.**

Edgar Cayce was a strong believer in the virtues of hydrotherapy and frequently prescribed it in some form or combination . . .—**H.J.R.**

there is the daily activity of the alimentary canal there is not need for flushing the system. But whenever there is the feeling of sluggishness, have the treatments. It'll pick the body up. For there is a need for such treatments when the condition of the body becomes drugged because of absorption of poisons through alimentary canal or colon, sluggishness of liver or kidneys, and there is the lack of coordination with the cerebrospinal and sympathetic blood supply and nerves. *For the hydrotherapy and massage are preventive as well as curative measures. For the cleansing of the system allows the body forces themselves to function normally, and thus eliminate poisons, congestions and conditions that would become acute through the body.* [Italics added.] (257-254)

To another individual he explained it as follows:

As we find for this body, the Hydrotherapy Bath would be well; which would be to lie in great quantity or a tub of water for a long period—this being kept a little above the temperature of the body; then followed by a thorough massage by a masseuse. This would be better than adjustments *or* deep treatments, though it will be found that with the massage along the spine, with the body prone upon the face, these would—with the knuckle on either side of the spinal column—tend to make many a segment come nearer to normalcy, by being so treated *after* having been thoroughly relaxed for twenty to thirty minutes *in* the warm or hot water, see? (635-9)

Some disturbances are indicated in the digestive forces of the body. These are from lack of proper eliminations even though there are regularities . . . the eliminations need to be increased from these angles. This may be done in no better manner than by having colonic irrigations occasionally and by including in the diet such things as figs, rhubarb and the like.

Hydrotherapy and physical exercise, combined with these, should bring the better conditions for the body. These are the manners in which the body, or any individual body may keep better activities. (4003-1)

In reading 2602-2, Cayce explains further:

As indicated—see—there are channels or outlets for the eliminating of poisons; that is, used energies, where there is the effect of the activity of the circulation upon foreign forces . . . These all, by the segregating of same in the system, produce forces which are to be eliminated. We eliminate principally through the activity of the lungs, of course, and the perspiratory system, the alimentary canal and the kidneys . . . The headaches are the signs or warnings that eliminations are not being properly cared for. Most of this, in this body, comes from the alimentary canal, and from those conditions that exist in portions of the colon itself, as to produce a pressure upon [these] . . . Hence the suggestion for the osteopathic corrections, which aid but which do not eliminate all of these conditions which are as accumulations through portions of the colon. Consequently, colonic irrigations are necessary occasionally, as well as general hydrotherapy and massage.

Conditions for Which Cayce Recommended Hydrotherapy Treatments

acidity	debilitation	palsy (cerebral)
adhesions	dermatitis	Parkinson's disease
alcoholism	ear-deafness	pelvic disorders
allergies	eliminations	plethora
anemia	eyes	polio (aftereffects)
aphonia	flu (aftereffects)	prolapsus
appendicitis	glands	prostititis
arthritis	glaucoma	pruritus
assimilation	headache	psoriasis
asthma	hemorrhage	rejuvenation
blood clots	(intestines)	relaxation
bronchitis	hives	rheumatism
cancer	Hodgkin's disease	sciatica
catabolism-metabo-	hypertension	spine (slipped disk and
lism (incoordina-	injuries	subluxations)
tion)	intestines	strains
catarrh	lesions	streptococcus
cholecystitis	mesenteritis	stricture
circulation (incoordi-	nervous septenis	toxemia
nation and impaired)	nervous tension	tuberculosis
cold congestion	neurasthenia	ulcers
colitis	neuritis	
colon engorgement	obesity	

Cayce at various times recommended for the patients he sent to the Reilly Health Service bubble baths; Epsom salt baths; Finnish baths; foot baths; fume baths (given with a variety of aromatic substances such as Atomidine, witch hazel, etc.); hot-mustard (foot) baths; pine-needle-oil baths; salt-water baths; sand baths; sitz baths; bicarbonate-of-soda baths; sponge baths; steam baths; sun baths; Scotch douche; and Turkish and sal-soda baths, among the hundred-odd baths that we featured at the institute.

Fume or vapor baths and colonics were prescribed more frequently than any other modality—often in tandem and combined with castor oil packs and massage to effect thorough cleansing of the system and removal of toxins. Colonics and castor oil packs will be discussed in detail in the next chapter.

Cayce also made liberal use of tub baths, especially those with Epsom salts or aromatic substances added. And during his lifetime, when the Reilly Institute was flourishing, he also frequently recommended our bubble baths (alone or with aromatic oil of pine), needle showers, and Scotch douche. The bubble bath, by the way, had no relationship to the effervescent soap bubbles in which

Cayce also made liberal use of tub baths, especially those with Epsom salts or aromatic substances added. And during his lifetime, when the Reilly Institute was flourishing, he also frequently recommended our bubble baths (alone or with aromatic oil of pine), needle showers, and Scotch douche.—**H.J.R.**

many women like to luxuriate, but was a device for forcing air bubbles into the water, simulating a gentle massage. The whirlpool bath has a similar function and is used chiefly for relaxation and to stimulate circulation.

However, since this book is designed to help you stay healthy and fit at home, we will stick to those beneficial procedures that you can manage comfortably in your own bathroom.

Let us first turn our attention to the most common use of water—for drinking. To a patient suffering from toxemia (and that probably applies to everyone in modern life), Cayce had this to say:

> Drink plenty of water at all times—and preferably—no matter where the water may be taken from—*boil* the water before it is used; then cool and add ice to same, around rather than in it. (515-1)

> Drink *plenty* of water. No stimulants, as tea or coffee . . .
>   The care of the body in general—keeping plenty of water for the system, internal and external . . . will build the body to its normal resistance. (583-4)

In general I would recommend six to eight glasses of water for the average person each day unless he/she is suffering from a specific illness in which this is contraindicated or where more may be desirable.

Try to use spring water or distilled water for drinking and check to see that the brand you buy is what the label claims—not bottled tap water. Ice should also be made from sterile water. You can also take fluids in the form of herb teas.

In an interesting case that Cayce diagnosed as arising from poor assimilation and elimination, he analyzed the importance of water as an aid to digestion and assimilation:

Edgar Cayce on Water

In the matter of diet for the body—these, we find, are quite varied under circumstances and conditions over which the body often hasn't the control [due to being a traveling man?]. Most of all, train self never to bolt the food. Take *time* to assimilate, masticate, so that *assimilation* is well—and we will find that with these kept, with an *even* balance between those that produce acid and those that make for the alkaline, if well balanced will digest under most all circumstances. Well to drink *always plenty* of water, before meals and after meals—for, as has oft been given, when any food value *enters* the stomach *immediately* the stomach becomes a storehouse, or a medicine chest, that may create all the elements necessary for proper digestion within the system. If this *first* is acted upon by aqua pura, the reactions are more near normal. Well, then, each morning upon first arising, to take a half to three-quarters of a glass of *warm* water; not so hot that it is objectionable, not so tepid that it makes for sickening—but this will clarify the system of poisons. This well especially for this body. Occasionally a pinch of salt should be added to this draught of water. (311-4)

One of the most enthusiastic devotees of the Reilly Health Institute and physical fitness was the previously mentioned David Dubinsky, who headed the International Ladies Garment Workers Union. I had the honor and pleasure of taking care of him personally for over forty-five years. He was deeply interested in health programs for his workers. In fact, when he autographed his book for me, he wrote, "A healthy worker is a good worker."

One day he asked me to drive with him to Bushkill Falls, Pennsylvania, where Unity Camp, which was to serve as a vacation and health spa for union workers, was adding new buildings. Mr. Dubinsky asked me if I would be willing to work with their architect on the design for the baths, steam rooms, massage rooms, gym, and other physical-fitness facilities. They adopted some of the ideas I gave them.

I suggested they face the steam and treatment rooms with glass blocks on the sunny side of the building so that sunlight could illuminate the rooms during daylight hours. Then we installed fluorescent lighting in such a way that it would illuminate, not reflect. We arranged the layout so that the massage therapists could look through portholes into the steam rooms while they were working, in order to keep an eye on everybody there; therefore, in case someone fainted or was overcome by the heat, he or she could be taken out immediately. This was an important safety precaution.

The highest heat in a Turkish bath or sauna is always at the top of the room. People generally sit or lie on the bottom or middle tiers, and when they stand up, as their head reaches the hottest layer of air, they can faint, especially if there is a tendency to a cardiovascular condition that they are not aware of.

There had been some accidents in New York City Turkish baths, resulting in several fatalities at one of the most famous institutions. A man had fainted and no one had missed him or looked for him. When the attendants returned in the morning, they found him on the floor—dead. A similar fatal accident happened to another man in a steam room at one of the famous hotels in New York City.

It is always most important to take proper precautions and to have someone around when using extreme heat—whether in tub baths, steam, or sauna. This is one of the reasons I prefer the sweat cabinets, where the head is exposed to the air.

A factor of absolute and prime importance in hydrotherapy is the different reaction that can be induced by changing from one temperature to another. We can use water at Fahrenheit temperatures of 40-120 degrees. The extremes are rarely used, but there are unlimited possibilities for the therapeutic effects in this wide range, with the added variant of the bath's duration. Water pressure is another beneficial therapy: Scotch douche, whirlpool, bubble, oxygen, and Nauheim or carbon dioxide baths. Taking these baths at home is difficult, if not impossible; they require expensive modern apparatus. What can be taken at home most effectively, at no cost, are warm baths for relaxation; very hot baths to relieve aches and pains; and short, cold baths for stimulation. The effectiveness of these baths—especially the hot ones—can be increased by adding Glauber's or Epsom salts; different combinations of sulphur; or herbs of

The highest heat in a Turkish bath or sauna is always at the top of the room. People generally sit or lie on the bottom or middle tiers, and when they stand up, as their head reaches the hottest layer of air, they can faint, especially if there is a tendency to a cardiovascular condition that they are not aware of.—**H.J.R.**

A factor of absolute and prime importance in hydrotherapy is the different reaction that can be induced by changing from one temperature to another.—**H.J.R.**

If you are trying to relieve stiffness and soreness, after the bath, don a toweling bathrobe, go to bed, and cover up. If the bath has been very hot, you will continue to perspire.—**H.J.R.**

many descriptions, such as tannin, pine, etc. Hot–air or steam baths are used to stimulate elimination through the skin, for they open the pores and release perspiration. Quite frequently volatile substances such as pine oil, benzoin, eucalyptus, or chlorine are vaporized for inhalation.

For the most effective use of water it is necessary to have a precise knowledge of temperature, both centigrade and Fahrenheit. In the United States we are more familiar with Fahrenheit. The range is 32 degrees, at which water freezes, to 212 degrees, at which it boils. These temperatures apply when you are based at or near sea level.

Temperatures used in tub baths usually run from 55 to 110 degrees. Never neglect using a bath thermometer to determine temperature, for our own judgment of degrees of heat and cold can be very misleading. When taking baths, regulate your room temperature to 68–74 degrees. For active exercise it can be a bit lower, 65 degrees. Tub baths for relaxation are best at 98–100 degrees, taken from ten to thirty minutes, averaging twenty.

Hot Baths

To "soak out" pains and aches, 100–106 degrees are necessary. If you are unaccustomed to very hot baths, I would suggest that you acclimate the body slowly, starting at 101 degrees and carefully graduating up to 104 degrees. Though 108 degrees and higher are very effective, it is best to have someone on call "just in case," for faintness can overtake the neophyte. Even the Japanese, who "boil out" before they "bail out" at 120 degrees, take these baths in mobs—in public, as it were. These baths have value in raising body temperature, inducing short fever therapy, and cleansing the skin of fungus and vermin. But, to repeat, unless you are thoroughly accustomed through long practice with high bathing temperatures, don't try for the Lobster Jackpot. The Japanese can take it; they've been boiling themselves for centuries. The average hot tub at 102–106 degrees is usually taken from twenty to thirty minutes.

If you are trying to relieve stiffness and soreness, after the bath, don a toweling bathrobe, go to bed, and cover up. If the bath has been very hot, you will continue to perspire. The bed rest can continue from thirty minutes to two hours, depending on your reaction to the bath, how long you continue to perspire, and the degree of your restlessness. If, when you rise, you are still perspiring, dry yourself with a towel and gently rub the entire body with a towel dipped in alcohol or cold water. Then dry again slowly.

Do warm baths before the cold high–energy baths.

Cold High-Energy Bath

The water should be from 40-55 degrees. Cayce recommended some cold baths at 46 degrees; the cool at 65-85 degrees; and tepid 85-95 degrees. The cold bath increases energy and it should be short—about one and a half minutes to begin with, increasing to two or three minutes. It has a tendency to stimulate the heart rate, to increase respiration and metabolism, and is refreshing to the nerves.—**H.J.R.**

Cold Sitz Bath

Cayce and I both recommended sitz baths extensively and I have found them to be one of the most rewarding uses of water—one that is well worth the trouble. It speeds up circulation and relieves congestion of the glands and the organs of the lower abdomen. It is one of the best methods of invigorating the sex organs and extending their life, especially for men. The cold sitz bath also

oil of balsam or pine

counteracts fatigue and stimulates elimination. Indirectly, this bath is an aid in relieving headaches and if taken before bedtime has helped many get a good night's sleep.

In our hydrotherapy department we had two specially built tubs for taking this simple yet wonderfully effective bath. This double-bath intensifies the reaction by quick changes from the hot to the cold tub, sometimes once, twice, or sometimes even three times. But you can also get a very good effect in your own tub at home.

Fill the tub to a depth of six to nine inches of water, up to the navel in sitting position. Have this water at about tap temperature, 60–65 degrees. Cover your shoulders and back with a towel, step into the tub, and (remembering that most accidents happen in bathrooms) sit down! Don't think it over or rationalize about it, just sit in it. Be sure to brace your feet up out of the water on the inside end of the tub; you can buy or make a metal or plastic foot-rest for this purpose of keeping the feet up and extended above the water. Then count slowly up to sixty, the equivalent of a minute. Carefully rise from the tub and wrap a towel about your middle—the one you had around your shoulders if large enough—or jump into a toweling robe. Then take to bed and freedom from tension for at least thirty minutes, or if it is bedtime, go to sleep. If work or pleasure is calling, take ten or more, then dry off slowly and dress the same way.

When the body is warmed up by exercise, the reaction to the sitz bath is much more effective. In fact, one should never take a cold sitz bath if the body feels cold. You can warm up by exercise or lying in bed under blankets, but if you are not warm enough, in no case take a cold sitz bath. After you have followed this bath program about six times and the reaction is good (that is, the body has a warm, relaxed glow after the bath), you can increase the sitting time to two minutes or a slow count of 120. After the twelfth sitz bath you can increase the count or sit-in time to 180—three minutes. For most people using the home-tub method, this seems to work best for optimum reaction.

The Shower

A substitute for a sitz bath is the alternating, low-back shower bath. Stand with your back to the shower and let the warm water run over the lower back. Bend over a little and "back into" the shower so that the water hits the desired area. Gradually increase the temperature up to the limit of your tolerance, for some three to five minutes. Then turn on the cold, full cold, rather quickly. Let the cold water hit the warm parts for a slow count of forty. When acclimated, you can take it up to twice as long or a count of eighty. After this bath, wrap up in a towel or toweling robe and relax in bed. Any rest from ten minutes up will do a lot of good. If in a hurry to get out, finish up this bath with a cool or cold shower. Then dry slowly, dress slowly, and take off—thoroughly refreshed.

While most of us think of an ordinary shower only as a cleansing procedure, it can and does have a very good circulatory and tonic effect. A long, hot shower followed by a short, cold one is very stimulating to circulation, and it

Warm Baths
These are used for relaxing (taken at 90-101 degrees for ten to twelve minutes). Quite often Cayce added oil of balsam or pine to these baths for relaxation. Although we do not know what the oils do physiologically, they are pleasant psychologically. Step into a toweling bathrobe and go to bed.

Warm baths lower the blood pressure, dilate the blood vessels, and relax the nerves.—H.J.R.

Cayce and I both recommended sitz baths extensively and I have found them to be one of the most rewarding uses of water—one that is well worth the trouble. It speeds up circulation and relieves congestion of the glands and the organs of the lower abdomen.

—H.J.R.

Hot Bitz Bath
The hot sitz bath has many therapeutic uses, but as an exercise equivalent it is chiefly used for relaxing and warming up the body, especially before bedtime. It also can be used to warm up the body before taking a cold sitz bath, and to relieve the discomfort of rectal conditions.—H.J.R.

While most of us think of an ordinary shower only as a cleansing procedure, it can and does have a very good circulatory and tonic effect. A long, hot shower followed by a short, cold one is very stimulating to circulation, and it helps relieve fatigue.—**H.J.R.**

helps relieve fatigue. In changing from hot to cold, avoid having the cold water hit the head or upper part of the body at first; let the cold water first hit the legs or lower abdomen, then work up to the shoulders, neck, and head, and finish off all over the body.

In a newspaper interview a while back I stated that taking cold showers in the morning during the winter months was a good way to catch cold, especially for the hurry-up, always-tired businessperson. As many of my friends know, I advocate the general use of cold water to toughen and condition the body. But again I say, "Don't take a short, cold shower—especially after a hot one—and then go out into cold weather." When you take a short, cold bath your metabolism is speeded up and the body grows warm. If you then dress and romp forth, your pores are open. Outdoors, perspiration continues (though hardly noticeable).

Unless you are well conditioned and acclimated to sudden changes, it is best not to try to be hardy in six lessons. A tepid bath or shower is sufficient for when you are going out into cold weather. Or you might try a cool sitz bath of three minutes. You can also finish up a hot or warm bath with a slow, cooling shower, which conducts the heat away from the body without too much effect on the metabolism. Remember: *slow* and *cool*.

Epsom Salts Baths

For therapeutic purposes, Cayce prescribed Epsom salts baths for many cases of arthritis. He also recommended Epsom salts baths for circulation, glandular disturbances, incoordination, injuries, lesions, impaired locomotion, lumbago, neuritis, paralysis, prolapsus, rheumatism and rheumatic tendencies, scleroderma, toxemia, sciatica, and venereal disease (aftereffects).

His directions to many people for taking an Epsom salts bath could differ quite radically. In Case 349-12 he directed a secretary who had been injured in an accident as follows:

> We would have *every day* at least one bath with a good amount of Epsom Salts in it, following this with a good rubdown along the whole cerebrospinal system . . .
> The Epsom Salts bath would be taken during the day. Put a pound of salts to about ten to twenty gallons of water; not too hot but rather a tepid bath, but remain in same so that the absorption and reaction to the whole nerve system is received. Add a little hot water to keep this warm . . . from 20 to 30 minutes.

Another person was told:

> Have this [Epsom Salts bath] about once each week . . . Use about 10 lbs. of Epsom Salts in about 40 gallons of water, and this pretty warm . . . [each week] for 3 weeks . . . [omit] for 6 weeks, another, then, would be taken but increase the amount of Epsom Salts to [15 pounds. Massage over spine dur-

ing the bath. Afterward, massage with peanut oil]. (5169-1)

Epsom salts baths are contraindicated in cardiovascular or high-blood-pressure conditions. Ask your doctor, in such a case, whether you may take the bath.—**H.J.R.**

To another patient with arthritis he gave directions to use three to five pounds of salts to twenty gallons of warm water. The patient was told to remain in the water as long as he could stand it and then to rest for eight to ten hours after such ministration.

Other patients were advised to use varying amounts of five to twenty pounds of salts. I tried the different amounts on myself and when I reached the twenty-pound limit, I swear I could taste the salts in my mouth.

Directions

I generally advise five pounds for a modern tub (about twenty gallons) or eight to ten pounds for an old-fashioned tub of water—which generally holds about thirty gallons of water—at a temperature beginning at about 102–104 degrees working up to 106 degrees.

One time a patient came to me and said that he had been taking the Epsom salts baths and they weren't doing him much good. I asked him how hot he was taking them, and he said about 100–104 degrees. Then I asked him how much Epsom salts he was using and he replied, "A few spoonfuls."

Start with six to eight inches of water in the tub at about 101–102 degrees. Be sure to use your thermometer. Add five pounds of salts to an average-size bathtub and be sure to stir the salts thoroughly so they do not remain in a lump at the bottom. Gradually add hot water as you immerse yourself so that you keep the temperature even, and progressively raise the temperature to 106 or 108 degrees by adding fresh, hot water until the bath is deep enough to cover your back; then soak. If you are trying to relieve chronic pain, eventually, as you take the baths over a period of time, you may be able to get the water temperature up to 110–112 degrees. As I said before, the Japanese can take their baths at 118–120 degrees and they are particularly free of skin disorders and skin parasites. But if you are trying to compete, go slowly and increase the temperature a few degrees at a time. To relieve pain, you should remain in the tub ten or twelve minutes to start, and gradually increase to twenty minutes. An ice bag or cold washcloth or sponge to the forehead or back of neck will help you bear the heat. DON'T OVERDO—EASY DOES IT. This is a particularly good therapy for stiff joints, muscular pain, arthritis, and rheumatism; for increasing the metabolism and the work of the heart; and for raising body temperature and relieving pain.

Epsom salts baths are contraindicated in cardiovascular or high-blood-pressure conditions. Ask your doctor, in such a case, whether you may take the bath.

CAUTION: When taking hot baths of all kinds, be sure to have someone nearby in case you are overcome by dizziness or faintness. It is also best to set a timer for accuracy, for your sense of time may not be accurate.

I have used fume baths for over sixty years with great effect. Cayce increased their effect with the use of aloe, alum, Atomidine, tincture of benzoin, camphor, balm of Gilead, iodine, oil of lavender, tincture of lobelia, myrrh, oil of pine needle, witch hazel, balsam of tolu, sulphur, and wintergreen.—**H.J.R.**

Epsom Salts Hand Baths for Arthritis and Rheumatism

Where there is crippling of the joints of the hands, pain of arthritis, or inflammation of the tendons, considerable relief can be gotten from an Epsom salts hand bath and massage. Not long ago a seamstress was sent to me by a doctor from New York. I told her to use the Epsom salts hand bath and massage for two weeks, and after this time she was able to close her hand, something she had not been able to do two weeks before.

Many years ago I used the same treatment with Fannie Hurst's husband, who was a pianist, and since then on a number of instrumental musicians. Make a hot Epsom salts solution, adding about one pound of salts to a basin or bowl, which should be half full of hot water. Soak the hand for five minutes and then massage the fingers and the hand with the other hand under water and work the fingers and hand, rotating the joints. Then soak again for another five or ten minutes. After about twenty minutes of soaking take the hands out and massage peanut oil into one, continuing up the arm. Then reverse the hands and repeat. This same procedure can be used for the feet.

Fume Baths

You will recall, I earlier discussed the important role of the skin in elimination. Since elimination must take place through the skin as well as through the colon, kidneys, and lungs, Cayce made liberal use of fume baths—which at times he referred to as "sweats"—as well as Turkish and Finnish baths (the most common variety in America is the sauna). These "sweats," or fume baths, are an absolutely essential element when you embark on any of the cleansing routines. (The apple diet, colonics, or other cleansing procedures will be discussed in the next chapter.) The skin and the lungs help to throw off the toxins that otherwise can cause considerable discomfort, such as headaches, dizziness, gas, acidity, and nausea. Fume baths are also very valuable in bringing down cholesterol levels. Recent research has revealed that soaping the body after sweating stops the cholesterol from coming out through the pores, so don't use soap in hot baths, steam baths, or vapor baths.

I have used fume baths for over sixty years with great effect. Cayce increased their effect with the use of aloe, alum, Atomidine, tincture of benzoin, camphor, balm of Gilead, iodine, oil of lavender, tincture of lobelia, myrrh, oil of pine needle, witch hazel, balsam of tolu, sulphur, and wintergreen. His directions for using these substances were in many instances very precise; and these are usually followed by an oil rub or massage. To a man fifty–four years old with a total lack of the ability to assimilate food and who was suffering from asthenia he gave this advice:

> As we find, the greater help would come from the massage following, at least every other day, a hydrotherapy treatment which would be given with Fume Baths or a cabinet or an open container in which there would be a pint of water and in this two teaspoonsful of Witch Hazel. Let this boil. No other

heat, but the fumes from this which may settle over the body. Then have a thorough massage and rubdown using equal portions of Olive Oil, Tincture of Myrrh and Compound Tincture of Benzoin. These should be massaged in and along the cerebrospinal system, especially, always away from the head.

(5372-1)

The wife of an English insurance executive, suffering from pains thought to be arthritis, pains in the arms, pelvic disorders, and digestive trouble, was referred to Mr. Cayce. He identified much of the trouble as arising from an old injury to the lower end of the spine in the coccyx area, and recommended a course of treatment that included vapor baths, referred to in one part of a sentence as "sweats" and in another as "fume baths":

We would find first, then, that there should be the use of the sweat baths; those that carry not a raising of the temperature of the body to a great extent . . . but rather *fume* baths, where there is used in same an alternation of Oil of Wintergreen and the Tincture of Iodine—or that of Atomidine full strength; one used one day of the treatment, the other at the next treatment . . . with the thorough rubdown after same. (1302-1)

One of the earliest forms of internal cleanliness was the sweat bath. The Turkish bath is actually a dry-heat hot-air bath that runs about 160–180 degrees. In addition we have the Russian-Finnish steam bath, which runs about 150–160 degrees, and the Finnish sauna, which may run as high as 190–200 degrees. In the Finns' authentic version of the sauna, water is thrown on hot rocks, which creates a vapor that is in some respects similar to the fume bath that Cayce recommends so often. Then we have the typically American sweat bath invented by Dr. Kellogg—the electric cabinet. In the electric cabinet the heat does not go much beyond 110 degrees, but the radiant action of the light on the skin does produce sweat. The Kellogg model that I am still using is particularly useful for giving the Cayce fume baths and for people who cannot tolerate too much heat, since the head is not enclosed and has free access to oxygen or cold compresses, ministered by a member of the family or friend.

It is possible to take a vapor or steam bath at home. There are many home saunas and inexpensive steam devices and cabinets on the market. Some, more elaborate, come in sections to be set up like a box; others are portable and are usually draped from the shoulders and zipped up from the inside, allowing you to put it on while sitting on a stool or chair. Under this chair or stool (preferably of wood) an electric steaming unit is placed; a large towel or small blanket is folded several thicknesses and then placed partly on the seat and hanging down in front and on each side to protect the back of the legs and buttocks from excessive heat. (We are not referring here to the sauna-type garments that are supposed to reduce you overnight, but to an apparatus that encloses the entire body except for the head.)

Some of the portable units are advertised for under fifteen dollars. However, for those who are counting their pennies to cope with inflation and taxes, here are some instructions for a satisfactory homemade device for taking steam and fume baths.

Instructions for Homemade Fume Bath

Sew several blankets or shower curtains together, leaving an opening about a foot in diameter. Ready a stool or chair. For a steaming unit, you can use a croup vaporizer, one of the inexpensive jar vaporizers sold to moisturize air or treat colds, or an old electric coffee pot or tea pot. Half-fill the container with water to make the steam. If you are going to use Atomidine, be sure not to place it in a plastic or metal container, which will corrode. Use glass or ceramic. Other substances, such as witch hazel, pine, benzoin, eucalyptus, or other volatile oils, can be placed in a container of any material. Place over the water so that the steam vaporizes the substance. Drape towels or blankets over the stool or chair so that you do not burn the back of the legs or the buttocks. Then climb in, drape the tent around you, and close it. Use a large bath towel around your neck to prevent steam from escaping. If you wish to inhale the vapor or to steam the face, remove the towel and bend the head forward into the opening. Fume baths are an essential accompaniment to colonics, to an apple diet, or if you embark on one of the other cleansing procedures described in the following pages. They help to throw off toxins that otherwise can cause considerable discomfort (such as headaches, dizziness, nausea, etc.) during internal cleansing.

One woman, suffering from arthritic–like pains, reported great success with her homemade vapor unit used in conjunction with massage, osteopathy, and the other therapies Cayce had recommended:

> For the witch-hazel vapor baths, which were recommended, I did not find any place where they would give this, or in fact knew what it was. So I found a vaporizer which is used for treating croup, etc., a little electric gadget which will make steam out of water and whatever other liquid is put into it. The tent I made by hanging a sheet up over a line. This made low enough that I could sit on an ordinary kitchen chair, which would not be harmed by the steam bath . . . The opening in the tent allowed me to leave my head outside and read a book, which I managed to rig up à la Rube Goldberg. Of course, I did put the little electric steamer under the tent along with me and the chair. I used a mixture of half and half witch hazel and water.
>
> Altogether the results have been very good . . . (2970-2 Reports)

It is also possible to take a vapor bath in your tub. First, cover the top of the tub with a blanket, rubber, or plastic sheet. Then run water as hot as possible into the tub. When you have it up to maximum heat, fill the tub a quarter full of this very hot water. Let this stand steaming a few minutes and then run some water as cold as possible. When the bath temperature is down to your usual hot-bath temperature (104–106 degrees), try getting into the tub with a minimum opening of the cover to conserve the vapor. Be sure enough of your body is out of the water and exposed to just the steam. If necessary, remove the stopper and run off some of the water.

Another old-time method recommended by Priesnitz is to have a platform of wood set about two inches above the bottom of the tub. It can have a small opening in the platform or narrow spaces left open between the boards. Then, one end of a hose is attached to the hot-water faucet and the other end is run to the bottom of the tub farthest away from the drain. Now let the full hot water run, the steam or vapor coming up through the sides and openings in the platform. It is surprising how little hot water will give you a vapor bath, and if the tub is well covered, you can shut off the hot water in a few minutes and the vapor will continue on the job for quite some time. A fine spray-nozzle on the end of the hose will produce a more rapid vapor.

Foot Baths

A hot foot bath is an excellent palliative for sore, aching feet or for a congestive headache at the first sign of feverishness or a cold. When such is used as therapy for a cold or congestion, its effectiveness can be increased by adding one or two tablespoons of mustard to the water. Wrap the patient well in blankets and have him or her sip hot water or lemonade.

For a hot foot bath, use a large basin, pail, or foot tub. The water should be above the ankle and the temperature should be about 110 degrees to start with. As the water cools, keep adding hot water. The bath should be continued from five to twenty minutes.

The hot leg bath needs to be taken in a deeper container—or it can be taken by filling the bathtub with sufficient water to cover the legs up to the knees—with the patient sitting on the side of the tub. This can be used when it is desirable to induce perspiration, to break congestion, or for aching legs, muscle strain, or leg cramps.

As I noted earlier, in arthritic or rheumatic cases, Epsom salts can be added to the water and the feet massaged like the hands, as described on page 210.

Mustard

Cayce recommended mustard foot baths for aching and burning feet to increase circulation (3776-9):

[It would be] well if the feet and limbs be bathed in very warm water, to increase the circulation in this portion of the system, putting mustard in the water when this is done . . .

And for colds and grippe:

Keep the feet bathed well with mustard water; this extending to the knees, even to the hips—even sitz baths of the mustard water would be well if not made too heavy; but rather sponge off across the small of the back, down the

Baths for Skin Conditions

For general dermatitis, poison ivy, and hives that cover a large area of the body, the following baths bring relief for itching:

1. Dissolve one pound of laundry starch in boiling water and add to the tub (twenty gallons of water) at 104-106 degrees.
2. Place two pounds of bran in a closed muslin bag in a hot tub at 104-106 degrees.
3. Use eight ounces of bicarbonate of soda to a tub of water (twenty to thirty gallons of water). This is particularly good for alkalizing an acid-skin condition.
4. If you've been exposed to any poison plant—ivy, oak, sumac, etc.—or already have a rash, lather affected areas with brown borax soap. Let the lather dry and then rinse in a hot tub.—**H.J.R.**

Hot packs or fomentations have traditionally been used to relieve muscular pains and aches from overexertion or other causes, and cold packs, which constrict the blood vessels, can ease congestion of the head and relieve headaches, fever, insomnia, and indigestion.—**H.J.R.**

limbs and then bathe the bottoms of the feet with a combination of equal parts of Mutton Suet, Spirits of Turpentine, Spirits of Camphor and Tincture of Benzoin. Heat these each time before the combination is applied, not to boiling but so that they may be stirred thoroughly together. Massage into the bottoms of the feet and under the knees, back of the neck, across the face, especially the upper antrums and just under the eyes or around those portions of the body. We will find these will help materially. Do this two, three times a day. (1005-15)

Coffee Grounds

Cayce recommended this foot bath to a lady of middle years who complained that her feet "bothered her so much":

As for the limbs—each evening, or at least three to four evenings a week, soak the feet and the limbs to the knees in a fluid made from boiling old coffee grounds. It is the tannic acid in this that is helpful, which can be better obtained from boiling the old grounds (but not soured) . . . Following such a foot bath, massage Peanut Oil thoroughly into the knee and under the knee, through the area from the knee to the foot, and especially the bursa of the feet . . . This done consistently will relieve these tensions. (243-33)

(Q) What will relieve the pain in the feet?
(A) This, as we see, is produced from poor eliminations through the system, and the impaired circulation . . . [It would be well] if these [feet] were bathed occasionally in saturated solution of Sal-Soda. Not Bicarbonate, Sal-Soda. This . . . will gradually correct this portion and will relieve the strain on the body. Have this as warm as the body can stand when the baths are taken . . . rubbing same along the limbs to the knees. (325-7)

(Q) What will stop the condition that occurs between the toes occasionally?
(A) Use occasionally witch hazel in its full strength to reduce this [itching]. Bathe—when feet are bathed, and bathe them often—in *salt* water. (903-16)

Water Packs

Hot packs or fomentations have traditionally been used to relieve muscular pains and aches from overexertion or other causes, and cold packs, which constrict the blood vessels, can ease congestion of the head and relieve headaches, fever, insomnia, and indigestion. A large number of naturopaths have reported great success in their use of packs in serious diseases.

Those old enough to remember the success and attention paid to Sister Kenny, in her revolutionary treatment of the aftereffects of polio, may recall that her therapy consisted largely of the application of hot–water vapor packs to relieve the muscle spasms, followed by massage. Back in the days when I served a term of learning and experience in the Benedict Lust Sanitarium, cold- and hot-water packs were part of the standard therapy.

Cold-Water Packs

These packs are very effective in relieving insomnia, indigestion, gas, headaches, congestion, sore throat, temperature, sprains, and bruises, and for fast first-aid application in a large variety of injuries. There are three types of cold packs: immediate, relaxing, and derivative. The immediate is left on a short time, from five to fifteen minutes, to produce a fast movement of blood to the surface in cases of temperature, injury, sprain, or bruise. A cold pack for fever will heat up in five to eight minutes and should be changed frequently. The relaxing cold pack is useful in nervous conditions such as nervous indigestion, insomnia, etc., and can be repeated every two hours. The derivative is left on for several hours or overnight and is a most effective treatment for sore throats and bringing down edema, particularly water on the knee.

The first effect is the contraction of the blood vessels from the cold water. The second effect is to start normalizing the circulation, and after twenty minutes to a half-hour, the pack becomes heated and increases the metabolism of the patient.

To prepare a cold pack, use four or five thicknesses of linen or toweling; wring it out in very cold water; apply to the throat, ankle, knee, or other area; cover with a piece of plastic and another towel, and wrap it tightly so that the pack is airtight. For edema or sore throat leave it on overnight.

Abdominal Cold Pack for Insomnia

An abdominal cold pack will relieve insomnia when all else fails and is excellent for the stimulation of the liver, kidneys, and other organs.

Cover the bed with a rubber sheet, oilcloth, or plastic or waterproof material about 18–24 inches wide and 48–60 inches long crosswise on it. Prepare a towel or cloth long enough to wrap around your middle. For the average person this should run about 24 by 40 inches. Then thoroughly soak a small cloth or large towel in cold water below 65 degrees. Wring it out loosely and fold lengthwise to a 9-inch width or thereabouts and place it on the larger cloth or towel. Or you can tuck the cold pack around the abdomen while standing up, if you first put it on the dry pack and wrap it about your abdomen when you lie down. Be certain it is tight and in contact with the skin at all points. If too long, it can overlap in front of the abdomen. Be sure that the pack is airtight for proper reaction.

Other hydrotherapy remedies will be described in succeeding chapters (see also index).

11

Internal Cleansing: Colonics and Packs—and a Cure for the Common Cold

M.B.'s hands trembled visibly as he lit up a cigarette, drawing and inhaling deeply. "You see, Dr. Reilly, the doctors tell me I am finished. They told me to get my affairs in order because I won't be walking around much longer. I'm only forty-four years old. It isn't easy to face whatever is left of my life in a wheelchair."

The man sitting before me was obviously desperate. He was an executive of a successful radio station in Charleston, West Virginia, and had exhausted the medical resources of his own state. His present difficulty stemmed from the blockage of circulation in the veins and arteries of his lower limbs—it sounded like the start of Buerger's disease. The dictionary defines this as chronic inflammation of the arteries and veins of the lower extremities, thought to be most prevalent among heavy smokers.

"So when I read about you in Jess Stearn's book and the success you have had with the Cayce treatments, I just had to try before I give up and settle for that wheelchair," he went on, adding brightly, "You know, I had a terrible hacking cough which really interfered with my broadcasting work and the Cayce cough remedy [see end of this chapter] was just wonderful—just wonderful. So I do believe."

I examined him. "Are you a heavy smoker?" I asked.

"Oh, yes," he replied, "I smoke two or three packs of cigarettes a day. Sometimes more."

"Didn't the doctor warn you about smoking?"

The doctors had already explained this danger to him.

I explained to the patient that the stoppage in his circulatory system could result in gangrene and amputation, especially if he ever had even the slightest injury to his feet or legs.

M.B. wanted to try the four-day apple-diet cleansing routine and was literally begging me to try this therapy on him.

"I won't take you unless you promise that you will cut out your smoking," I

Consistently heavy smokers have a tendency to develop antibodies which counteract the effect of the cigarette chemicals to the system. If a nonsmoker were to smoke one or two packs of cigarettes at one time, it is possible he or she might die from the aftereffects. **—H.J.R.**

told him. "You can't do it any other way. You will have to follow a new routine—a new lifestyle that will consist of diet, exercise, and elimination therapies, including sweat baths and massages. If you can follow that after the apple diet, I will lay out a program for you."

Consistently heavy smokers have a tendency to develop antibodies which counteract the effect of the cigarette chemicals to the system. If a nonsmoker were to smoke one or two packs of cigarettes at one time, it is possible he or she might die from the aftereffects. The body of a heavy smoker gradually builds up a protective device, and part of the craving is a result of the body's effort to balance the intake. It is a chemical craving as well as a psychological one. If we can cleanse the body thoroughly—which we can do with hydrotherapy (colonic irrigations with sweat baths or fume baths)—with a nonstimulating and corrective diet, the body in time can throw off the chemical antibodies, and the craving for tobacco won't be as strong. Even a heavy smoker will be able to resist it until it finally disappears.

M.B. came to me every three months for colonics, massage, and sweat baths, and for checkups on his exercise and diet, which he practiced faithfully, until he had an almost complete recovery. He was so grateful and excited that he made a recording that was a glowing testimonial to the Cayce therapy and played it on his stations in West Virginia and then wanted to distribute it nationally.

Another dramatic case that is well documented medically and that testifies to the benefits of the Cayce regimen is that of Mrs. M.M. of Atlanta, Georgia.

Mrs. M.M. had a long history of glandular malfunction dating back to her early teens that caused her to have periodic attacks of dizziness, profuse sweating, and a feeling that unconsciousness was imminent. She also developed a tumor on her thyroid gland, which was surgically removed (thyroidectomy) when she was twenty-nine years old. All of these symptoms became increasingly severe during each of her four pregnancies, and it was not until she was six months pregnant with her fourth child that her condition was diagnosed as hypoglycemia. She was put on a diet requiring six meals a day and several ounces of glucose before going to bed at night; however, when she was about eight months pregnant she awoke at approximately three o'clock one morning with the familiar symptoms of dizziness, clammy perspiration, etc., which she knew preceded shock. Several months after the birth of her fourth child she was sent to one of the most famous endocrinologists in the United States for a complete diagnosis.

"I was there in Augusta [Georgia] for about two weeks," she said, "and when he ran the endocrine tests it was found that my thyroid and estrogen levels were very, very low and my adrenal function practically nonexistent. His diagnosis was 'mild hypo-pituitarism.' My pituitary was not stimulating the adrenals, thyroid, and other glands properly, and I was told that I would probably need treatment with steroids for the rest of my life. Then, some years later I found out about Edgar Cayce, and my husband and I went to see Dr. Reilly in New Jersey. We went through the whole regimen—exercise, colonics, fume baths, the apple diet for three days, massage and spinal adjustments daily—we stayed four days. I was not miraculously transformed afterward but I felt better.

"Slowly in the following months as I continued the regimen Dr. Reilly and Betty Billings had outlined for me, I continued to improve and felt a little more energetic. But now I come to the best part of the story. I was having some abnormal bleeding and my gynecologist thought I should have a D & C. Well, because of my hypo–pituitary condition it was thought to be a little dangerous to give me an anesthetic without preoperative steroid treatment—my blood pressure was low and there was some risk of circulatory failure. So they scheduled me for a series of endocrine tests before surgery—particularly the one where they test adrenal function. The first surprise came when they took my blood pressure: it was normal—120 over 70. It had usually been around 90 or 100 over 60. The surgeon had the test results from the doctor in Georgia, and other internists who had treated me over the years and had given me follow-up tests, and they all were about the same—some showed a slight improvement but all were still subnormal. After the new series of tests, the doctor called me and said, 'Mrs. M.M., we don't know how to explain it, but your tests are all normal now. I am in a quandary because, with your past medical history, you should be given hydrocortisone therapy before undergoing general anesthesia and have it administered intravenously during surgery, but these tests indicate that these procedures would not be necessary.' It was so unexpected, even to me, that I asked him to let me think about it a little while. I decided to ask the doctor to let me try it without the hydrocortisone and he agreed—but he had a doctor standing by to administer the hydrocortisone in the event I should need it. When I awoke in the recovery room, the doctor told me that my blood pressure had remained stable throughout and no hydrocortisone had been given to me.

"Well, when I went to Dr. Reilly for therapy, I hadn't expected it to produce a cure for a lifelong condition—I thought it would just improve my general health because all the doctors have told me that my condition was not curable. I have been taking the apple diet regimen once or twice a year and having regular osteopathic treatments, colonics, massage, and trying to follow the diet routine outlined for me by Dr. Reilly and Betty (which stressed low sugars and starches as well as other important changes in my diet). Other than a slight relapse several years ago when I went through a period of great stress along with menopause, I have remained normal ever since. As a matter of fact, I had all the tests run routinely several months ago and they were all completely normal! When I left my doctor's office he said, 'Just keep on with what you are doing—I don't know what it is but it is working!'"

Another case on which we have medical documentation is that of an eighty-year–old patient, whom I sent to a New Jersey physician for a series of tests. Her cholesterol was 296. After four days on the apple diet with her daily exercises, colonics, fume baths, and massage, she went back to Dr. A. for checking. When he retested her, he found her cholesterol was down fifty points.

I have mentioned that after I closed the institute in Rockefeller Center and embarked on the first of my four "retirements," I continued what I hoped would

Another case on which we have medical documentation is that of an eighty-year-old patient, whom I sent to a New Jersey physician for a series of tests. Her cholesterol was 296. After four days on the apple diet with her daily exercises, colonics, fume baths, and massage, she went back to Dr. A. for checking. When he retested her, he found her cholesterol was down fifty points.—**H.J.R.**

be a limited practice for some of my longtime patients—labor leader David Dubinsky and Alex Rose; John Harris, whose real-estate firm built Rockefeller Center; David Sarnoff; and a few of their friends. One day one of my patients prevailed upon me to see a friend of his, R.M.C. When the man walked in, I saw that he was in a bad state. His letter to Hugh Lynn Cayce of October 3, 1968, describes his condition more graphically than my memory can, as well as the results he got from a cleansing regimen and a disciplined way of life:

"It is now eighteen months since I first joined the A.R.E. and began treatment with Dr. Harold J. Reilly here in New York City. The following is a progress report of the remarkable, lasting results of the treatments with Dr. Reilly.

"In my original correspondence I stated my age as forty, married, and having been treated with antibiotic drugs for over twelve years (almost continually) for chronic prostatitis, from time to time infecting the entire genito-urinary system—which was the case at that time. I also had a long-standing infection of the eyes, blepharitis, and of the face, sycosis barbae (staphylococcus)—both having been intensively treated by specialists for over two years, but without much success.

"At the very first treatment with Dr. Reilly he set up a schedule of therapeutic exercises for me, taking about twenty minutes a day. This was gradually increased until my home program extended to about one hour when exercises were done (as in my case) very slowly.

"A series of colonic irrigations was started almost immediately, as were cold sitz baths at bedtime. Changes in diet were suggested by Dr. Reilly, and his assistant, Betty Billings, was most helpful in providing precise recipes for food preparation according to the 'readings.'

"About one month after starting treatments of every two weeks, there was enough improvement in the prostatitis to stop the antibiotic drugs. They have never been taken since. The drugs for the face and eyes had been stopped even sooner.

 " . . . For the blepharitis, raw potato poultices were used on the eyes, followed by Glyco-Thymoline rinses. This proved to be of great help and the only treatment to bring relief in over two years. Although this treatment has given great relief, the blepharitis recurs from time to time, whereupon I return to the Glyco-Thymoline eye baths and, if necessary, the raw potato poultices.

"The sycosis barbae was being treated by a new specialist when I started with Dr. Reilly, and that condition cleared shortly thereafter, not returning again.

"In conclusion, although not being completely free of the original symptoms all the time, my overall general health has dramatically changed for the better without the use of any antibiotic drugs, and has been maintained by the program set up by Dr. Reilly through guidance of the 'readings.'

"My wife and I now follow much of the dietary advice outlined in the 'readings' and are avid 'Cayce enthusiasts' with interests in many fields.

"Of course, it is to Dr. Harold J. Reilly I feel we owe so much for these remarkable results. It is true, he does not do this 'alone,' but he does serve rich and poor alike with a knowledge and dedication unsurpassed in these times, and an enthusiasm undimmed by his years of service.

"I feel I have been given a new chance to return to a healthful life. Indeed Dr. Reilly has done this for perhaps thousands of people—a record for service to God and humankind."

What is the secret of this miracle therapy?

Since most people are toxic to a greater or lesser degree, I have found that a good cleansing routine with the apple-diet regimen is the first step toward improving assimilation and elimination for anyone. If one is reasonably well, the detoxification will bring about an almost euphoric feeling of well-being and provide inexpensive and effective insurance against disease. If one is not well, the apple-cleansing regimen is an excellent beginning of a therapeutic program.

Cayce advised as follows:

> We would use first the apple diet to purify the system; that is, for three days eat nothing but apples of the Jonathan variety . . . The Jonathan is usually grown farther north than the Delicious, but these are of the same variety, but eat some. You may drink coffee if you desire, but do not put milk or cream in it, especially while you are taking the apples.
>
>   At the end of the third day, the next morning take about two tablespoonsful of Olive Oil. (780-12)

> (Q) What should be done to remove the seeming toxic condition in my system, which would cause me to be more alert physically and mentally?
> (A) As indicated, keep nearer to the alkaline-reacting foods, and these will overcome toxic forces . . .
>
>   Balance the diet as indicated. Have a great deal of the stimulations from the whole wheat, citrus fruits, and vegetables that are green and raw. Not too much of the meats. No raw apples; or if raw apples are taken, take them and nothing else—three days of raw apples only, and then olive oil, and we will cleanse all toxic forces from any system! Raw apples are not well unless they are of the Jenneting variety. (820-2)

"Jenneting" variety is an obsolete word that refers to those apples of a sheep-nosed nature such as Delicious, Oregon Reds, Arkansas Black, Jonathan, and Sheep Nose.

These are the preferred varieties, but in our experience, the most important element is that the apples be "organic" and free of chemicals, since it is the purpose of the regimen to cleanse the system.

Cayce recommended the apple diet for a wide variety of ailments too lengthy to enumerate here, but in all cases where toxemia or toxicity could be a cause or contributing factor to such problems as headache, debilitation, neuritis, arthritis, constipation, incoordination of assimilation and elimination, subluxations, anemia, stroke, pinworms, and so on.

At other times but far less frequently Cayce advised a four-day grape mono diet or a five-day citrus-fruit mono diet for cleansing. For some people, he

Colonics, together with castor oil packs and manipulation, are truly the distinctive hallmark of the Cayce drugless therapy. Certainly in my own practice and experience they have produced some of the most dramatic and fantastic healing results.—**H.J.R.**

recommended, in conjunction with the apple–diet therapy, that castor oil packs be taken to stimulate good elimination: " . . . first the system needs cleansing with the [castor] oil packs and then the apple diet, before beginning to build up." (1409–9)

In the very beginning, we encountered reports that some patients simply could not handle the apples—they got cramps, toxicity, headaches, and other symptoms. Gradually, with experimentation, we combined the apple diet with other Cayce therapies, and finally Miss Billings and I laid out a regimen for people who came to stay with us for the Cayce apple diet that included colonics, fume baths, and other hydrotherapy when called for, daily massage, and castor oil packs as a preparation before they came and as a follow–through when they left.

The results deservedly spread the fame of the Cayce apple diet, but we must caution anyone who decides to try it to adhere to the instructions at the end of this chapter, after first checking with a doctor (a good checkup before and after the diet will generally show health improvement, particularly in cholesterol and blood–pressure levels).

However, the apple diet itself is not the only, or even the principal, factor in the cleansing and therapeutic process. I have seen many cases respond in a highly satisfactory way where the main therapy has been the colonics and the castor oil packs with exercise and massage.

Colonics, together with castor oil packs and manipulation, are truly the distinctive hallmark of the Cayce drugless therapy. Certainly in my own practice and experience they have produced some of the most dramatic and fantastic healing results.

Stressing as he did the vital role of elimination in health, longevity, beauty, sexual vigor, and joy in living, it is not surprising that Cayce gave this reply when asked about colonics:

When these are necessary, yes. For *every one*—everybody—should take an internal bath occasionally as well as an external one. They would all be better off if they would. (440-2)

In another reading he said this:

One colonic irrigation will be worth about four to six enemas. (3570-1)

Cayce gave precise directions for the administration of the colonics:

. . . have a good hydrotherapist give a thorough, but gentle colon cleansing . . . In the first waters, use salt and soda, in the proportions of a heaping teaspoonful of table salt and a level teaspoonful of baking soda [both] dissolved thoroughly—to each half gallon of water. In the last water use Glyco-Thymoline as an intestinal antiseptic to purify the system, in the proportions of a tablespoonful to the quart of water. (1745-4)

Glyco-Thymoline

Glyco-Thymoline is an inexpensive mixture readily available at most drugstores, and it was used by Cayce in over a hundred readings covering such ailments as:

cardiovascular disorder	hemorrhoids	incoordination
catarrh	herpes simplex	lumbago
cirrhosis of the liver	hives	Parkinson's disease
colitis	hypertension	pelvic disorders
dropsy	hypochondria	prolapsus
eliminations	hypotension	toxemia
engorged heart	impaction	

We have found the salt-and-soda mixture useful in constipation, cholecystitis, general debilitation, dropsy, eliminations, prolapsus, sciatica, and toxemia, among other ailments.—**H.J.R.**

The colonic is given to stimulate the bowels, but it also has a tendency to stimulate the kidneys. The main difference between an enema and a colonic is that an enema is a relieving process and a colonic is a stimulating and corrective process.—**H.J.R.**

At the institute, we had four rooms in which colonics were given with the Duerker machines. Once in a while we had some irregularity with the mercury gauge that registered pressure. We then knew that there was a condition that required the immediate attention of a doctor. Invariably the physician found tumors or polyps, because the gauge was so sensitive it would show a blockage. The Duerker also creates a water wave that stimulates the peristalsis in the colon and is very effective. We use between six and ten gallons of water in and out, some of the water being used to siphon the other water out. I would say of the six gallons of water, three go in and out of the patient and the other three are used for the suction effect.

The colonic is given to stimulate the bowels, but it also has a tendency to stimulate the kidneys. The main difference between an enema and a colonic is that an enema is a relieving process and a colonic is a stimulating and corrective process. Quite frequently there will be extra bowel action for a day or two after the colonic, showing stimulation, and this, combined with the proper diet, exercise, and all the other adjuncts, has proven to be a valuable and effective method of elimination.

Colonics unfortunately cannot be administered at home either to one's self or to another person. For this treatment you must visit a professional, and many communities do not offer this service. We have found the Duerker machine—invented by an engineer who was suffering from high blood pressure and had tired of having long fifty-feet tubes put into him—the most satisfactory. The Duerker has a series of levers and mercury gauges that register the pressure of the water and the pressure in the intestine. There are other, newer models on the market, but they are not an improvement and do not really do the job as well.

Cayce used colonics in many cardiovascular conditions or rather more accurately in conditions thought to be cardiovascular. Many of those he sent to me were cleared up with the colonics, castor oil packs, and the other procedures, for improper elimination with abdominal-gas disturbances often masquerades as heart trouble and many other diseases.

One of my patients, a very successful real-estate operator in his middle forties, would go into a toxicoma, and specialists at one point predicted that he had only one year to live. He took colonics at the institute for over thirty years and lived to be eighty-one.

A fifty-year-old man suffering from too much uric acid, albumin in the system, and symptoms of cardiac disturbances was told by Edgar Cayce that " . . . as we find in the ascending colon there is a plethoric condition that causes the extension even of the abdominal area, and naturally a prolapsus in the lower part of the descending colon. This pressure causes the slowing of the circulation between liver and kidneys. It also causes a pressure that tends to fill the aorta artery to such an extent as to cause the thrombose to be more oft too full. This gives the shortness of breath, as well as the fullness about the heart." (2489-2)

Then Cayce recommended a "series of colonic irrigations so as to disseminate this plethoric condition."

The rest of the reading advised certain osteopathic adjustments and diet correction. " . . . and don't ever eat too much. Better get up from the table hungry than to be hungry a long time without being able to eat."

With these corrections the symptoms of heart trouble disappeared.

Another of my patients, Mrs. V.K., a lovely young housewife married to a chiropractor, was brought to me suffering from terrible headaches. In the past months she had become torpid, sluggish, and progressively unable to do her housework or perform any of the normal functions of living. Her husband had tried all the adjustments that could be given her without any response or improvement. She went from doctor to doctor, one of whom pronounced her a mental case and suggested to her husband that she be sent for psychiatric treatment.

I gave her a checkup and a thorough massage, to familiarize myself with her condition as well as to help her. She did not feel any better during the week. The next week she had a colonic, and thereafter she took two colonics a week.

Miss Billings reported that the improvement began after the second colonic. The color of her complexion started to change. Before this she had been too nauseated by food to eat anything. She just took to her bed. She had given up her job in August, six weeks before she came to us in September, and as we have said, couldn't cook, do the housework, or anything. Then after about the third colonic, her husband called Dr. Reilly and reported that when he came home he found that his wife had cooked a most delicious dinner. He couldn't believe it. A week later, he said he had come home and found that his wife had had everything in the apartment moved around. After the sixth colonic she went out to see many people who had not seen her for some time and they all told her how well she looked and wanted to know what she was doing. In one month, this woman had shed about twenty years. She was only about thirty years old when she came to us but she looked fifty. After only eight colonics she was really a transformed person. All that was wrong with her was that she was loaded with toxic material. We suggested she stay on the Cayce nontoxic diet and some Reilly exercises.

Another striking case was the wife of Dr. R. Mrs. R. was sitting in the steam cabinet having a fume bath after her colonic one day and told Miss Billings, "I always went around telling everybody that I was yellow because of my Chinese reincarnation. I came to find out it was only toxins, and since I have had the fume baths and the colonics I have had to buy new lipstick because the shade of lipstick I had used to go with my yellow color looked terrible with my new white skin."

It is an interesting fact that the skin of the patients who undergo the cleansing routine of the apple diet, colonics, fume baths, and castor oil packs routine begins to lighten. If they are blonde or redheaded, the skin will take on an almost alabasterlike translucence; if brunette, the skin tone is many shades lighter and very clear. The color of the iris of the eyes becomes much brighter and the whites of the eyes very clear.

Another patient, Mrs. D.S. of Rockland County, New York, came to me originally at Rockefeller Center for a frozen arm and shoulder, which we treated successfully, restoring total function with massage and manipulation, hot and cold packs, and diathermy. It was not until some time later that I discovered that Mrs. D.S. also had been suffering for over thirty years from heartburn and regurgitation of bile in her throat.

"I had been going to doctors for years for this burning which I felt came from a gallbladder condition," she told Mrs. Brod. "Nothing ever showed up in X-ray and they would give me medicines. I must have swallowed tons of antacids—you name it—I took it . . . None of them helped . . . I kept changing. The taste in my mouth was awful. The heartburn, too, and this awful bitter stuff—the gall was coming up in my mouth all the time and I had to throw up.

"Dr. Reilly put me on the apple diet, the colonics, and the fume baths, and it is the only thing that worked. I got relief, and as long as I watch my diet and come periodically for the therapy I am fine."

Enemas

When colonics are not available, take an enema each day when on the apple diet or one of the other cleansing routines.

In the case of a sixty-three-year-old woman suffering from Bright's disease (381-2) who was bedridden, Cayce gave the following directions for the administration of a daily enema:

We would in the present begin, surely—gently, but each day[—]with tepid water high enemas, gradually dilating the lower portion of the colon and anus . . . . It will be necessary that this be done gradually, but in a five day

It is an interesting fact that the skin of the patients who undergo the cleansing routine of the apple diet, colonics, fume baths, and castor oil packs routine begins to lighten.—**H.J.R.**

B. P.

While the medicinal properties of the oil of the castor bean have been known to physicians and folk healers for thousands of years, Cayce's use of castor oil in packs seemed to be distinctively his.—H.J.R.

period the blood pressure should be reduced at least 30 or 40 points—or more. Begin as in this manner, with the water for the enema:

To three quarts of water add a level teaspoonful of salt and a heaping teaspoonful of baking soda.

We would also use the oils in the last portion of the enema, that to remain [the oils] in the bowel as much or as long as possible. The [last] quart of water we would use at least a heaping tablespoonful of the Petrolagar. Stir this thoroughly as it is injected. (381-2)

(See my directions for taking enemas at home at the end of this chapter.)

Castor Oil Packs (The Palma Christi)

Almost everyone who has ever heard of Edgar Cayce has also heard of his extensive use of castor oil packs. The A.R.E. library index in Virginia Beach shows that he used this therapy—usually in conjunction with colonics—in hundreds of cases for over fifty different ailments, among them aphonia, appendicitis, arthritis, cancer, cerebral palsy, cholecystitis, cholecystalgia, cirrhosis of the liver, colitis, constipation, epilepsy, gallstones, gastritis, hepatitis, hernias, Hodgkin's disease, hookworm, intestinal impaction, lymphitis, migraine, multiple sclerosis, neuritis, Parkinson's disease, pelvic cellulitis, ringworm, sluggish liver, stenosis of the duodenum, sterility, strangulation of kidneys, stricture of the duodenum, and uremia. In addition, there are many cases listed under "lesions," "incoordination," "intestines," "toxemia," "eliminations," and "adhesions."

While the medicinal properties of the oil of the castor bean have been known to physicians and folk healers for thousands of years, Cayce's use of castor oil in packs seemed to be distinctively his. Dr. William McGarey does report that one patient mentioned that her mother, who was born in Yugoslavia and who emigrated to the United States in 1901, had told her daughter that the castor oil packs were a standard treatment "back in the old country" for all kinds of stomach and kidney disorders and baby's colic.

The external use of castor oil to cure warts, for body ulcers, to clear up liver spots, to increase the flow of milk when applied to the breasts of a nursing mother, and for a number of other minor disturbances is mentioned in Dr. D.C. Jarvis's excellent book, *Folk Medicine.* Cayce used castor oil, too, but use of castor oil for the treatment of epilepsy and serious diseases I believe is a true Cayce trademark. Dr. McGarey also points out that Edgar Cayce first recommended the use of castor oil packs in Case 15-2 (September 20, 1927) for a woman suffering from a tumor in the upper bowel.

The directions for making the castor oil pack run pretty much the same in most readings, but the frequency of use, the length of time they should be kept on, and how much olive oil to take with them orally differs among readings. A typical example is that of Case 5186-1, a woman forty-four years old, suffering from gallstones:

to clear up liver spots warts or body ulcers

For Gall Stones

Have at least three to four thicknesses of old flannel saturated thoroughly with Castor Oil, then apply an electric heating pad. Let this get just about as warm as the body can well stand—cover with oil cloth to prevent soiling of linen. Keep this on every afternoon or evening for an hour. Then sponge off [the oil on the body] with soda water. Do this for at least seven days without breaking. One hour each day, same hour each day. After and during those periods take small doses of olive oil two, three times each day. These [small doses of olive oil] should not be so severe as to cause strain, but be careful after about the 3rd or 4th day to observe the stool, and there should be indications of the gall ducts being emptied, and should be gravel, and there should be some stones. (5186-1)

In another case, that of a man sixty years old suffering from cholecystitis with resulting gastroduodenitis creating a "lack of assimilation and digestion for the system," Cayce recommended as follows:

. . . Castor Oil Packs. Take these each evening for three days in succession, and then the large dose of Olive Oil. Leave off three to four days, then take another series. Continue in this manner until the condition has entirely cleared. Then leave off three to four weeks; then [repeat] . . . regularly—in series—even though there is not the severe pain. (294-199)

In my own practice, Miss Billings has worked out a system for patients that simplifies the procedure for handling the packs. The directions will be found at the end of this chapter.

Mrs. A.P., a socially prominent Connecticut woman related to a member of the late President Roosevelt's cabinet, was suffering from a uterine tumor. Her own physician had once researched the Cayce readings and recalled that in a similar case Cayce had recommended treatment with ultraviolet rays along with other physical therapies. Her search for help finally led Mrs. A.P. to my door. I administered the treatments as outlined in the readings, and gradually the tumor diminished and finally disappeared altogether. Her supervising physician confirmed her progress and the happy result that obviated the need for surgery. This same grateful patient contributed a grant of $3,000 to the A.R.E. Clinic in Phoenix to initiate a research program on the castor oil packs.

When Mrs. J.M. came to me she had been suffering for thirteen years from excessive bleeding of the uterus. She had combined a career as an opera singer, singing mainly in Europe, with her roles of wife and mother. Now her physical disability was threatening her career and her ability to function in her personal life. She consulted four leading gynecologists in New York City, all of whom recommended some kind of surgery, from a simple D & C to a complete hysterectomy.

Mrs. J.M. told Mrs. Brod: "Dr. Reilly found every place that I hurt and some places of pain I didn't know I had. And when he told me, 'I think we can help you,' I could have cried. I was so sure and confident that he was right."

Mrs. J.M. started a regimen that began with the colonics and castor oil packs four nights on, three nights off.

I administered the treatments as outlined in the readings, and gradually the tumor diminished and finally disappeared altogether. Her supervising physician confirmed her progress and the happy result that obviated the need for surgery.—**H.J.R.**

"Betty found that I had so much gas that I could have supported all of Con Edison," Mrs. J.M. recalled. "Betty said she had never had such a *lack* of reaction to a colonic in all the years she had been giving them. I hadn't connected up the two symptoms—but I always had a very bloated feeling after I ate, and frequently had heartburn and other discomfort, but I didn't think too much about that because I had had a GI series and they didn't find anything. Well, that was where the trouble was. All that gas was pressing on the organs in my pelvic region and causing all that bleeding.

"After the first two nights of the castor oil packs . . . the spotting stopped and this was remarkable because it was just after my menstrual period and usually that went on and on and on. By the end of the week I sang a concert and felt fine.

"Dr. Reilly had given me the exercises to do too—lying on a striped towel on the floor (so that I'd be sure my body was in a straight line) and touching my knees to elbows and then the left knee to the right side and then both knees, etc. One was particularly effective. He said it would help to get my womb, uterus and all that back in place. You get down on all fours—on hands and knees. Then first you crouch back on your heels and then you stretch your arms out as far as you can go and cough hard two or three times. That is supposed to be for the pelvic organs and it seemed to help. He calls it the 'Chinese Kow-Tow' or the 'Praise Allah' exercise. [See Chapter 7.]

"I had one setback when I started to bleed a little again after menstrual periods, and he and Miss Billings told me to take the castor oil packs seven nights straight. I did that (just for one period of seven nights) and it has since been many months now and still no spotting or bleeding. (I continued four nights on, three off, for three months.) I had three series of colonics and they helped, too, because I have no more gas and my digestion has improved tremendously. So has my singing. Of course, I changed my diet—avoiding all spicy foods—but the castor oil packs are really wonderful. They cured me of my insomnia, too, and I have much more energy now. They are so relaxing. I felt well enough at this time to take a singing engagement which would necessitate my being away for nine weeks. Dr. Reilly told me I could leave off the packs for six weeks and then start again, if necessary; but I felt so well I have never had to return to them to this date [March 1974]."

Mrs. J.M.'s dramatic recovery inspired her close friend, Mrs. R.C., to come to me. She had a terrible pain from an inflamed ovary, which doctors had told her required surgery. She had bad pockets in her colon—her entire abdominal and pelvic areas were distended and so painful she could not bear to be touched. Mrs. R.C. was the daughter of a physician and was half-afraid to tell her family that she had come to me for help. After a series of colonics and castor oil packs her improvement was so dramatic that when she returned to her own internist, he declared an operation unnecessary.

Dr. William A. McGarey, who heads the A.R.E. Clinic in Phoenix and was the director of the Medical Research Division of the Edgar Cayce Foundation, has done a marvelous job of research on the subject of castor oil packs, particularly the use of packs in the treatment of epilepsy. His preliminary findings, based on a study of 81 patients with 101 complaints, were published some years ago in *Edgar Cayce and the Palma Christi*, a book available through the A.R.E. ("Palma Christi," meaning "Palm of Christ," is the botanical name of the castor oil plant, from whose bean the oil is derived.)

I have found the castor oil packs to be invaluable in all cases of constipation, a variety of gallbladder, kidney, and liver disorders, pelvic disorders, inflammation, gallstones, and kidney stones.

I have also found that the application of castor oil will accelerate healing of any wound, broken bones, and especially damage to mucous membranes. When Mrs. Brod was mugged, her mouth was severely lacerated by the assailants. She called me from New York for advice on how to handle this and other injuries sustained during her ordeal. I advised her to wash her mouth with Glyco–Thymoline and to apply castor oil directly to the inside of the lips as well as exterior. She reported that the mouth healed in twenty-four hours.

In my own experience, I recently had a bad hemorrhage of the eye that did not respond to any of the treatments I tried—including Glyco–Thymoline eye baths and packs and raw potato packs. The castor oil packs did it, and I have since learned that Cayce recommended castor oil to dissolve the film of cataracts.

Letters are constantly arriving from doctors who are trying the Cayce therapies and readers of *Edgar Cayce and the Palma Christi* and other Cayce books that mention the castor oil packs, confiding their personal experiences with them and expanding our knowledge of their versatility and effectiveness.

A woman from Pennsylvania wrote, "I happened on Jess Stearn's book *Adventures into the Psychic* and read about the castor oil pack and its many cures. I made a poultice of the flannel soaked in castor oil, and for three afternoons in a row laid with the castor oil pack and the heating pad on my side. (I've had a pain in my left side and back, around the ribs, for two years. It was gradually getting worse, and the spot was so tender that I could barely lay on that side at night. It was like a jagging pain.) This I did for one–and–a–half hours each day. After that time the pain went away entirely and there is no soreness in that spot. It is like a miracle!"

A man from New York had an extraordinary experience with the castor oil packs and wrote to Dr. McGarey: "Being a letter carrier for over twenty–five years (I am fifty–one years old), my feet and legs are my livelihood. I developed a sprained Achilles heel of the right foot. I suffered many months walking on it. After reading your book (*Edgar Cayce and the Palma Christi*), I decided to try your packs—not on the sprained heel, but for a spastic muscle of neck and shoulder. I applied the pack on the neck–shoulder area, with a heating pad held in place by a towel. I made myself comfortable and was watching TV. After about an hour (and without ever thinking about it), I noticed that I felt a soothing heat develop on my right heel, and it felt so good I left the pack on for an hour–and–a–half and then removed it.

"The final result has been that I now have no pain on my right heel. I am wondering if the pack did it, and in such an odd way. In your book, most of the areas where the pack was applied was either the part afflicted or the stomach area. Yet I got the desired results from placing the pack in the neck–shoulder

Books on the Edgar Cayce Remedies

The Oil That Heals: A Physician's Successes with Castor Oil Treatments by William A. McGarey, M.D. (A.R.E. Press, 1999).

Edgar Cayce on Rejuvenation of the Body by John Van Auken (A.R.E. Press, 1999).

The Edgar Cayce Remedies by William A. McGarey, M.D. (Bantam Books, 1983).

area. I would like to have your comment on this."

Dr. Robert McTammany, a surgeon in Shellington, Pennsylvania, tells the following story about a postvaginal hysterectomy patient who developed a fever and a large pelvic abscess, which improved on antibiotics and proteolytic enzymes, but which persisted as a large mass that remained tender. She refused further surgery, and after several weeks of malaise, fever, low abdominal tenderness and pain, and no general improvement, she was then convinced she should begin applications of castor oil packs for one hour daily. She improved remarkably, and examination in one month showed almost complete resolution of the pelvic abscess. The patient reported, "The packs always put me to sleep and make me feel good all over." Dr. McTammany felt that these packs might be beneficial in postoperative patients to improve wound healing and reduce the incidence of infection.

Dr. Ernie Pecci, whose field is mental retardation, has been doing basic work with castor oil packs applied to the abdomen of infants and children of all ages, at his two multipurpose centers near Oakland, California; he wrote the following to Dr. McGarey:

"In what I would call a major breakthrough, a UC medical researcher wants to conduct some research studies on the use of castor oil packs based upon our previous success. They are especially interested in investigating my hypothesis that 'minimal brain damage' is really an endocrine dysfunction which might be helped with the use of the castor oil packs. They have set up an elaborate EEG monitoring system which can be linked to computers which would indicate whether learning is really enhanced after treatment. I will be sending you details soon."

From a woman who was stationed with her husband and children in Germany comes a story that involved Elsie Sechrist. It seemed that when Elsie traveled, she lectured, and when she lectured, the simple remedies that Cayce advocated were well covered:

> When Elsie Sechrist was here in May 1970, my husband told her about Richard's bleeding from the kidney, and the doctors had given no medication, only bed rest, and were soon to do a biopsy. Elsie suggested the castor oil packs, which we did on three separate occasions, and each time the tests, taken before and after, showed marked improvement, and finally, normal kidney functioning after the third application. How we thank God for that simple solution![1]

 A research report[2] returned from an A.R.E. member in Irvington, New Jersey, tells a story in itself. He had palpitation of the heart, which apparently had not responded to anything. He used hot castor oil packs three days each week for an hour-and-a-half over his abdomen following this on the third day with one teaspoonful of olive oil by mouth. He continued the therapy for four weeks. The symptoms cleared up for eleven months, then recurred when he underwent some psychological shock. After another four-week course of therapy, they disappeared again and have been absent for over a year now.

The late Dr. Mayo Hotten of California reported that he has used castor oil packs over the eyes in two cases to reduce the inflammation of pterygium (a growth of mucous membrane over the inner portion of the conjunctiva of the eye)—perhaps sufficiently to prevent surgery. Recently I received a report about a twenty-four-year-old housewife, the mother of two small boys, who was found to have a golf-ball-sized cyst on her left ovary when she underwent a routine examination. She was scheduled for a return visit, but in the meantime applied castor oil packs to her lower abdomen for one hour a day, four days each week. She noticed that she received welcome relief from the old nagging problem of the menstrual cramps from which she had suffered for a long time. When she was again examined for the cyst, it had entirely disappeared.

Another story of interest to mothers is that of a young couple who wrote me that for five to six months their year-old boy had been subject to chronic, persistent diarrhea. Having known them for several years, Dr. McGarey wrote to them about the castor oil packs and the possibility of using Glyco-Thymoline packs also. They recently informed me that the boy, now twenty-two months old, has no problems with his GI tract—it cleared up completely on just the castor oil packs.

The "Case of the Curly Hair," related by Dr. McGarey in *Edgar Cayce and the Palma Christi*, is noteworthy because of its humor and serendipity. Dr. McGarey was treating a young woman (Case 36) who, after the use of oral contraceptives, was having difficulties, including uterine hemorrhage, elevated blood pressure, cramps in her legs, and great personal tension heightened by a tense domestic situation.

"She noted when she washed her hair," Dr. McGarey wrote, that "for the first time in her life, she could not make her shampoo develop suds. She changed shampoos three times to no effect, and the beauty parlor met with the same results—no sudsing."

Dr. McGarey began treating her for the blood pressure and uterine condition after other doctors had failed to produce notable and lasting improvement. She was given some medication for the hypertension and castor oil packs were prescribed. After one week of packs the patient reported that her hair was sudsing, as it hadn't for nearly ten months, and became curly again.

For home use, I would advise the castor oil packs for chronic constipation, gallbladder trouble, sluggish liver, and many types of abdominal conditions, but check with your doctor first, for discomfort or pain may be the symptom of a serious ailment. However, if you do not require medical care, you may follow the directions at the end of this chapter. (The method has been somewhat simplified from the way it appears in the Cayce readings.)

Next we come to grape packs. During the 1920s Johanna Brandt of South Africa created a sensation in the United States when she arrived from Germany and challenged American doctors to operate on her to validate her claims that she had been cured of cancer by a grape diet and grape packs. I was introduced to her by Bernarr MacFadden and Benedict Lust, M.D., N.D., D.O. Mrs. Brandt made little headway with the medical establishment, although her records in South Africa and Germany were impressive. We find that grapes—

*For home use, I would advise the castor oil packs for chronic constipation, gallbladder trouble, sluggish liver, and many types of abdominal conditions, but check with your doctor first, for discomfort or pain may be the symptom of a serious ailment.—**H.J.R.***

for tumors + some cancers

During the 1920s Johanna Brandt of South Africa created a sensation in the United States when she arrived from Germany and challenged American doctors to operate on her to validate her claims that she had been cured of cancer by a grape diet and grape packs.—**H.J.R.**

both as a monodiet and in packs—have figured in therapy for over six thousand years. They seem to be particularly helpful with tumors and some cancers.

Cayce prescribed grape packs for colitis, eliminations, gastritis, glands, incoordination, injuries, intestines (gas), nervous systems, pelvic disorders, peritonitis, food poisoning, Recklinghausen's disease, rheumatism, streptococcus, tuberculosis, tumors, typhoid fever, and ulcers.

In one case, that of a forty-five-year-old woman (757-6), he did prescribe grape packs and the grape diet for her skin cancer along with the use of animated ash, and ultraviolet, violet-ray, and infrared treatments.

When asked: "How long should I follow these treatments before another reading?" he replied:

We would let at least a week to ten days be between the three day grape diet, you see, and we would have at least three series of the grape diet before a recheck. This will give the opportunity for the proper balance.
(Q) In making the grape poultice, should the grapes be heated or anything mixed with them?
(A) Nothing mixed with them and *not* heated. Let them make the heat from the body by drawing onto the system in a normal manner. Well that they be rolled you see, retaining the hull *with* the pulp. Any type of the grape is well, at the present season. (757-6)

In two tumor cases Cayce said this:

We find it would be helpful to have three or four days each month when *only* grapes would be used as the diet and during those 3 to 4 days we would apply the grape poultices across all the abdomen itself.

(Q) The kind of grapes—does that matter?
(A) Concord grapes are preferable. (683-3)

Or the body may, under the existent circumstances, go on an entire grape diet—see, *entire* grape diet, for at least three day periods; then to the regular normal diet that has been indicated. Quantities of grapes! And should there appear any disturbance in the stomach and duodenum through those periods, make a poultice of the grape hull and pulp—between cloths and apply over those areas; or over the abdomen and liver area, you see. Make this about an inch and a half thick—that large a quantity, you see, all over. Plenty of water, but just grapes for three days—*quantities*—all that the body may eat. (757-6)

He also used the grape therapy for ulcers:

ulcers
– inflammation in caecum

For as we find, there are both ulcers in the stomach and duodenum (or thickening tissue) as well as an inflammatory condition in the caecum and appendicial area . . .

As we find, the body should rest for at least a week or ten days, first; and during that period be in the open air as much as is practical.

Also have the *heavy Grape Poultices each day over the abdominal and stomach area.* Leave these on for at least two hours each day, changing them about once during the two-hour period, see? Have them at least half an inch thick. Crush the grapes and apply, raw; the Concord Grapes being preferable.

And *live practically on grapes during that period, or grapes and milk*—with a little curd or crackers in same. The Concord grapes are preferable to be eaten also, but not the same ones that are used for poultice, to be sure! Of course, other types of grapes may be eaten also, but preferably and principally the Concord or the colored grapes rather than the green, see?

After there have been the Grape Poultices used for at least three to four days, then we would have a colonic irrigation—very gently given; and do not attempt to do this by self! Have it done rather by a professional, with the warning as to the disturbance in the caecum area! Rest during this whole period, you see, but especially remain quiet during the period the colonic is given—just one, gently but thoroughly done, but after the Poultices have been used for three to four days as indicated.

Beware of any temperature, or too much of night sweats, or the poor eliminations through the respiratory system. Hence we would rub the body down with alcohol—whenever there is any tendency in this direction. [Italics added.] (1970-1)

I have had a few cases where the patients were sent to me with instructions to try the grape therapy in conjunction with the colonics, hydrotherapy, electrotherapy, and other modalities. In a number of them there was significant shrinkage of the tumors and in one case there was a complete elimination of the tumor. Of course, these were all benign, but I have observed patients undergo grape therapy in naturopathic institutes where the therapy was applied for cancer. This would suggest that perhaps some systematic medical research might be justified and undertaken.

Cayce also used a variety of other packs with great effectiveness. Many years ago, I had an automobile accident and smashed up my left leg. At that time I had a reading from Cayce and he advised massages and packs every day with a combination of apple cider vinegar, iodine, and salt, and this would restore a near normal use of my leg. In my eightieth year I can still jog a mile or more.

In Case 304–3, that of a sixty–nine–year–old man, Cayce prescribed a salt and vinegar pack for the ligaments about the knee.

We would massage well almost a saturated solution of pure apple vinegar and common table salt, preferably the very heavy salt than that carrying too much of . . . ingredients to prevent the sticking.

Last April I had been doing a tremendous amount of manipulation and massage; I was on my feet a lot and found it extremely difficult to climb stairs

Then there is another recommendation from the Cayce readings on the use of grated potato for the eyes. It is a very effective treatment, and I wish doctors would do more research in it.—**H.J.R.**

Knees, joint stiffened joints, tendinitis sprains

and had to use the rail to pull myself up. I decided to look up my old Cayce reading, which mentioned salt and vinegar. I thereupon used a pack with a couple of thicknesses of gauze or muslin soaked with cider vinegar. In many readings, I noticed Cayce recommended kosher salt—heavy, coarse salt—and I put the salt thickly on the muslin and wrapped it around my knee, wound plastic around it to make it airtight, and kept it on for about four or five hours, and several times during the night. I did this for eight days, and at the end of the eighth day I was running up and down stairs. I have used it a lot since then, for stiffened joints and sprains, and especially tendinitis and inflammation of the knee joint. For ordinary loosening up of tendons and the joints, the Cayce salt and vinegar therapy is very effective:

> In the area of the knee, where ligaments have been torn, use about twice each week this combination: moisten table salt (preferably iodized salt) with pure apple vinegar, not having [it] too liquid, but that it may be gently massaged into the knee cap [and] the end of the ligaments. While this will hurt a few times at first, if this is kept up each day for quite awhile we will get better results here. (3336-1)

Then there is another recommendation from the Cayce readings on the use of grated potato for the eyes. It is a very effective treatment, and I wish doctors would do more research in it. Take old Irish potatoes (white potatoes as opposed to sweet potatoes). Get them unsprayed—in an organic state. Grate the potatoes, peel and pulp, and scoop up a large spoonful and put it directly on the eyelid and over the entire eye. Place a piece of gauze over the eye and keep the pack on one or two hours. Several years ago I used the raw potato eye pack on a trip I made to a medical symposium in Phoenix. I drove about 6,000 miles, continuing on to California after the meeting. I felt considerable eye-strain, but I put the potato pack on and it was extremely effective. It is also good to alleviate the feeling of "sand" in your eyes or pressure on the eyeball or bloodshot eyes. But again, be sure you are using organic potatoes for an eye pack!

Another distinctively Cayce pack is made by soaking three thicknesses of cloth in Glyco-Thymoline. As explained previously, Glyco-Thymoline is an inexpensive preparation available without a prescription at drugstores that is both soothing and antiseptic for mucous membranes. It is often used as a gargle and mouthwash and Cayce even recommended a few drops of it taken internally to keep the system alkaline.

Glyco-Thymoline packs have been found to be particularly effective in relieving sinusitis, as Cayce recommended:

> We would use the Glyco-Thymoline packs over the nasal passages, or sinus passages. Saturate 3 to 4 thicknesses of cotton cloth, or gauze, in warm Glyco-Thymoline, and apply over the passages, allowing such a pack to remain on for 15 to 20 minutes at the time—and keep up until the passages are clear. Apply such packs whenever there is any distress—either in the sinus or in the

digestive system. Such packs may also be applied over the abdominal area to advantage as well as over the face, see?

Also we would take Glyco-Thymoline internally, 2 to 3 drops in 1/2 a glass of water about twice a day (and drink a glass of water afterwards) until the system has been purified.

Then—when the system has been purified—begin taking those vitamins that will stimulate better building of resistance; the B-1 Complex. Also as an aid to resistance building, take beef juice daily as medicine—and prepare this at least every other day. This will be a stimul[us] for strength and resistance through the body. Make only a small quantity at the time, you see, do not try to keep it over two days. (2794-2)

Case 808 wrote the following:

"In 10 to 15 minutes I obtained relief from using the Glyco-Thymoline packs for sinusitis. The pain is relieved completely, when condition is acute. I use the infrared bulb as a source of heat. This treatment alone pays for my A.R.E. membership in doctor bills saved. The eyes are rested and strengthened. Since breath control is important in meditation, this system is extremely valuable to me in relieving bad sinus conditions.

"In February 1948 I received extracts from 2794–2 regarding Glyco-Thymoline packs when I was suffering with an awful attack, the fourth that winter. It was rather messy, but . . . it opened the congestion in my sinuses, and it was the first time I felt any relief. I continued for about a week and it cleared up completely.

"This past winter whenever I'd feel an attack coming on, I'd heat the Glyco-Thymoline in a glass custard dish set in boiling water and use the packs as hot as I could stand over the temple. Then I put a piece of oilcloth over that, and the heating pad on top of that. I used this for ¾ of an hour. It would clear up immediately any persistent pain in that area and would require several days' treatment to clear up a severe sinus infection.

"I purchased Glyco-Thymoline and began to use same to eliminate the catarrhal condition within the body. After a period of several weeks I noticed a change within the body, the catarrh not being as heavy and frequent as in the past.

"My teenaged daughter is troubled with a sinus problem [see 2794–2], and after sending for the bulletin on health, she tried out the Glyco-Thymoline treatment internally twice a day and externally twice a day. After the third day the stuffiness let up completely and she feels she has had very good results from it." (2794–2 Reports)

The Apple Diet: Directions

Check with your doctor to see if there is any contraindication.

Obtain organic apples, if possible. The Delicious are the easiest of the recommended varieties to find. Both the red and the yellow may be used, although most people prefer the yellow, which contain the most pectin, a

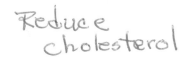

substance that helps to reduce cholesterol. Try to get a colonic on the first day if that service is available in your area.

First Day

Eat as many apples as you like. Most people consume around six to eight apples the first day, four to six the second, and two to four the third. Some people continue to eat eight to ten a day; others as little as one.

If organic, the apples may be eaten with the peel; if not organic, be sure to peel the apples. If you don't like the whole apple, they can be mixed in a blender into uncooked applesauce; this way they are quite tasty and easy to consume. Preferably at the end of the day, have your first colonic, although it can be taken any time the first day.

If there is no colonic service available in your area, you must have an enema at the end of the first or during the second day. Otherwise you may begin to reabsorb the toxins you are throwing off from the lower colon. Be sure to take a fume or steam bath, and try to get a massage and do some general exercise.

Second Day

Have colonic or enema and any number of apples.

Third Day

Continue with apples, another colonic or enema in the evening, if possible.

Olive Oil

Cayce recommended three ways of taking olive oil, but I use only two of them. You may have one tablespoon of olive oil each night and if you prefer you may mix it in hot water, which makes it easier to take if you don't like oil.

The other way is to take two tablespoons of olive oil at the end of the third day.

If you have a history of gallbladder trouble or a liver condition, take the minimum amount of olive oil each day.

gall bladder or liver trouble

Enemas

For directions on how to take the enemas, see below.

Take the first two enemas with salt and soda solution; for the last, use Glyco-Thymoline.

Also it is very helpful to take a fume or steam bath, since the skin is a major organ of elimination. (Consult Chapter 10, on "Hydrotherapy" for directions on how to make a homemade fume bath.)

For my patients, I prefer to use Atomidine in the vaporizer; but some respond equally well to witch hazel or one bath with Atomidine alternated with one with witch hazel.

How to Take an Enema

Prepare the enema can or bag setup. Sterilize the nozzle or tube. For a simple enema, use l quart of lukewarm water and 1 teaspoon each of salt and soda. If we are using the apple diet regimen and wish to obtain results comparable to a colonic, a three-stage enema will be required.

For the simple enema, lie on your left side. Use Vaseline either on the rubber coot that fits over your finger or on the tube, and gradually dilate the rectum, working the Vaseline around.

Control the speed at which the water enters to prevent cramping. If you feel you cannot hold the water, take deep breaths and close the valve until the intense feeling subsides.

After the quart of water has entered, hold as long as possible before expelling. If you do not get satisfactory results, it will be necessary to repeat the procedure until there is evacuation of the descending colon.

Recommended method: Take the first quart of water, as above, on left side. Second stage: Get in a knee-chest position on all fours on the floor and take a second quart of water with the salt and soda mixture. Third stage: After expelling the second stage, rest a moment and then take a third quart, in which you have added one tablespoon of Glyco-Thymoline instead of the salt and soda. Take the last enema lying on your right side.

Get up and walk around before you expel the last enema. It will give you a more thorough cleansing and the Glyco-Thymoline is very good for the mucous lining of the colon and entire intestinal system.—**H.J.R.**

Castor Oil Packs: Directions

Place the cloth in a disposable aluminum baking pan or Pyrex glass or enamel baking pan. Pour castor oil over the cloth until it is well saturated. The pack can be kept permanently in the pan and reheated when and as needed for use. For storage, either the pan or pack can be slipped into a plastic bag. Heat the pan and pack in oven or on electric plate. Be careful to get it only warm—not hot—it will burn easily.

Spread the plastic sheet on the bed to protect the bedclothes. Cover with an old towel or cloth. Apply the pack to the area of the body to be treated. *If it is being used on the abdomen for liver and caecum and ascending colon, be sure to cover the right side as well as the entire abdominal area. If for the spleen and descending colon, favor the left side.*

Next apply a plastic covering over the soaked flannel cloth. On top of that place a heating pad turned up to "medium" and gradually increase to "high" as the pack cools. Wrap a towel folded lengthwise around the entire torso and fasten it with safety pins—big bath or beach towels are excellent for this purpose. The pack usually should remain in place at least one hour, and preferably from one-and-a-half to two hours.

Materials Needed for a Castor Oil Pack

1. Wool flannel cloth (do not use cotton flannel). The size depends on the size of the person and area to be covered when folded in four thicknesses. It should be large enough to cover the area involved. (You can use old wool socks, blankets, or underwear, if light colored wool flannel is not available or is too expensive by the yard.)

   For an abdominal pack: On the average person this would be about 10 inches wide by 12 inches to 14 inches in length. For other parts of the body, the size should be altered, but it must always be four thicknesses of cloth.

2. Plastic sheet—medium thickness (old shower curtain, rubber sheet, or any waterproof material will do).

3. Electric heating pad.

4. Bath towel.

5. Two safety pins.

6. Old plastic covers (those returned by cleaners are excellent).

The skin should be cleansed afterward by using water prepared as follows to avoid a rash, which affects some people. To a quart of water, add two teaspoons of baking soda. Use this to cleanse the abdomen or other treated area.

Store the pack in a baking pan or a plastic bag and reuse. A pack must never be washed. Just add additional castor oil as it dries out from use. It can last for six months to a year. Make up a pack for each member of the family and label each for reuse for the appropriate person. Be sure you use the same pack on the same person once it is made up to the correct size.

Frequency: For general use it is desirable to use the packs three or four nights consecutively, and then not use for three nights.

When taking a series of packs, take two teaspoons of olive oil nightly or two tablespoons after the third night.

Glyco-Thymoline Packs

Use two to three thicknesses of cotton cloth well saturated with Glyco-Thymoline as you purchase it from your druggist. Apply this over the affected areas or those areas specifically directed in your particular case. An electric pad may be used to keep the pack warm. The saturated cotton cloth should be applied first, then a piece of plastic to prevent soiling, and then the heating pad over that with perhaps a towel on top to hold it in place.

This should be applied for twenty to thirty minutes or longer if directed. Do not apply the pack when the Glyco-Thymoline is cold, as in chilly weather. Rather, you might place the bottle of Glyco-Thymoline in a pan of hot water to take the chill off before using it for the pack.

In my experience I have found that in most cases it is unnecessary to heat the pack. Put it on at room temperature.

Mullein Stupes (Packs)

In 1943, Cayce sent me a lady who had been given a reading for a series of hydrotherapy treatments, massage, and electrotherapy with green glass. The lady, about fifty years old, with a close friend, had come from Utah for a series of readings with the "sleeping prophet of Virginia Beach." I was interested in noting in the reading she brought me (5089-1) that Cayce recommended the application of mullein leaves stupes to her legs for her acute phlebitis—just one of a complex of complaints exacerbated by the menopause:

If there continues to be a great deal of trouble with the phlebitis or the swelling, apply Mullein stupes over the limbs once a week and take Mullein tea once a week. This will aid in eradicating the trouble but the pressures that cause same must be removed also.

I have had occasion to be grateful for that advice many times in the intervening years. Besides the mullein tea I have applied the mullein leaves to my own legs for varicose veins with grateful appreciation for the prompt relief they bring. The mullein plant is a velvety broad-leafed weed that we gather along the roadside in the spring; dried mullein as tea is also available from health food stores. The broad leaves are applied directly to the skin.

Cayce Directions for Making Mullein Stupes

We would apply the Mullein Stupes now more to those areas that are the *sources* from which the limbs receive their circulatory activity, and those positions about the limb to reduce the swelling. Apply these about once a day, and for about an hour. The Mullein made into a tea would also be well, but not of the same leaves used on the leg of course! About two ounces of this would be taken each day. (1541-6)

NOTE: If and when mullein stupes are used, use a crock or enamel or glass container for preparing them (*not* tin or aluminum or such.) Also, when applied, use cotton—layers of cotton over same, to preserve the heat—then gauze over that.

These instructions were given in another reading (1541-7) which gave the mullein stupes, so I'm sure they wouldn't hurt here.

Bruise the leaves very thoroughly and dip them in hot water until wilted (usually for one to three minutes). Apply directly to the skin and cover as directed above.

Turpentine Stupes

Instead of Glyco-Thymoline packs for painful menstruation, cystitis, and other vaginal pains, Cayce sometimes recommended turpentine stupes:

. . . over the pubic bone area. This will relieve these tendencies for the stricture in the clitoris and remove the disturbance there; easing the pain when activity of the bladder is desirable. There should be at least 4 or 5 thicknesses of cotton flannel dipped in water in which turpentine has been put; the proportions being a teaspoonful of turpentine in an ounce or two ounces or three to four ounces of hot water. Wring out cloths in this and apply low down over the pubic center. (243-35)

Cayce had a versatile repertoire of packs—many of them are just as rewarding to use as the castor oil for the specific purposes for which they were designed.

Epsom Salt Packs

Dissolve as much Epsom salts—about a pound in a small basin or pot—as will dissolve in the amount of water necessary to saturate a bath towel. Apply as hot as possible over the area indicated. Keep repeating the hot applications for two or three hours at each treatment.

Directions for Making Mullein Tea

Take 2 oz. of the mullein leaves and bruise very thoroughly if the green leaves are used, or 3 oz. of the mullein leaves if the dried leaves are used, and put into a quart of nearly cold water. Let it come to almost a boil, but very slowly. As it comes to the boil, take off. (See 1541-7.)

If possible, instead of repeating the hot applications, use an infrared lamp and then use an electric pad to keep the pack warm until the Epsom salts have completely dried or have become caked in the pack.

(See following pages for appropriate uses of Epsom salt packs.)

Partial List of Other Packs and Their Uses Recommended by Cayce

Alcohol (grain): arthritis, assimilation, asthma, cancer, carbuncles, tuberculosis.

Epsom salt: (used for most cases) adhesions, arthritis, childbirth (aftereffects), colitis, digestion, eliminations, enteritis, feet, fistulas (womb-vagina), flu, gastritis, hemorrhoids, infections, injuries, kidneys, lesions, liver (about twenty-six cases), lumbago, muscles, neuralgia, neuritis, paralysis, rheumatism, sciatica, sinusitis, spine, tic douloureux, toxemia, tumors, uremia, uterus.

Eucalyptus oil: tuberculosis.

Fig: teeth infections.

Fig and milk: dentistry.

Fuller's earth (mud): spine subluxations, tuberculosis.

Glycerine: pelvic disorders.

Glyco-Thymoline: adhesions, arthritis, bronchitis, cataracts, catarrh (nasal), cold congestion, cystitis, cysts, epilepsy, eyes, glands, goiter, hay fever, herpes simplex, injuries, intestines, kidneys, lesions, migraine, paralysis, Parkinson's disease, pelvic disorders (over forty cases), ptomaine poisoning, sciatica, sinusitis, subluxations, throat, tonsillitis, toxemia, tumors.

Grape: colitis, eliminations, food poisoning, gastritis, glands, incoordination, injuries, intestines (gas), nervous systems, pelvic disorders, peritonitis, ptomaine, Recklinghausen's disease, rheumatism, streptococcus, tuberculosis, tumors, typhoid fever, ulcers.

Honey: cysts, hands, infections.

Hot: adhesions, arthritis, assimilation, baldness, cancer, cholecystitis, circulation, dermatitis, elimination, incoordination.

Hot salt: acidity, adhesions, apoplexy, arthritis (sixteen cases), cholecystitis, circulation, colitis, congestion (cold), cystitis, cysts, debilitation (general), dysmenorrhea, ears (abscessed), edema, eliminations, epilepsy, eyes, feet-ankles, gallstones, glands, headache, hemorrhoids, injuries (twelve cases), intestines, iritis, kidneys (ten), lesions (fourteen), liver-kidneys (incoordination), lumbago (eight), lungs, menopause, multiple sclerosis, muscles (sprains), nausea (vomiting), nephritis, nervous system, neuralgia.

Ice: fever.

Kerosene: mumps.

Laudanum: kidneys (strangulation), sinusitis.

Lavoris: cataracts.

Linseed oil: injuries.

Partial List of Other Packs and Their Uses Recommended by Cayce, cont.

Liver: eyes.
Lobelia oil: spine subluxations.
Milkweed: blepharitis.
Mud (boncilla, clasmic clay): acne, complexion.
Mullein: abrasions, boils, cancer tendencies, circulation, dermatitis, femur cancer, lymph, varicose veins.
Myrrh: spine subluxations.
Onion: asthma, bronchitis, common cold, congestion, lungs, pneumonia.
Pine needle oil: epilepsy.
Plantain salve: cysts, injuries, tumors.
Potato (raw): blepharitis (fourteen), blindness, cataracts, eyes (about fifty).
Salt: arthritis, bites, rheumatism.
Salt and apple vinegar: colitis, elimination, injuries, strains.
Salt and spiritus frumenti: general debilitation.
Sand: arthritis, circulation, colitis, debilitation, elimination, lesions.
Sassafras oil: arthritic tendencies, cysts, fistulas, liver, tumors.

The Common Cold

Prevention

The best way to cope with the common cold is to avoid catching it in the first place. If the body is maintained in an alkaline condition (as described in Chapter 5), it will be resistant to cold germs, which, in fact, require an acid environment.

In hundreds of readings Cayce said:

> . . . a body is more susceptible to cold with an excess of acidity *or* alkalinity, but *more* susceptible in case of excess acidity. For, an alkalizing effect is destructive to the cold germ. (902-1)

In addition to wrong eating, fatigue, worry, stress and strain, and other emotional upsets help to produce the acid condition that invites attack from cold germs and other infections.

The controversy concerning the merits and/or demerits of utilizing massive doses of vitamin C for the prevention and cure of colds strikes me as being a tempest in a teapot. This therapy is another effort at restoring the alkaline balance in the body, which should be achieved through correct and balanced diet (see Chapter 5).

There is no mystery or magic about getting rid of a cold once it has been contracted. All therapy aims at alkalizing the body in one way or another and relieving the symptoms of discomfort brought on by the infection.

Cold Therapy

1. Rest is a primary factor in treating a cold, because during rest and sleep, balance is restored to the autonomic nervous system.
2. Stop eating for two days and drink as much liquid as possible—up to one gallon a day. This should be largely citrus fruit juice that is freshly squeezed with the addition of a lemon to orange or grapefruit juice (as described in Chapter 5).

    In addition we have had remarkable success with a folk medicine remedy popularized by Dr. D.C. Jarvis of Vermont. Part of the liquid consumed during the day should be four glasses of water, taken at mealtimes and before going to bed, to which has been added one or two tablespoons of apple cider vinegar and two tablespoons of honey. Also drink large quantities of fenugreek tea.
3. Another good alkalizer, recommended by Cayce, is one teaspoon of baking soda in a glass of water, sipped slowly every hour.
4. Bowel elimination must be complete—either through a colonic or a series of three enemas, two with baking soda and salt, one with Glyco-Thymoline. (Follow directions of the correct positions and proportions described in this chapter.) A half-teaspoonful of a herbal laxative taken every hour until the digestive tract is cleared can also be administered.
5. Percussion massage is very useful in breaking up a cold (a technique we often used on famous singers who had to perform with colds). (If you cannot get to a physiotherapist or massage therapist, a member of the family or friend can administer it following directions in Chapter 9.)
6. Fume baths with Atomidine are most useful in breaking up congestion and stimulating elimination through the lungs and skin. And foot baths, especially mustard foot baths, are useful in colds, grippe, and flu (see Chapter 10, pp. 213-214).
7. Glyco-Thymoline makes an excellent gargle for the throat and spray for the nasal passages, being a natural treatment for mucosity.

For Sore Throat

Apply a cold compress, wrapping it with plastic to keep it airtight and leave on for at least four hours or overnight.—**H.J.R.**

Need your own chickens or purchase from a chicken farm.

Cayce Cough Remedies and Expectorants

Cough Mixture 1:

For any flu or cold, *this* would be well as an expectorant and as an eliminant, and to cause the clearing of hoarseness—made in this way and manner:

Take an egg that has *not* been in the refrigerator or cold storage. Take the white of same. Beat it.

Then, to this white of egg, add:

Juice of one lemon, dropped very slowly into same. About a teaspoonful of Honey, dropped slowly into same also. About *three* drops—one at a time—of Glycerine.

Beat thoroughly together. Of course, it would be worked in together when the Glycerine is added.

Take a teaspoonful every two or three hours.

We will find this will clear a cold, relieve stress through the throat and the nasal passages, bronchi and larynx, and be most helpful for this body.

It would be well for *this* body that sweats be set up by the use of hot pads across the abdomen and across the lower portion of the lung area. These, as we find, should bring the better conditions for this body. Use hot pad or electric pad on the spine or back, and either heavy cloths or a hot water bottle across the abdomen . . .

(Q) Why does flu affect people differently?

(A) Attacks different portions of the body, as just indicated! One may be intestinal flu, or it may be the bronchials; another may be nasal, and one may be lungs, one may be stomach, one may be through the colon. We have all types of same!

Do these for this body. (845-3)

Cough Mixture 2:

As a cough medicine, an expectorant, and for a healing through the whole system, prepare:

Put 2 ounces of strained pure honey in 2 ounces of water and let come to a boil. Skim off the refuse, then add 1 ounce of Grain Alcohol. To this as the carrier, then, add—in the order named:

Syrup of Wild Cherry Bark	1 ounce
Syrup of Horehound	½ ounce
Syrup of Rhubarb	½ ounce
Elixir of Wild Ginger	½ ounce

Shake [the solution] well before the dose is taken, which would be about a teaspoonful—and this may be taken as close together as every hour. It will allay the cough, heal those disturbing forces through the bronchi and larynx, and make for better conditions through the eliminations. (243-29)

Cough Mixture 3:

In making applications for the body in the present, we would take this as an aid for the cold and for assistance in expectoration; this to be taken about

---

The Cayce Inhalant for Clearing Nasal Passages and Throat

To 2 ounces of pure grain alcohol, add . . . *in the order named:*

Oil of Eucalyptus	20 minims
Compound Tincture of Benzoin	15 minims
Rectified Oil of Turp	5 minims
Tolu in Solution	20 minims
Rectified Creosote	3 minims

Shake the solution together, inhale through the nostrils and through the mouth, two or three times, through each, two or three times a day.

(1992-3)

three to four times a day, or at night when there is the tendency for spasms of coughing.

Dissolve 1 ounce of Rock Candy, as a syrup, in a pint of good rye whiskey.
Then add, in the order named:

Syrup of Horehound .... ½ ounce
Glycerine .... 10 drops
Elixir of Lactated Pepsin .... 10 drops

Shake these well together before the dose is taken. (303-25)

Part III

The Cayce/Reilly Beauty Handbook

12

It's Better Off (Excess Weight)

. . . the greatest danger to the health of the American people is obesity.
—**Dr. Louis M. Orr, former president of the American Medical Association**

The longer the belt, the shorter the life.—**Anonymous**

(Q) How may I prevent gain in weight?
(A) This may be done by keeping down the calories, and by the general workout once a week with the masseuse and the hydrotherapy treatment. Also for weight reduction we would follow the grape juice way. (1567-3)

One day, Phil Baker, the well-known comedian of theater and radio, was heard to remark from his perch in a radiant-heat cabinet, "That Reilly lives off the fat of the land."

There was a lot of truth in what he said. The Reilly Health Institute was always filled with professional performers who were motivated by the demands of their careers to keep slim, vigorous, and energetic. They had a public to please.

Today, in our youth-conscious society, everyone has to be a "star"—has to please, not only the public, but also one's own ego, in order to maintain self-respect. Fat in modern America is not funny. Fat is frustrated and rejected, and is very unhealthy.

In my fifty-five years of active practice, I have observed that the same people always seem to be reducing. I often wonder how they and thousands of others manage to remain overweight, in view of all the "miracle" diet books and the thousands of magazine articles published on the subject, reducing salons and spas, clothing and belts that reduce you while you sleep, and other home gadgets, reducing doctors, pills, and diet clubs that abound.

The answer is that they don't. They are eternally taking it off and putting it back on—off and on, off and on—in what Dr. Neil Solomon, secretary of health and hygiene for the state of Maryland and a respected endocrinologist, has labeled aptly the "yo-yo syndrome."

Despite our national preoccupation with youth and slimness, Americans are constantly getting fatter. According to public health reports, we now have 79,000,000 overweight Americans who have generated a $10-billion industry to fight fat. An article in *Esquire* magazine by Grace Lichtenstein[1] reports that Weight Watchers, now an international conglomerate, weighs in at $14.9 million; the various networks of health spas and reducing salons at $220 million; the exercise-equipment market at $1 million; the legal diet-pill market at $54 million; the diet-food market at $1 billion.

Most of the commercially success-ful devices—whether books, gad-gets, pills, or whatever—adver-tise: "no diet, no exercise, no harmful drugs." The fads in re-ducing change so fast that I am sure by the time this book is pub-lished, a host of new books, gad-gets, creams, baths, and other quick, no-effort nostrums wilt be flooding the marketplace and some of those mentioned here will be all but forgotten.—**H.J.R.**

I have before me a collection of a few of the bestselling books of recent times, such as *Dr. Atkins' Diet Revolution*, which has sold millions of copies in hardcover and paperback editions, despite the fact that the American Medical Association has denounced the diet as unsound and potentially dangerous to health; and Dr. Charles Roland of the Mayo Clinic says that its thesis rests on unproven assumptions. Dr. Atkins' "diet revolution" consists of unlimited con-sumption of proteins and fats and virtually no carbohydrates. Patients are instructed to purchase a Ketone stick to test their urine on a daily basis to make sure they are in a state of "ketosis"—a state described in medical diction-aries as "acidosis," occurring sometimes in severe diabetes.

Another bestseller is *The Doctor's Quick Weight Loss Diet*, by Dr. Irwin Maxwell Stillman, often called the "water diet" because the dieter, while permitted to eat unlimited quantities of protein foods and nothing else, must drink eight glasses of water a day to keep from damaging the kidneys or producing other side-effect illnesses.

Dr. Solomon has tried to inject a few medical facts and some common sense into the scene with *The Truth About Weight Control*,[2] and his book has enjoyed a respectable success. But the runaway bestsellers are still the "get-thin-quick and eat-all-you-want" books.

Overweight people can be an optimistic breed, and I could go on and on. *The Ladies Home Journal* and *McCall's* magazine both ran a different diet every month for a year. And other women's magazines feature a diet article in almost every issue. All these diets work—for a while—until the dieters slip back to their old living habits.

As for the sauna belts and garments that are supposed to reduce you effort-lessly as you loll before your TV set or take a nap—they do help you lose water through perspiration, but that will return when you take your first sip of liq-uid. The reduction to the contents of your pocketbook, unfortunately, will be permanent.

Most of the commercially successful devices—whether books, gadgets, pills, or whatever—advertise: "no diet, no exercise, no harmful drugs." The fads in reducing change so fast that I am sure by the time this book is published, a host of new books, gadgets, creams, baths, and other quick, no-effort nostrums will be flooding the marketplace and some of those mentioned here will be all but forgotten.

How many people can recall the 900-calorie drink that was the popular answer to the overweight problem some years ago? Since I am older than most of my readers, I can remember the vogue for machines that jiggle or vibrate the fat off hips and abdomen; the special reducing foods or tablets (eat all you want and this, too); chemicals or salts to put in the bath (drop a spoonful or wishful in the water); powerful laxatives and various types of reducing medi-cation that are now being banned by the FDA. Many of the models who posed for the various reducing advertisements used to keep themselves trim, svelte, and lovely at the Reilly Health Institute with exercise in the gym, massage, baths, and Spartan diets.

A powerful drug was widely advertised some years ago. It was given alone or mixed with other drugs or foods. Without much clinical experimentation, especially of the aftereffects or side effects, this drug was launched on an unsuspecting public. Reducing without effort or diet has an irresistible appeal, except perhaps to a few cynics who "don't believe in Santa Claus." This new drug did have a powerful effect in stimulating the metabolic rate. It did reduce fat—and quickly. It also harmed people who took it. It upset glandular function, caused extreme toxemia, and in some cases resulted in blindness; in other cases, deaths resulting from the use of this reducing drug were reported. It is a sad commentary on human nature that, for the sake of a few dollars, unscrupulous people will use such drastic and fraudulent procedures to fool the uninformed and optimistic overweight public.

Another danger is involved when any inexperienced person operates a therapeutic electric machine. If the machine is on the safe side, it is usually too inadequate to effect much reduction. However, should you follow the diet which comes with most of these machines, you will then be able to give a testimonial to the many pounds you lost. You could very possibly lose the same number of pounds on the diet without the machine. (Also substituting the use of the machine by ten to twenty minutes of active exercise would increase the weight loss and decrease the financial one.)

There are exercising machines that are used for stretching and pulling–and-pushing movements. Some of these are conceived without much knowledge of anatomy. Others offer some help, but they must be used under proper supervision or they can cause back sprain, tearing of the muscles, and rupture of the abdominal wall. They can also influence the breaking down of the valves of the veins. Under proper supervision or when people are physically conditioned to use them, these machines can be of some value. But many people, even after the novelty has worn off and they find they don't reduce as easily as the advertising and literature led them to believe they could, will still have an occasional final fling at reducing. Every few weeks they take the machine from under the bed or from the closet, dust it off, and try it again. The bending and stretching does give them some exercise, and the psychological effect of having a gadget might persuade one to indulge in some physical activity rather than neglect all exercise. This is why this kind of technique can produce results and glowing testimonials. The users' faith in the gadgets or techniques has kept them exercising consistently, and I am all for it. But as long as it is within the range of the capacity of the person, I still say that the best exercises for reducing are the ones you *do*—not the scientific and complicated ones you read about but never attempt. Most medical preparations that you run across or see advertised for weight reduction are a pure gamble, for along with your weight you can lose your health or even your life.

There is actually no easy way to "take it off" once you have put it on. If you wish to stay reduced after taking off excess weight, it requires a radical change of habits and lifestyle, and discipline and know-how. The body is like a bank, and the caloric input must be balanced to the energy outgo for both reduction and maintenance of weight.

The Dangers of Gimmick Weight Loss

One of the greatest hazards to health in trying easy fat reduction is the use of the more powerful drugs and glandular extracts for easy and rapid weight reduction (or should I say destruction?). Some of these preparations contain iodides in various forms. Except in a pathological condition of the goiter (and this is for your physician to decide), the iodides usually damage health as well as reduce weight. The thyroid extracts could, in sufficient quantity, stimulate weight reduction by increasing metabolism. However, this can cause general irritability and severe nervousness and can be an even more serious menace to health. There are also drugs for lessening the appetite, but these have many serious side effects and are not usually recommended by *authoritative* medical sources. Most are unproven as to any benefit, but we know their use can cause very serious negative effects on both the body and the mind.—H.J.R.

There is actually no easy way to "take it off" once you have put it on. If you wish to stay reduced after taking off excess weight, it requires a radical change of habits and lifestyle, and discipline and know-how. The body is like a bank, and the caloric input must be balanced to the energy outgo for both reduction and maintenance of weight. —**H.J.R.**

In looking over the Cayce readings, we seldom find a case in which the problem of obesity is the only etiology. Cayce treated the obesity syndrome in conjunction with cases of toxemia, lack of elimination, poor elimination and assimilation, allergies, psoriasis, diabetes and diabetes tendencies, hypertension, kidney disease, glandular disorders (including incoordination), neurasthenia, heart and vascular disorders, and many other diseases. Cayce probably regarded obesity as a symptom of the malfunctioning of the body that was in the process of causing other diseases as well. —**H.J.R.**

That the public continues to spend billions of dollars to lose weight must mean something. Certainly there are many reasons why it is undesirable to carry excess weight around. Many experiments have established that cutting one's calorie intake and keeping weight down can prolong the life span by 20 percent. Dr. Roy A. Walford, professor of pathology at UCLA, reported to a science writers' seminar that laboratory rats have been kept alive and active for twice their normal life span by reducing their calorie quotas. He said that repeated experiments have determined that low-calorie diets slow down deterioration of body functions, retard the normal loss of immunological factors, and have delayed the well-established high susceptibility period to cancer—from the present sixty-to-seventy age bracket to the late eighties. Overweight and obese individuals not only have a shorter life span, but they are hosts to a wide range of diseases brought on by their lifestyle.

This is why, in looking over the Cayce readings, we seldom find a case in which the problem of obesity is the only etiology. Cayce treated the obesity syndrome in conjunction with cases of toxemia, lack of elimination, poor elimination and assimilation, allergies, psoriasis, diabetes and diabetes tendencies, hypertension, kidney disease, glandular disorders (including incoordination), neurasthenia, heart and vascular disorders, and many other diseases. Cayce probably regarded obesity as a symptom of the malfunctioning of the body that was in the process of causing other diseases as well.

The role of fat in premature death and disease is so acute that Dr. Louis M. Orr, when he was president of the American Medical Association, was quoted in a newspaper interview as saying, "Cancer is the most dreaded disease in the United States. But the greatest danger to the health of the American people is obesity."

The problem is so widespread that it has been estimated that 25 percent of men in their thirties and 35 percent of men in their fifties are about twenty pounds overweight, making them prime victims for heart attacks, strokes, emphysema, and diabetes. The incidence for women is higher, with about 40 percent becoming obese by the time they reach forty. In addition, the AMA points out that, in the overweight, high blood pressure is found twice as frequently as in others; hardening of the arteries occurs three times as often; and diabetes and arthritis are more common.

Corinne H. Robinson, whose *Normal and Therapeutic Nutrition* is a standard textbook for nutritionists and nurses, states: "The prevention and treatment of obesity are among the most perplexing problems facing the physician, the nutritionist, and most especially, the patient himself. The incidence and mortality from degenerative diseases are significantly greater for those who are obese than those who are lean. The popular saying, 'The longer the belt, the shorter the life' is far too true."

Overweight is a physical handicap as well as a primary health hazard. Obese people are more uncomfortable during warm weather because the thick layers of fat serve as an insulator to hold in the heat of the body. More effort must be expended to do a given amount of work because of the increase in body mass. Because of their lessened agility, obese people are more susceptible to accidents. Fatigue, backache, and foot trouble are common complaints of the obese.

Surgery is a double hazard for the overweight and obese.

I have been called in by surgeons to give massage and manipulative therapy to patients who could not heal properly because of their fat. In one particularly memorable case, I was summoned by a surgeon to the Pierre Hotel to help a Mrs. Fernandez. The doctor said in a European accent: "We took her kidney out and the operation was very difficult but successful. But now she can't heal. She is quite heavy and her fat keeps pulling the incision open."

I went to the Pierre, to a magnificent suite with quite a few servants running around, all of them worried and communicating in whispers. There were beautiful hangings and rugs draped over everything. I wondered who Mrs. Fernandez was. It turned out that she was the Dowager Queen of Egypt, King Farouk's mother.

The queen was a Syrian and her face was quite lovely. She had a beautiful bosom, a tiny waist, slender legs, and delicate feet. But she ballooned out at the hips and abdomen like an Oriental vase and the weight of fat was just tearing the wound apart every time she breathed or moved.

Every day for a month and a half, I gave her special massage and manipulation two and three hours at a time to promote circulation. Gradually, the wound started to heal. After that, because I was too busy to keep up this schedule, I sent my sister Violet to look after her. Violet saw her every day and finally the queen wanted to take Violet back to Egypt with her.

Another case was that of Marie Rippe, sixty-eight, who had been bleeding with increasing frequency and volume for eight years. She had been to gynecologists, but they were afraid to operate because of her large pendulous abdomen. The cancer tests were negative. I saw her in March 1973 and she had been bleeding without a stop since January. I came to the conclusion that the bleeding was being caused by the pressure of the fat on her internal organs. She weighed 180 pounds and her height was only five feet—and she carried most of her excess weight in the lower abdomen. I told her that she would have to reduce and she said that was impossible. She had tried almost every known method and just couldn't lose weight.

I was very firm with her and said I would not see her again and could not help her if she did not lose at least a pound a week. I could not give her exercises because of the bleeding, but I gave her special massage and manipulation and instructed her how to prepare and use the Cayce castor oil packs. As for her diet, we had her keep a "diet diary" and then we made an evaluation of it and started to cut down her food intake. Instead of two slices of toast in the morning we cut to one slice. We cut the desserts—in general the quantities of food she was used to eating—and substituted salads for lunch and other modified menus. By August she had lost thirty-two pounds at the rate of one pound a week and she has been able to keep it off. She healed inside and the bleeding stopped. Only occasionally does a spot of blood appear when she stands on her feet too long. Surgery is no longer necessary.

Excessive weight is closely associated with cardiovascular and renal diseases, diabetes, degenerative arthritis, gout, and gallbladder disease. The obese frequently have elevated blood triglycerides and cholesterol, and a reduced carbohydrate tolerance. Obesity entails a respiratory cost in a normal person by increased work of breathing, a decrease in lung volume, and pulmonary hypertension. (In any person with chronic pulmonary disorders, such as emphysema and asthma, obesity greatly increases the respiratory stress.) The hazards of surgery and of pregnancy and childbirth are multiplied.[3]

—Corinne H. Robinson

Why Am I Overweight?

The causes of excess weight are many and varied. Besides the most common causes, overeating and underexercising, it can also be influenced by heredity and geographical environment, racial body type, social and economic conditions, and—less frequently—disease.

The best way to avoid becoming obese is to choose thin parents. Studies reported by Dr. Jean Mayer indicate that it "has been repeatedly shown that obesity runs in families with genetic as well as environmental factors involved. Studies in the U.S. have shown that less than 10 percent of the children of parents of normal weight are obese, but that the proportion rises to 50 percent if one parent is obese and to 80 percent if both parents are obese. Studies of identical and fraternal twins have shown that food habits are not the main factor. Instead of denying the facts of heredity, it would be more intelligent and effective to use them to detect and identify overweight-prone persons and more important to try to prevent the development of obesity in susceptible children. Obesity is more malignant when the onset is early."[4]

Corinne Robinson writes, "The pattern of obesity is often set in infancy when the mother overfeeds the baby in the erroneous belief that a 'fat baby is a healthy baby.' Sometimes overeating becomes a habit with a child . . . during adolescent years food is often used to submerge the many problems that face the boy and girl. The best hope for the prevention of obesity is through greatly expanded programs of nutrition education directed particularly to schoolchildren, teenagers, and mothers."[5]

The tragedy of the "fat-baby myth" is that studies by Dr. Jules Hirsh and his associates at Rockefeller University have demonstrated that it is possible to make an actual count of the number of fat cells in the human body. Dr. Hirsh has concluded that the actual number of fat cells is determined in the first few months of life, and Dr. Jerome L. Knittle, a physician and nutritionist at the National Institutes of Health, has confirmed Dr. Hirsh's work by showing that obese people have a higher number of fat cells than the nonobese and the fat cells are generally bigger than in the nonobese.

According to the work of Doctors Sims and Horton at the University of Vermont School of Medicine, the mother who overfeeds her infant condemns her child to a lifelong sentence as a "fattie" or a life sentence of dieting, hard exercise, and watchful discipline. As the individual gains weight, the fat cells increase in size like a wet sponge. When the sponge is wrung out, however, or the person reduces, although the number of holes in the sponge (or fat cells in the person) remain the same, they gradually empty of water, and fat-cell size is reduced.

Because of our survival pattern, most people have the capacity and the ability to increase the storage content of their fat cells. Those who are born with good digestion have to watch their intake and keep more active physically to maintain normal weight, and as a rule men and women who are born in a favorable environment require less physical activity in their daily living. Environment can also influence weight. If you are raised in a family of hearty eaters and are continually exposed to a bountiful variety of tempting foods, human nature being what it is, you are very likely to overeat. The capacity of the body for assimilation of food also varies with the individual. If your environment offered you a greater variety of food, while it might be conducive to a well-balanced diet, it could also easily encourage you to overeat. The stomach can be conditioned to accept less. Eat less and your stomach will shrink.

Another weight factor can be the geographical formation of the country. The people of countries that are very hilly are usually less obese than those of flat, level countries. Food is generally more abundant and varied in the latter countries and there is a great deal less physical activity. Living in a rough, hilly, or mountainous section usually requires a great deal of strenuous and varied physical activity. While the chest of the mountaineer is usually larger to accommodate more oxygen as the air becomes lighter, there is seldom excess fat on his body—unless an iodine deficiency exists. People living away from the sea, where there is a lack of iodine in the water, soil, and air, will become obese due to lack of this important element. When iodine is lacking, the thyroid gland has a tendency to slow down and the person becomes fat and sluggish. This is called hypothyroidism. It can be prevented by using iodized salt in the daily diet. Medical tests can easily determine if deficiency exists and your physician can advise you on the proper corrective procedures.

Even with a people considered small, a great deal can depend on environment. Most American-born children of undersized and underweight foreign-born parents grow taller and heavier. It has been found that children of smaller and less-heavy races grow much larger in both height and weight when the environment is more favorable. Children of Japanese parents who are born in Hawaii are much larger and heavier than their parents, and Australian-born children of English parents are larger.

With a change from the regimented life of the Old World and the teeming, struggling masses of most of Asia, the minds and bodies of these children have expanded upward and outward.

Another contributing factor in the overall problem of weight control is bone structure. A large, heavy-boned person may register overweight according to the charts, when actually there is not too much fat. Allowances must be made for this on a height-weight chart. However, when these people do put on fat, they usually become very heavy because of the large bone foundation, so they must make special efforts to prevent any accumulation of fat.

Then there is the asthenic type, with a short body and long legs. These people can be within the normal weight range and still have an excess of fat, especially on the abdomen. In the same way, the short-legged, long-bodied type can easily be overweight without having too much fat.

Does this mean that because of your genes and early feeding patterns, which permanently endowed you with more fat cells, you can do nothing about it?

Nonsense. It is harder, to be sure, and you will have to persevere, perhaps work at it for the rest of your life. This is why crash or fad diets and quick-reducing gimmicks are not for you. It is precisely because of the factors of genes and fat cells that you have not been, and will not be, able to stay thin

Environment can also influence weight. If you are raised in a family of hearty eaters and are continually exposed to a bountiful variety of tempting foods, human nature being what it is, you are very likely to overeat. The capacity of the body for assimilation of food also varies with the individual. If your environment offered you a greater variety of food, while it might be conducive to a well-balanced diet, it could also easily encourage you to overeat. —**H.J.R.**

Another contributing factor in the overall problem of weight control is bone structure. A large, heavy-boned person may register overweight according to the charts, when actually there is not too much fat. Allowances must be made for this on a height-weight chart. However, when these people do put on fat, they usually become very heavy because of the large bone foundation, so they must make special efforts to prevent any accumulation of fat. —**H.J.R.**

We all know of people who eat or drink through sheer boredom or as an escape from an unpleasant situation. An unfortunate love affair can cause people to put on a great deal of weight. People who are unhappy or frustrated or lack security find an outlet in the so-called retreat or reward foods. These are usually sweet, fat, rich foods or alcoholic drinks. They simulate the reactions of pleasure that love, affection, and success would supply.—H.J.R.

once you reduce—that is, unless you change your entire lifestyle.

There is a tendency nowadays to blame much of our obesity on our psychological or emotional state. This theory is supported by the fact that the hypothalamus, sometimes referred to as the middle brain, has much to do with our automatic control mechanisms. The hypothalamus is the part of the brain that controls the appetite, known as the appestat. It is interesting that many scientists also believe that it is the part of the brain that acts as a switchboard, translating ideas and emotions into physical action through nerves and hormones.

We all know of people who eat or drink through sheer boredom or as an escape from an unpleasant situation. An unfortunate love affair can cause people to put on a great deal of weight. People who are unhappy or frustrated or lack security find an outlet in the so-called retreat or reward foods. These are usually sweet, fat, rich foods or alcoholic drinks. They simulate the reactions of pleasure that love, affection, and success would supply.

Dr. William McJefferies, a Cleveland endocrinologist and researcher, says, "It is tempting to say, 'Well, because a specific person tends to have overresponsive adrenals this explains his tendency to be a stress eater.' When these people get under tension, they feel better when they eat because their system puts out more of an adrenal secretion called hydrocortisone which tends to increase the appetite. It could also explain the fact that these people seem to prefer carbohydrate foods rather than protein foods. On the other hand, you could turn it around and say, 'This might not be the cause; it might be an effect.'"

If a person is overweight, it may alter his or her body's metabolism so that the adrenals tend to be overresponsive. It is similar to the situation with regard to insulin, a hormone produced by the pancreas. Obese persons, as a group, tend to have overresponsive pancreas glands and produce excessive quantities of insulin. When they eat a certain amount of carbohydrate, they get a higher rise in insulin than a person who is not obese. Which is the cart and which is the horse? It is important to understand that when the obese person, through a normal well-balanced diet, returns to his or her ideal weight, the excretion and the production of adrenal hormone returns to normal.

So when certain individuals blame their overweight or obese condition on their glands, there is a certain amount of truth in their complaint. Their glands are affected, and so are their organs, the coordination of their nervous systems, and everything else in their body processes. But except in rare cases where there is a serious organic malfunction of the thyroid, adrenals, or pancreas, attaining and maintaining normal weight will correct the disorders. In fact, a restricted but balanced diet and adequate exercise are the usual medical treatment for hypoglycemia and other glandular disorders.

The role of exercise and physical activity is often overlooked by the overweight, misguided by bits and pieces of incomplete information.

A discouraged dieter might say, "Well if I can only walk off two calories in one minute, what's the use of bothering?" The two calories become 120 in an hour, and if you increase the speed of walking from 2.5 miles per hour to 3 or 4 miles per hour, you will burn up 5.2 per minute, or 312 calories. (See the activity calorie table at the end of this chapter.))

Moreover, the effect of physical activity on the body chemistry and the appestat mechanism, which affects our feeling of hunger or satiety, is considerable and is now being explored by eminent researchers with interesting results.

Dr. Williams points out in *Nutrition Against Disease:*

> Most of us are born with appestat mechanisms that are, or can be made, entirely serviceable. When they are not serviceable, something may have intervened to make them faulty. Lack of exercise has a crippling effect on appestat mechanisms . . .
>
>   Why is exercise so important for health? We do know that we are built to strive physically for food and other necessities, and that to get these necessities without any striving is not in accord with our biological background. It is probable that improved circulation, which is induced by exercise, is an important factor in promoting well-being. It is also probable that exercise promotes an improvement in the quality of our blood. *Valuable hormonal substances may be released as a result of exercise, and these substances may contribute to an improved cellular environment for the appestat and other mechanisms.*[6])

In any event, the fact remains, as Dr. Yudkin has pointed out, that "the appestat only works well with at least a moderate amount of physical activity. What might be adequate exercise for one individual might be inadequate for another."

Reports confirm the fact that prolonged vigorous exercise or activity can lower blood cholesterol levels. A Swiss physician, Dr. Daniella Gsell, and Dr. Jean Mayer compared the cholesterol levels of the population of a remote Swiss village with those of a control group of Basel, a modern industrial Swiss city. The people of the Swiss village had a high fat intake and, moreover, ate 100 calories more each day than their city cousins. However, they worked very hard and were physically very active, as all supplies into the village had to be carried in by mule or by the residents themselves. Dr. Mayer reports that "the serum cholesterol levels of the physically active men and women in the village were much lower than those of the Basel residents."[7]

The story is the same on this side of the Atlantic. A study comparing mortality from heart disease among railroad employees again showed the importance of activity. The section hands, who do the heavy labor of repairing the roadbed, had a much better record than switchmen (light activity, walking), who, in turn, did much better than the sitting clerks.

Despite the well-known and well-advertised health hazard of excess weight and our cultural preoccupation with youthfulness and slimness, it seems to require very strong motivation to make a person reduce and then stick to a lifestyle that will keep the weight off permanently. If fear were enough of a deterrent, there wouldn't be a cigarette smoker left in the United States today.

Motivation is the key.

I remember one of my first important reducing assignments—with Metro-

Despite the well-known and well-advertised health hazard of excess weight and our cultural preoccupation with youthfulness and slimness, it seems to require very strong motivation to make a person reduce and then stick to a lifestyle that will keep the weight off permanently. If fear were enough of a deterrent, there wouldn't be a cigarette smoker left in the United States today.

Motivation is the key.

—H.J.R.

politan Opera star Beniamino Gigli. He was convinced that he had to have a big stomach and lots of fat to get volume for his voice. Then one day, in *Romeo and Juliet*, he knelt on the stage before his fair Juliet and couldn't get up. That did it. The impresario of the Met at the time told him to reduce—or else. Getting Mr. Gigli to exercise wasn't easy, and to curb his appetite for pasta was a truly Herculean job. I had to shrink him from 245 pounds, at five-foot-nine, to 195, and hold him there so that he could continue to sing the romantic parts he loved.

I kept him in shape for eleven years, and during that time, while reducing, he also cured himself of the arthritis that had forced him to miss many of his performances.

I made Gigli arise at a certain time. If he was still asleep, I'd grab a handful of his midriff and start working then and there. He punched the bag, walked the treadmill, and rode the mechanical horse. Sometimes I had him saw and chop wood, which we gave away to the poor. I sometimes went on tour with him and sat next to him at banquets. When he was eating too much, I'd nudge him with my foot under the table as a gentle reminder that it was time to pause for station identification.

Now, all this was fine for an opera star or other professionals who must reduce for their careers, but what about Suzy Housewife and Joe Bookkeeper? What is their motivation? Each person has to discover what his or her own motivation is. It may be getting a better job—I can assure you if you reduce in a healthful, constructive way, you will have more energy, think more clearly, be able to cope and solve problems, and assuredly be better able to absorb the stress and strain of the competitive life.

It could be pleasing a man—or a woman.

For a long-married woman it could mean fitting into a sexy dress—the kind you have not been able to wear for many years or since your wedding. Go out and buy it—hang it up where you will constantly see it, and look forward to the day when you can wear it.

For husband and wife, the motivation could be a second honeymoon or a trip or the purchase of a new car—some reward that you will enjoy once you have achieved your goal.

Write it down—not only the weight you want to achieve but the reward that awaits you when you reach your goal. Paste it on the refrigerator door to remind you each time you are tempted. Also to inspire you, paste on the refrigerator—and the food-storage cupboards, too—a picture of yourself in your younger years, when you were slimmer.

If you meditate or pray, visualize yourself as you want to be and read some of the inspirational affirmations that abound in the Cayce literature or that of other seers.

Remember: anyone can reduce. Stop eating. In some sections of the world, many of the inhabitants are chronically underweight. The average person, if not panicked by fear, could find it possible to do without food for twenty to thirty days, and some records show that it can be for as long as seventy days. But we who have access to food of many tempting varieties that appeal to our vision, sense of smell, and other pleasant associations that go with eating must apply discipline somewhere along the line. Except in a very few cases of glandular abnormality we gain weight because of the simple fact that the intake is greater than the outgo.

Putting on fat is a storage mechanism of the body. It was useful in primitive times to tide the body over during famine, for in those times eating was largely a matter of feast or famine. The fat storage was necessary for survival when food was scarce, and no doubt the extra fat that forms on the well-rounded and pleasing contours of the female figure was useful for storing reserves for the mother and potential child. Methods of storing and preserving food have improved as civilization advanced, but the capacity of the body to store fat has remained and the physical energy formerly required to obtain food is no longer necessary. Therefore, to reduce permanently you will have to increase your output of physical energy and decrease your input of food energy (which means calories).

First, check with your physician or a specialist in endocrinology to detect any abnormalities. If there are none, you are ready to begin your R[esolution] I[nformation] P[erseverence] reducing program. Cayce and I will supply the "information." You must provide the "resolution" and the "perseverance."

It is important to have a scale on which you can weigh yourself the first thing every morning. Make each day a reducing day by careful attention to diet and exercise. Plan recreation that involves physical activity.

Start keeping a "diet diary." Write down every mouthful of food you normally consume and add up the calories, the carbohydrate content, and the content of other nutrients. Calorie and carbohydrate counters are widely available for a small cost at many stores. Nutrient charts can be obtained from the Department of Agriculture at the address given in Chapter 5.

Depending on your starting weight and general condition, a loss of from one to two pounds per week is a good goal to aim for. Greater reduction is possible but not desirable without supervision.

Remember, there is inside fat holding the abdominal organs in place. There is a structural factor to be considered in weight loss. If you reduce too rapidly, before you have had time to develop muscle tone to substitute for the fat, it can result in a prolapsis (dropping of the organs of the abdomen).

You will have to cut your calories by 3,500 a week to lose one pound; by 7,000 to lose two pounds. From this basic figure you can subtract the calories you spend on exercise and physical activity. Consult the table at the end of this chapter for the number of calories you burn in various physical activities. I have had patients take off as much as 108 pounds following the regimen described here.

You will also have to take your measurements to determine and type your figure.

Measurements can be taken about once a week at the beginning, and if the weight reduction is satisfactory, about every two weeks of the first six weeks. Taking your own measurements is a tricky procedure. You must always be sure to measure the parts at the exact spot and use the same amount of ten-

You will have to cut your calories by 3,500 a week to lose one pound; by 7,000 to lose two pounds. From this basic figure you can subtract the calories you spend on exercise and physical activity. Consult the table at the end of this chapter for the number of calories you burn in various physical activities. I have had patients take off as much as 108 pounds following the regimen described here.—**H.J.R.**

sion on the tape. It is very easy to let your enthusiasm get the better of your accuracy. In fact, you might even subconsciously cheat on an inch or so. Be sure to use what is known as a seamstress tape, which is made of oilclothlike material that won't expand or contract and is unaffected by heat, cold, wet-ness, or dryness.

Now for the facts on different types of figures that the tape measure will tell. Let's begin with the male figure. We consider a man to have a good figure when the chest is at least five inches larger than the waist and the hips one-half of that difference or two and one-half inches less than the chest. The abdomen should not be over two inches larger than the waist, and one inch would be better. This would produce the following average measurements:

| Chest | 40" | Abdomen | 37" |
| Waist | 35" | Hips | 37½" |

For a very good physique and figure we would like to have the chest eight to ten inches larger than the waist, with the hips in the same proportion as in the chart. This is not easy to attain, but we have accomplished this with a great many men, including some over the half-century mark in age.

Now for the women. The first is a composite form of several high-fashion models whose figures you may have seen hundreds of times dressed in the most glamorous creations of well-known designers:

Weight	117 lbs.	Bust	33"
Height	5' 9"	Waist	23"
Neck	12"	Hips	32"
Upper Arm	9"	Thighs	19½"
Wrist	6"	Ankle	8"

Then we have the more substantial figure that is fairly suitable for the young matron. She might try for a slimmer figure, but if she will retain the same measurements and proportions in relation to her height and weight to her eightieth birthday, it is all right with me:

Age	25 to 35	Bust	35"
Height	5' 6"	Waist	27"
Weight	133 lbs.	Abdomen	30"
Arm	11½"	Hips	37"
Ankle	9½"	Thighs	21½"

In the older-matron type, there are some measurements that will keep one looking well in clothes and even in a bathing suit. These figures have made some concession to age and the accumulations that are part of growing older, but if you condition into these measurements to start with, there is no law to prohibit you from working into the "young matron" or "fashion model" group:

Age	35 to ???	Bust	37"
Height	5' 5½"	Waist	28" to 30"
Weight	138 to 148 lbs.	Abdomen	32" to 35"
Arm	12"	Hips	39"
Ankle	10"	Thighs	22½"

On the basis of life-insurance statistics the most nearly ideal weight to maintain throughout life is that which is proper at age twenty-five for one's height and body build.

—H.J.R.

(The term "overweight" is applied to persons who are 10 to 20 percent above desirable weight. Obesity is applied to persons 20 percent or more over desirable weight.)

On the basis of life–insurance statistics the most nearly ideal weight to maintain throughout life is that which is proper at age twenty–five for one's height and body build. (Consult the accompanying tables from the Metropolitan Life Insurance Company and note that desirable weights under current conditions are somewhat lower than those shown in the tables prepared by the same company in the early 1940s.)

The Cayce readings have given us two superb reducing aids—the three–day apple diet and grape juice in water (taken four times a day, a half–hour before meals and before bedtime).

If there will be a change in the diet or the application of foods for reducing the weight, we will aid much in more normalizing the weight, for there is the tendency for high blood pressure throughout the body.

We would use first the apple diet to purify the system; that is, for three days eat nothing but apples of the Jonathan variety if possible. This includes the Delicious, which is a variety of Jonathan. The Jonathan is usually grown farther north than the Delicious but these are of the same variety, but eat some. You may drink coffee if you desire, but do not put milk or cream in it, especially while you are taking the apples.

At the end of the third day, the next morning take about two tablespoons of Olive Oil.

Then begin with taking . . . about one-half hour before each meal and before retiring at night, three ounces of grape juice in one ounce of plain water.

Do not take any carbonated drinks. Cut down on sweets, but if you wish, honey may be taken or honeycomb at times, but not too much of this either . . .

(Q) What about the remainder of the diet?
(A) Just a normal diet. Cut down on the sweets and do have more of the leafy vegetables. (780-l2)

Here in reading 1268-1 Cayce spells out the diet in greater detail:

Mornings—citrus fruits. Brown toast, whole wheat, of cereals (not at the same meal with the citrus fruits). Do not use cow's milk in same . . .
Noons—only vegetables; these may be combined.

Evenings—have either all leafy vegetables, well-cooked, or else have same with a little chicken, fowl, or fish, or potatoes and lamb. (1268-1)

In the Diet . . .

In the diet: Abstain from great quantities of starches. Most of the breads (if any are taken) should be of the Rye Bread or Ry-Krisp. One meal each day should consist of green raw vegetables. No potatoes with meats. No starches that have the greases should be taken at the same time with meats. Use grape juice rather than water; and whether this is two, three, four, five glasses a day, let it be taken with half water (not carbonated water) and half pure grape juice. (1339-1)

Edgar Cayce on Obesity

Other Cayce comments on obesity are consonant with current scientific and nutritional knowledge:

(Q) Are there any exercises that I can take to keep my weight down that will not be detrimental to my back?
(A) Take grape juice regularly four times each day, about half an hour before each meal and before retiring. Use three ounces of pure grape juice (such as Welch's) with one ounce of plain water, not carbonated water. This with the sweats or baths will keep down the weight as well as remove poisons.
(3413-2)

(Q) Why should the body take Grape Juice?
(A) To supply the necessary sugars without gaining or making for greater weight. (457-8)

(Q) Why is it hard to increase weight in portions [of the body] and decrease it in others?
(A) The natural tendency or trend in the development of the foetus forces in its inception, and then the general activities have been in these directions. This would go more into the psychological than the pathological conditions, to be sure, as we have indicated through these sources respecting the associations throughout the sojourn of the entity and its bodily forces in the earth. (288-38)

Preventing Weight Gain

Cayce recommended massage and hydrotherapy for keeping down weight:

(Q) How may I prevent gain in weight?
(A) This may be done by keeping down the calories, and by the general work-out once a week with the masseuse and the hydrotherapy treatment.
    Also for weight reduction we would follow the grape juice way; that is:
    Half an hour before each meal and at bedtime, drink two ounces of Grape Juice (preferably Welch's) in one ounce of plain water (not carbonated water).
    Keep away from sugars, pastries and the like.
    These will keep better conditions in the assimilation and elimination also.
(1567-3)

In my own practice I have found that repetition of the apple diet four times a year and a regimen of balanced, restricted eating, following the Cayce grape juice diet, exercise, baths, and colonics, invariably works. I have scores of patients who have reduced and who stay reduced, and I have kept my own weight down following my own advice.

Professor R.H. from Illinois was terribly overweight. She taught singing and had chronic trouble with her sinuses, a nasal drip, and a sore throat. She went to a doctor in New Jersey for the nose and throat condition and was told to reduce. She came to the Reilly Institute at Rockefeller Center and, after it closed, began coming to my New Jersey home two or three times a year for the apple-diet cleansing regimen to keep her weight down and her sinuses clear and fit, so that she could teach and sing. Now, after twenty-five years she is still teaching and says: "I feel younger and much more alert than in my forties. In the process of improving my health with the massage and exercise Dr. Reilly taught me, I was able to resolve a severe condition of diverticulitis."

I would like to take exception to a feature found in most reducing diets: permission to drink unlimited amounts of black coffee. This is counterproductive for the reducer who, by following such a course, will suffer more acutely than ever from hunger. Dr. E.M. Abrahamson in *Body, Mind, and Sugar* presents the scientific reasons why this is so:

> Overindulgence in sweets tends to sensitize the islands of Langerhans by subjecting them to repeated stimulation and exercise. Caffeine stimulates the adrenal cortex to produce more of its hormones, which in turn induce the liver to break down glycogen into glucose, which flows into the bloodstream. This is why a cup of coffee "gives you a lift." Trouble develops because the islands of Langerhans cannot distinguish between the effects of drinking coffee and eating food. They don't know and don't care whether the sugar has come from the food that is being digested or from previously stored glycogen, broken down by the action of the caffeine's stimulus to the adrenal cortex. To the islands of Langerhans sugar is sugar. They go to work to force the blood sugar to its normal level. In the course of time, because of their repeated stimulation, the islands become so sensitive that they overrespond to a normal stimulus.[8]

Obviously, then, anyone trying to lose weight who drinks black coffee to quiet the pangs of hunger is only making matters worse for him- or herself. The repeated stimulus to the islands of Langerhans makes them more sensitive, and the resultant low blood sugar only makes the rigid diet more onerous. Dieting to reduce is much easier if coffee, as well as caffeine in other forms (such as strong tea, chocolate, and soft drinks containing this alkaloid) is excluded.

In closing, I would like to share an amusing but significant conversation I once had with a multimillionaire client who had been coming to the Reilly Health Institute for about twenty years. He took colonics, sweat baths, massages, Scotch douches—all the passive therapies we offered. He had a low pot-belly, and one day while I was giving him a massage, he patted it and said: "Dr.

Preventing Weight Gain
Cayce recommended massage and hydrotherapy for keeping down weight:

(Q) How may I prevent gain in weight?
(A) This may be done by keeping down the calories, and by the general workout once a week with the masseuse and the hydrotherapy treatment.

Also for weight reduction we would follow the grape juice way; that is:

Half an hour before each meal and at bedtime, drink two ounces of Grape Juice (preferably Welch's) in one ounce of plain water (not carbonated water).

Keep away from sugars, pastries and the like.

These will keep better conditions in the assimilation and elimination also. (1567-3)

In my own practice I have found that repetition of the apple diet four times a year and a regimen of balanced restricted eating, following the Cayce grape juice diet, exercise, baths, and colonics, invariably works. I have scores of patients who have reduced and who stay reduced, and I have kept my own weight down following my own advice.—**H.J.R.**

H.J., I have been coming here for twenty years and I still have a potbelly. Aren't you ashamed? Why don't you do something about it?"

I replied, "Yes, Mr. X., but I could never get you to exercise. You are a very smart man and a great business executive and you have thousands of people working for you and your company, but there is just one thing you never figured out: how you could hire somebody to exercise for you."

No one can do it for you, but anyone can reduce. Just stop eating more than you work off—half of the world population is underweight because they don't get enough to eat.

Dieter's Food Choices

1. The following foods should be included in your diet:
   (a) All kinds of raw vegetables, such as asparagus, watercress, chard, mustard greens, kale, celery, lettuce (leaf or romaine), string beans, oyster plant (salsify), carrots, tomatoes, green peppers, radishes, etc.

   These may be eaten with gelatin. This should be Knox Gelatine, taken a minimum of three times per week, but better daily. Use the Knox Gelatine recipes; the gelatin may also be taken with tomato juice or other juices. (Gelatin has been called a catalyst in the body, helping it make use of the vitamins and other properties of vegetables and fruits.)
   (b) Black bread in limited quantity (pumpernickel, rye, or whole wheat; other whole or sprouted grain).
   (c) Nuts, especially almonds and filberts (raw nuts are better than those roasted and salted), seeds (such as pumpkin, sunflower, sesame), once a week as a meat substitute.
   (d) Fish and other seafoods, fowl, lamb, wild game, liver.
   (e) Vegetable juices, citrus fruit juices, at times when cereal is not eaten. Grape juice to be taken four times daily and at bedtime as directed later in this chapter under "Model Reducing Diet Plan."
   (f) Citrus fruits, berries.
   (g) Cooked leafy vegetables, oyster plant (salsify), parsnip, potato peelings from the baked potato, but not the bulk of it.
   (h) Jerusalem artichoke once each week (this is a root).
   (i) A great deal of watercress and beet tops (these especially help the eliminations).
   (j) Most fruits may be eaten, preferably fresh. (Apples should be cooked or baked except on raw apple diet.) Melons should be eaten alone.

2. The following foods should be avoided:
   (a) Fruits: raw apples, bananas.
   (b) Starchy vegetables.
   (c) Fried foods, fats, pork of any kind, including bacon.
   (d) Malt drinks, carbonated waters (i.e., in any soft drinks).
   (e) Alcohol, spices, or other stimulants.

Model Reducing Diet Plan, Based on Cayce-Reilly Principles of Diet and Nutrition

Grape Juice: Four times per day, thirty minutes before meals and at bedtime, drink at least 4 ounces of a combination of grape juice and water—3 ounces of grape juice to 1 ounce of water. Be sure the grape juice is natural and unsweetened, such as Welch's. When used over a period of time, this will help the digestion and the elimination and help one to lose weight.

Bread and Cereal: Limit bread to 1 or 2 slices daily or 1 slice of bread and one 3/4 cup serving of dry or 1/2 cup cooked whole grain cereal. Use *whole grain breads only.*

BREAKFAST Citrus fruits—combine 4 parts orange or grapefruit juice with 1 part lemon or lime, or one grapefruit or juice of two or three oranges. *Never combine citrus fruit with cereal.*

If having citrus fruit, have 1 coddled egg; 1 slice dry toast. If having cereal, have fruit juice or other fruits between meals.

Coffee substitute or Ovaltine or cereal drink. (Use very little coffee, tea, or milk. No coffee at all is better.)

LUNCH All raw vegetable salad with any oil dressing, or vegetable-gelatin salad (see recipe in Chapter 5, page 87)
                    or
Vegetable soup (no fat or starchy vegetables); herb tea.

DINNER Fish, fowl, occasionally lean lamb, nuts, or legumes, broiled, baked, roasted—never fried.

Cooked vegetables—no tuberous roots, although potatoes may be taken one or two times per week; eat only the skins and potato nearest the skin, discard the rest.

Have any of the green vegetables cooked that grow above the ground—cooked—use very little butter or fats. You may have two 3% carbohydrate vegetables and one small salad or one 5% carbohydrate vegetable and one 3% vegetable or salad.

DAIRY PRODUCTS: 4 ounces of buttermilk or yogurt daily—not taken with any food—eaten alone for a meal or between meals.

Once a week you may substitute one 3-ounce serving of ice cream for one milk and one fat. Herb teas may be taken with any meal—you may use 1 teaspoon of honey one or two times a week. Fruit or fruit juice may be taken between meals when not on breakfast menu.

FATS: One may have 1 tablespoon of oil (preferably seed oil) on salad one to three times weekly. You may substitute 1 teaspoon butter or nut butter for oil.

AVOID: Starches, fats, sugars, and sugar products (pastries, candy, syrups, honey, etc.), dried fruits, alcohol, carbonated drinks, spices (except herbs).

3% Carbohydrate Low-Starch Vegetables

Asparagus	Lettuce
Bamboo shoots	Mung bean sprouts
Beet greens	Mushroom
Broccoli	Mustard greens
Cabbage	Mustard spinach
Cauliflower	Okra
Celery	Radish
Chicory greens	Rhubarb
Cocozelle, zucchini	Snap beans
Collards	Spinach
Cress	Summer squash: yellow, scallop
Cucumber	Sweet pepper
Eggplant	Swiss chard
Endive (escarole)	Tomato
Fennel	Turnip
Green beans	Watercress
Kale	Zucchini, cocozelle
Kohlrabi	

5% Carbohydrate Starchy Vegetables

Beans: red, white, pinto, calico, lima, mung	Rice
	Rye grain
Chestnuts	Sweet potato
Corn	Wheat grain
Cowpeas	Winter squash: acorn, butternut, hubbard
Peas	
Potato	Yams

The Metropolitan Life Insurance Weight Table

Ideal, lowest mortality weight, ages 25-59

Height & Weight Table for Women

Height	Small	Medium	Large
	Frame		
4' 10"	102-111	109-121	118-131
4' 11"	103-113	111-123	120-134
5' 0"	104-115	113-126	122-137
5' 1"	106-118	115-129	125-140
5' 2"	108-121	118-132	128-143
5' 3"	111-124	121-135	131-147
5' 4"	114-127	124-138	134-151
5' 5"	117-130	127-141	137-155
5' 6"	120-133	130-144	140-159
5' 7"	123-136	133-147	143-163
5' 8"	126-139	136-150	146-167
5' 9"	130-142	139-153	149-170
5' 10"	132-145	142-156	152-173
5' 11"	135-148	145-159	155-176
6' 0"	138-151	148-162	158-179

Height & Weight Table for Men

Height	Small	Medium	Large
	Frame		
5' 2"	128-134	131-141	138-150
5' 3"	130-136	133-143	143-153
5' 4"	132-138	135-145	142-156
5' 5"	134-140	137-148	144-160
5' 6"	136-142	139-151	146-164
5' 7"	138-145	142-154	149-168
5' 8"	140-148	145-157	152-172
5' 9"	142-151	148-160	155-176
5' 10"	144-154	151-163	158-180
5' 11"	146-157	154-166	161-184
6' 0"	149-160	157-170	164-188
6' 1"	152-164	160-174	168-192
6' 2"	155-168	164-178	172-197
6' 3"	158-172	167-182	176-202
6' 4"	162-176	171-187	181-207

MetLife

THE ENERGY COST OF ACTIVITIES

Activity	Calories per pound per hour	Activity	Calories per pound per hour
Bedmaking	1.9	Piano playing (Mendelssohn's *Song Without Words*)	0.9
Bicycling (century run)	4.0		
Bicycling (moderate speed)	1.6	Piano playing (Beethoven's *Appassionata*)	1.1
Boxing	5.7		
Carpentry (heavy)	1.5	Piano playing (Liszt's *Tarantella*)	1.4
Cello-playing	1.1	Reading aloud	0.7
Cleaning windows	1.7	Rowing	5.0
Crocheting	0.7	Rowing in race	7.8
Dancing, moderately active	2.2	Running	3.7
Dancing rhumba	2.8	Sawing wood	3.1
Dancing waltz	1.9	Sewing, hand	0.7
Dishwashing	0.9	Sewing, foot-driven machine	0.8
Dressing and undressing	0.8	Sewing, electric machine	0.7
Driving car	0.9	Singing in loud voice	0.9
Eating	0.7	Sitting quietly	0.7
Exercise		Skating	2.1
very light	0.9	Skiing (moderate speed)	5.2
light	1.1	Standing at attention	0.8
moderate	1.9	Standing relaxed	0.7
severe	3.0	Sweeping with broom, bare floor	1.1
very severe	4.0	Sweeping with carpet sweeper	1.2
Fencing	3.8	Sweeping with vacuum sweeper	2.2
Football	3.6	Swimming (2 mi. per hr.)	4.1
Gardening, weeding	2.3	Tailoring	0.9
Golf	1.2	Tennis	2.8
Horseback riding, walk	1.1	Typing rapidly	1.0
Horseback riding, trot	2.5	Typing, electric typewriter	0.7
Horseback riding, gallop	3.5	Violin playing	0.8
Ironing (5-lb. iron)	1.0	Walking (3 mi. per hr.)	1.4
Knitting sweater	0.8	Walking rapidly (4 mi. per hr.)	2.0
Laboratory work	1.5	Walking at high speed (5.3 mi. per hr.)	4.3
Laundry, light	0.6		
Lying still, awake	0.5	Washing floors	1.0
Office work, standing	0.8	Writing	0.7
Organ playing (1/3 handwork)	1.2		
Painting furniture	1.2	Walking down stairs, calories per pound per 15 steps	0.011
Paring potatoes	0.8		
Playing cards	0.7	Walking up stairs, calories per pound per 15 steps	0.034
Playing table tennis	2.5		

Adapted from "Foundations of Nutrition," 6th edition, by Clara Mae Taylor and O. F. Pye.
Copyright © 1996, Macmillan Publishing Co., Inc.

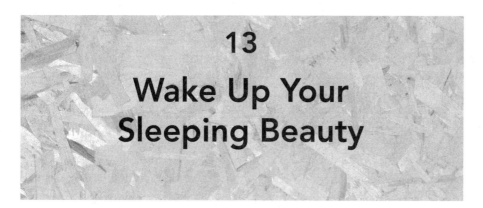

13
Wake Up Your Sleeping Beauty

If we would have life, give it. If we would have love, make ourselves lovely. If we would have beauty within our lives, make our lives beautiful. If we would have beauty in body or mind, or soul, create that atmosphere, and that which brings about life itself will bring those [same] forces [into the experience]. (2096-1)

While it is true that only God can make a tree or a great beauty, humanity's ingenuity, labor, and know-how have made deserts bloom. Similarly, every woman can become beautiful, every man attractive, if the desire, the will, the motivation, and the discipline are strong enough.

Marilyn Monroe, the idealized goddess of beauty and sex, was well endowed by nature and God to begin with. Nevertheless, plastic surgery helped to create a more harmonious contour for her face. As for her legendary bosom, there is a story about that which explains how Marilyn became an important pin-up girl at Reilly's Health Service and a source of inspiration to many of our clients.

During the time when author Maurice Zolotow was working hard with me at the institute to put some weight and muscle on his tall, angular frame and finally gained fifty pounds in all the right places, one of the ingredients in our mutual success was Marilyn Monroe's bosom—and this is how it happened.

Maurice came one day to Rockefeller Center and told me that he was flying to California to interview Marilyn Monroe—an interview that eventually led to the first full-length biography about her.[1] Maurice asked if I had any suggestions to offer for questions he might ask her. At that time I had never met Marilyn Monroe personally, but I was so sure of my surmise about her that I replied, "Yes, you might ask her to show you her gymnasium and the dumbbells or other equipment she uses to keep that forward look in her bosom and any other beauty secrets she would like to share with others."

Zolotow was a little surprised. "How do you know she uses dumbbells or does anything at all for the bosom?" he countered.

"Well, you just take my word for it and assume she does and ask her," I insisted. "I'll bet you anything you want that she does, and if I win you will have to stick with me until I put fifty pounds on you."

I won my bet, and Zolotow won his fifty pounds, for he did learn that Marilyn Monroe had a well-equipped gymnasium in her home and that she worked out with dumbbells of varying weights at least twice a day, paying particular attention to chest- and bust-developing exercises—a beauty secret we will share with you. Her example was a great psychological inspiration to Maurice with his own problem, and subsequently I used this story to encourage many other clients when flesh and spirit flagged.

While we acknowledge that true beauty comes from within, from the beauty of the soul—and, as Emerson said, "There is no beautifier of complexion, or form, or behavior, like the wish to scatter joy and not pain around us"—there is nothing wrong with beautifying the temple in which that soul dwells.

Edgar Cayce often admonished us that "the body is the temple" and that one need not be vain or frivolous in caring for it and making the most of it.

In reading 3350-1 he recommended the following for the teenager, particularly addressing himself to girls:

> . . . in such a program . . . include first, spiritual education, next physical—that of exercise, that of proper dress, proper tone of hair, proper care of hair, proper care of body, proper activities that will bring out the better attributes of each individual. For all may have heads and eyes, feet and arms, and a body, yet all may put them to different usages . . .
>
> Physical, mental, spiritual education, social activities all should be to one purpose, not too much of the satisfying of the emotions, but that the body as the temple of the living God may be a more beautiful place for thine own worship . . .

Moreover, the Cayce readings are replete with advice and remedies for all aspects of achieving and maintaining a more beauty-full body—care of the complexion; remedies for skin blemishes, hair, baldness, and dandruff; and care of the nails (even down to ingrown toenails) and the feet. In short, the Cayce readings offer a cosmetic guide that can enhance the beauty of any girl or woman who utilizes all the information of the Cayce CARE program outlined in preceding chapters to improve her health without which no one can achieve greater beauty, plus the beauty tips in this chapter.

To wake up your sleeping beauty and emerge as a new more beauty-full you, you will need to get out a notebook and pencil and take an honest inventory of your assets and faults. No matter what they are, your beauty program should begin with a thorough internal "housecleaning," utilizing the techniques outlined in Chapter 11. No one can have a glowing, clear complexion, gleaming hair, bright eyes, well-groomed nails, or a more beautiful figure when loaded with toxins.

Here I would like to remind you of Edgar Cayce's important admonition about taking time out to tend the body:

> . . . choose three days out of some week in each month—not just three days in a month, but three days in some definite week each month—either the first, the second, the third or the fourth week of each month—and have the general hydrotherapy treatments, including massage, lights, and all the treat-

thyroid problems

ments that are in that nature of beautifying, and [for] keeping the whole of the body-forces young. (3420-1)

Diet will play a very important role in helping your chrysalis of beauty emerge into a beautiful butterfly. Adequate protein, correct amounts of carbohydrates and fats, vitamins, and minerals are all needed to rebuild the trillions of cells of the body. Cayce pointed out time and again—and his theories have been confirmed by science—that lackluster hair, baldness, dull eyes, and brittle, breaking fingernails are due primarily to an improperly functioning thyroid gland and inadequate assimilation, elimination, and circulation:

From the unbalanced chemical forces through the system, or lack of sufficient iodine in the system, we find that the thyroids particularly are the upsetting disturbances.

All of these are the outgrowth, or disturbance through the glandular force causing portions of the body—or the functionings in the body, especially as related to the superficial circulation—to give disturbances. (2936-1)

So you see it is important to have a physical checkup by your doctor and have your thyroid checked with any one of the good current metabolic tests. Further, reread Chapter 5, on diet and nutrition, refer to its charts, and plan to change your diet habits so that you choose foods that feed your beauty as well as satisfy your appetite.

Posture

Recently a mass circulation weekly newspaper carried a feature asking a prominent male television star what would be the first thing he would notice about a young woman who would be waiting for him at the airport to escort him to the local CBS television station.

"I think there's nothing lovelier than to see a woman walking tall as though she had the whole world in the palm of her hand," the star replied.

I agree that true beauty announces itself with good posture. Posture proclaims to the world your own psychological image of yourself, and the world is all too ready to take you at your own slumping word and assist you in every way to realize the image of failure. Conversely, if you stand tall and carry yourself like a queen, the world will treat you like one.

Habits of good posture are best started in childhood. Correction of poor posture is especially important when the child has been subject to illness, malnutrition, or emotional setbacks. When any such weaknesses are corrected, or at least minimized, encourage the growing child to walk high, stand high, and sit high. (It might start him or her thinking high.) It will be a positive factor in a growing body, mind, and spirit.

Begin to instill a pride of posture in your children at the age of ten. It can be a very important factor in their general health and well-being as they grow into adolescence. Frequently, at this time, there is a sudden increase in height.

Cayce pointed out time and again—and his theories have been confirmed by science—that lackluster hair, baldness, dull eyes, and brittle, breaking fingernails are due primarily to an improperly functioning thyroid gland and inadequate assimilation, elimination, and circulation. **—H.J.R.**

I agree that true beauty announces itself with good posture. Posture proclaims to the world your own psychological image of yourself, and the world is all too ready to take you at your own slumping word and assist you in every way to realize the image of failure. Conversely, if you stand tall and carry yourself like a queen, the world will treat you like one.

—H.J.R.

While the muscles are being adapted and strengthened, try to help the child by encouraging the child to keep his or her head up, shoulders back, and spine straight and tall. Do this by explanation, example, and some postural exercise—not by criticism and nagging. Also, in these years, many girls think they are growing too tall and thus assume a sloppy posture to minimize their height. Please tell them to be proud of their height. You might even add that our finest and highest-paid models are the long-stemmed "American beauties," many nearly six feet tall. Parents should also warn the growing girl not to attempt to hide the natural development of her body. Hanging the head and crouching the body does terrible things to both appearance and spirit and retards the normal function of the glands and organs. At this time of their lives, providing an example while understanding and guiding these boys and girls in games and posture exercises will definitely improve their health, appearance, and morale. Assistance from a teacher might be required.

Point out to the boy the fine, manly appearance that good posture will give him; and to the girl how much more attractive she can be with her head held high, balancing a lovely straight, upright figure.

In Chapter 7, I discussed the subject of posture at some length and in the same chapter you will find the exercises that will help you achieve a regal posture. (See exercise numbers on page 275 of this chapter.)

Next we come to the figure contours. It would be foolish and impossible to lay down a rule of so many inches for your bust, waist, hips, legs, and arms, for we are somewhat restricted by the type of body we were born with. We have tried to give you some measurement guides for various figure types in Chapter 12 on weight control. However, busts can be enlarged, waists and hips and legs whittled, and height increased for a more harmonious whole. Kathleen Henderson of the Barbizon School of Modeling says that the ideal standard of proportions is that bust and hips should be the same; for a model's proportions, the waist needs to be ten to twelve inches smaller. For the average woman, eight inches smaller for the waist is quite adequate.

If you are overweight, you will have to begin an overall reducing program, cutting back on food and increasing exercise before working on your reshaping and recontouring.

Redesigning Figures

It is possible to increase or decrease any part of the figure, except the head. (I disregard figurative references to swelled heads and the like.) With most people, the body is extremely adaptable to physiological and psychological change. It is this adaptability mechanism that has enabled the human race to inhabit almost all parts of the world from the arctic wastes to the equatorial jungle.

Naturally, radical changes in figures take more time than minor changes, and in some individuals the changes take place more rapidly than in others. Also, the time factor of change is affected by the emotional, physiological, and psychological makeup of the different individuals. But change can be made with knowledge and perseverance.

Quite frequently I have been asked, "What is a perfect figure?" The answer depends on whether we mean feminine, masculine, classical, beautiful, or functional figure. Some women with beautiful figures could not stand up under farm work. But a woman who is strong enough to do heavy farm work might not look well on a calendar. (See the measurements in Chapter 12 for different figure types.) Of course, it is possible to combine both, and for perfection of figure even most women doing heavy farm work would have to do calisthenics and stretch–flexing exercises. It would be necessary to change the arc, the angle, or the rhythm of any repetitious heavy work. Sometimes all three changes would be necessary. Doing the same or similar work or very heavy exercise movements over and over tends toward an unbalanced figure. We can develop unnatural curves in the spine and build up large masses in our arms and legs, and we can create or accentuate bad posture.

If you try hard enough, you can even develop a bad figure from exercise. Let me explain this statement.

To start with, too much exercise with the same rhythm, too much practice of the same exercise movements, makes for bulges and bulk in the limbs that are thus exercised. Many ice skaters, for example, develop bulges, muscle, and fat in their legs. Dancers have the same problem. They are executing the same movements in the same rhythm for hours at a time. It perhaps makes for functional perfection in certain movements of dancing and skating, but it has little effect in creating a good figure. In fact, I know of many skaters and dancers who have a tendency to accentuate a bad figure with too much practice of regimented–type movements. This will cause an increase of bulk in legs already too heavy. I have also seen many dancers who have (and are continuing to accentuate) a lordosis, or exaggerated lower–back curvature, of the spine.

After fifty–five years of checking the figures of thousands of men and women, I am of the opinion that given time, intelligent cooperation, and a persevering spirit it is possible to improve or even change radically any type of figure. I can't guarantee making great changes in the length of your arms or legs, but I can lengthen your waistline or increase the line of the neck. From head to foot it is possible to increase or decrease any part of the anatomy by knowledge and perseverance.

Spot Reducing and Development

There are a few important principles to learn and remember when attempting to recontour your body. The same exercises can reduce you—or help you gain weight; can reduce a part of the body—or increase its measurements. It all depends on the speed and rhythm.

1. If you do exercises very rapidly, you have a tendency to increase the bulk of muscle above the movement. (If you move your arms rapidly, you tighten up the muscles in the shoulders and increase the bulk (consisting of hard fat and muscles) in the shoulders. If you move legs rapidly, you increase the bulk of the upper thigh and buttocks.)

2. The best way to reduce the measurement of any part of the body is to

If you try hard enough, you can even develop a bad figure from exercise. Let me explain this statement.

To start with, too much exercise with the same rhythm, too much practice of the same exercise movements, makes for bulges and bulk in the limbs that are thus exercised.—**H.J.R.**

Dr. Reilly Remembers Sonja Henie

Among my fond memories, the figure problem of Sonja Henie, the great skating star, comes to mind. Her weight was 138 pounds; her height, five feet two inches; and all was a mass of solid bunchy muscles. When she first came to me, she had tried in every way to reduce. She said, "I do six to eight hours of hard skating practice every day and my muscles grow bigger and bigger. You must do something for me." I learned that this young lady had a lucrative movie contract, which made it imperative that she slim down—and quickly. This was an interesting challenge. Here was a person whose diet was fairly normal, who exercised practically all day, yet still had a weight and figure problem. From past experience and knowledge, I could see we had two basic factors to contend with. The natural fat-contour deposits that normally differentiate the female from the male, and musculature that had responded to the natural movement economy of the body, were piling on more shortened muscles to be used in a regimented, repetitious, limited set of movements. While some of these movements were necessary for perfection, too many resulted in a heavy, unbalanced figure.

The first procedure was to limit the amount of skating practice and to substitute all-around exercise such as special stretching and leg movements given while lying on the back, side, and abdomen (see Chapter 7). General calisthenics for the entire body were advised. As time was important and our skater had many pressing professional appearances contracted for, we worked out a two-a-day special massage schedule. At midday a general invigorating tonic massage was given. A second treatment was given at night after the last performance. For the evening treatment I taught my masseuse some special manipulative techniques that are given with the person lying in a tub of warm water. This is to relax completely all the tense and fatigued muscles; it helps to speed up the elimination of toxins, to drain the lymphatic circulation, and to strip the muscles long and loose. These procedures, combined with the special exercises, produced a highly satisfactory result. The young skater reduced to 104 pounds and lost all the large, ugly, unsightly bulges in her calves and legs. Her flexibility and endurance were greatly increased, and more than forty years later, the skill, artistry, and figure of Sonja Henie are remembered and rank her among the top artists of the world.

perform the exercises at a moderate speed but try to increase the arc or angle a little each time you do them. Bring the leg up a little higher. If you are moving in circles, try to expand the circle.

3. Another point to remember is that you must relax the muscles completely between the movements of the exercise and then contract them. The pause and relaxation gives you a double action. If you hold the muscles contracted between movements, you get only one-half the action.

4. If you wish to develop and firm the body, perform the exercise slowly—

and you must use weights: dumbbells, books, sacks of sugar or flour, cans of food, or anything you can hold comfortably and that permits you to increase the weight gradually.

Since they are fairly inexpensive, I recommend that the earnest beauty-seeker invest in dumbbells. These can be used to toughen the body, improve musculature, and build up the physique. By increasing the resistance or progressively using heavier weights, it is possible to increase the size of the body either in its entirety or in any individual part.

5. In order to bring about a substantial alteration in measurements, you will have to perform the exercises more times each day than would be necessary for general tonic purposes.

6. Remember to "take it easy" and increase gradually. If you are starting with two- to four-pound dumbbells, don't do too many movements with them; and increase the number of times you do the exercise by about two a week. Then when you feel thoroughly at ease performing the exercise twenty-four times with the four-pound dumbbell, you can start all over again with a six-pound dumbbell. However, go back to doing the exercise six times with the heavier weight and gradually increase until you are doing the movement twenty-four times (twelve times twice daily) with a six-pound dumbbell. This is heavy enough for the average woman.

7. Begin all routines by checking your posture, by deep breathing, and by stretching as described in Chapters 6 and 7.

8. To increase the size of any part of the body, exercises must be performed *very slowly*, with complete relaxation between movements.

9. Check with your physician for a possible cardiovascular condition, for hiatus or other hernias, or other cautionary parameters.

Exercise Guide for Refiguring Your Figure

The Bust
Massage, combined with exercise, can help to enlarge or reduce the bust. For each respective goal, therefore, we have listed a valuable massage aid inherited from Edgar Cayce.

To Enlarge Bust
EXERCISE: If one is seeking to enlarge the bust, it is helpful to begin by *stretching and expanding the chest frame:*

Lie flat on the floor, bend your knees up, keeping the feet flat on floor. Lift your buttocks and chest frame up, keeping your head on floor; rest your weight on the shoulders, and hold to the count of six. Then lower to the starting position. Repeat three to six times in the beginning. Increase to twelve.

Also increase practice of the Push-Pull exercise: Chapter 7, V6 (Fig. 15). Work up to twenty-four times twice daily.

Circle the arms with palms up and thumbs back—start with a backward motion, doing it slowly, starting with twelve and increasing by two a week until you are doing it about twenty-four to thirty times.

If you wish to develop and firm the body, perform the exercise slowly—and you must use weights: dumbbells, books, sacks of sugar or flour, cans of food, or anything you can hold comfortably and that permits you to increase the weight gradually.—**H.J.R.**

After this you can start using light dumbbells of two pounds and then three to four pounds, doing these exercises six times and working up two a week until you are doing them twenty-four to thirty times. Then you can go on to a heavier weight, four to six pounds. Take your time so as not to strain your shoulder muscles or develop bursitis.

Hold one dumbbell with the back of hand facing forward. Lift the right hand high over your head, keeping the arm as stiff as possible. While the right-hand dumbbell is coming down, bring the left-hand one up. Besides raising and firming the bosom, this exercises arms, shoulders, chest, and back; and firms flabby underarms. Start with two-pound dumbbells and work up to four pounds.

Holding dumbbells in each hand, bring the arms out at sides and extend full length at shoulder level. Then flex the elbows and bring forearms and dumbbells as close to the shoulders as possible.

Start with six times and increase at the rate of two a week, twice daily, up to twenty-four times. This will bring out the pectoralis major and minor (the major muscles of the chest).

Also do:

The Frame-Up: Chapter 7, V7A and V7B (Figs. 16A and B).
The Hallelujah: Chapter 7, V8 (Fig. 17).
The Windmill, without dumbbells: Chapter 7, V10 (Fig. 19).

Massage:

This is a little bit late in beginning [the woman was aged thirty-two] but if there is the massage of the mammary glands with cocoa butter—not on the breast itself, but under the arm and lower and in the area between the breast—you can get 'em as big or as little as you wish. (934-13)

To Reduce Bust

EXERCISE: If a large bust contains a great deal of fat, the Windmill exercise (V10–Fig. 19), combined with the following massage and the general shoulder, arm, and back exercises in Chapter 7, can be helpful in normalizing the size without the use of dumbbells.

Massage:

Use a solution of cocoa butter with a little Alum in same; which would be a pinch of Alum mixed *thoroughly*—thoroughly mixed, of course—this with a [mortar] and pestle would be the better. To an ounce of the cocoa butter. Massage this solution over the bust itself, you see; not close to the tip of the breasts, of course, but more to the *glands* and the *base* of the bust; very gently, but sufficiently that it may be absorbed so that there is the natural contraction from these combinations [acting] upon same. This will not only give form, but the proper normalcy for the bust and proper position. (275-45)

The Rest of the Body

To Improve Posture (and Increase Height)

Check your posture against the wall as instructed in Chapter 7, p. 115, and then place a book on your head and walk around the room balancing the book on your head. As you improve, use a heavier book or a paper cup filled with nuts and bolts as described under "Posture," p. 149, then a glass half-filled with water. When you can move easily without spilling the water, use a pitcher of water. If you have ever seen pictures of women in developing societies carrying water or large loads of laundry, kindling, or produce on their heads, you must have noticed their graceful carriage.

The main trouble with women's posture is that they have a tendency, when trying to achieve a better posture, to thrust their chins up and forward to improve the jaw line. This places a great strain on the cervical spine. Note the posture of a West Point or other military school cadet. The chin is pulled in and back. This may produce a double or triple chin, but this can be eliminated with the facial exercises that follow. Balancing something on your head will make you hold your head in the correct position.

For Round Shoulders

The shoulder and arm exercises in Chapter 7 can correct round shoulders: see V4A, Shoulder Shrug; V4B, Shoulder Circles; V5, Arm Circles (Fig. 14); V6, Push-Pull (Fig. 15); V7A and B, Frame-Up (Figs. 16A and B); and Windmill, V10 (Fig. 19).

For Lordosis (Sway-Back)

Do: The Pelvic Tilt, H12A and B (Figs. 21A and B); Elbow-Knee Kiss, H13A (Fig. 22); Double Elbow-Knee Kiss, H13B (Fig. 23).

For a Strong Spine and Back

It is impossible to have good posture without a strong spine and back and feet to support the body weight, so practice the following:

The exercises in Chapters 6 and 7; the Cayce cat crawl and the head-and-neck exercises in Chapter 7 (Figs. 3A, B, C, and D); and the back exercises in Chapter 7: H25, Back Leg Lift (Fig. 40); H26A, Arm and Shoulder Lift (Fig. 41); H26B, Everything-Up Lift (Fig. 42); and H27, Reverse Back Bend (Fig. 43).

For Strong Feet

Do:

The foot exercises in Chapter 7: H28, Ankle Circles; H29, Ankles Aweigh; H30, Ankle Stretch (Fig. 44); H31, Tendon Stretch (Fig. 45); H32A, Charlie Chaplin Walk (Fig. 46); H32B, Pigeon-Toed Walk (Fig. 47); H32C, variation; H33, Foot Roll; H34, Pick-Up; and H35, Toe Wiggle.

To Increase Height

Do:

Point Stretching, V11 (Fig. 20); Hallelujah, V8 (Fig. 17); and Indian Rope Trick, V9 (Fig. 18).

To Reduce Arms

Use all the towel exercises and verticals: T1, Standing Kick (Fig. 7); T2, Pendulum (Fig. 8); T3, Wood Chopping (Fig. 9); T4, Knee Bend (Fig. 10); T5, Trunk Twist (Fig. 11); T6, All-Around (Figs. 12A, B, C, and D).

Also:

V4A, Shoulder Shrug; V4B, Shoulder Circles; V5, Arm Circles (Fig. 14); V6, Push-Pull (Fig. 15); V7A, Frame-Up (Figs. 16A and B); V7B, variation; V8, Hallelujah (Fig. 17); V9, Indian Rope Trick (Fig. 18); V10, Windmill (Fig. 19).

To Reduce the Waist

The important thing to remember is that movement that lifts the waist up from the rib cage tends to slim the waist. This is why the Point Stretching is so important. It will not only increase your height but also whittle your waist down by inches.

Use the Cayce morning exercise—rising on toes and stretching up—Chapter 6, pp. 105-106; the Cayce Trunk Circles, Chapter 6, p. 105 (Figs. 1 and 2) and T5, Trunk Twist (Fig. 11); Point Stretching, V11 (Fig. 20); Knee-Over Twist, H14A, B, and C (Fig. 24); Double Knee-Over Twist (Fig. 25); variation (Fig. 26).

To Reduce the Abdomen

Do:

The Horizontal Abdominals, H12A and B, Pelvic Tilt (Figs. 21A and B); Elbow-Knee Kiss, H13A and B, and Double Elbow-Knee Kiss (Figs. 22 and 23); Knee-Over Twist, H14A, B, and C; Double Knee-Over Twist, variation (Figs. 24, 25, and 26); and Sit-Back, H15 (Fig. 27).

The Scissors (H19) is good for the lower abdomen and thighs if done slowly.

When these exercises have been mastered and the number of times performed daily increased to twenty-four, you may add the following two exercises:

1. Lie on floor face up. Place legs on small hassock or stool, raising them from floor. Then extend arms and hands full length over head; sit up and touch toes and then return to original position and rest. Start with three or four times, increase by two a week until you can do twelve. (If there is any back pain when you try this exercise, do not use it.)

2. The Victory V. Sit on floor. Raise both legs and arms until your body forms a V and rock back and forth. This is also good for the legs and back as well as the abdomen.

To Reduce the Hips

Percussion massage is very useful in reducing hips. If you do not have a willing relative or friend to beat your hips, you can do so yourself by forming a fist and beating and kneading fat on hips. Also practice some wall-beating—hitting the fattest bumps against the wall.

All the exercises in Chapter 7, performed while lying on the side, will help to reduce hips.

To Reduce the Thighs

Use the exercises in Chapter 7:

Standing Kick, T1 (Fig. 7); Heel–Toe Leg Circles, 2 variations H16A, B, and C (Figs. 28, 29, 30, and 31); Leg Raise and Double Leg Raise, H17A and B (Figs. 32 and 33); Double Leg Circles, H18 (Fig. 34); Scissors, H19; Side Leg Raise and Back Leg Raise, H20A and B (Fig. 35); Double Leg Side Raise, H21 (Fig. 36); Side Knee-Chin Kiss and Double Side Knee-Chin Kiss, H22A and B (Figs. 37 and 38); Side Leg Circles and Double Side Leg Circles, H23A and B; and Side Scissors, H24A and B (Fig. 39).

To Firm the Flesh of the Inner Thigh

This is the hardest place of all to keep youthful and firm, for it must resist a strong gravitational pull that causes it to have a crepey, drooping appearance.

For this you will need a medicine ball of about four to six pounds in weight, or a hassock.

Sit on a straight chair, preferably one with side arms. Sit well forward, place the medicine ball or hassock between your thighs and then holding it tightly with the thigh muscles, raise and lower legs. Use the arms of the chair and your own arms to find maximum leverage. Begin by doing this exercise six times twice a day and increase by two a week until you are doing twenty-four movements, twice a day, for lovely, firm, slender thighs.

To Reduce the Calves

If you have a problem with heavy calves, avoid skipping rope and bicycle riding. These have a tendency to develop large calf muscles.

The leg exercises in Chapter 7, particularly those that change the position of the heel and toe, if performed carefully with great emphasis on the change can stretch and elongate the calf muscles, resulting in a slimmer, more graceful line.

See Chapter 7 for the following:

Heel–Toe Leg Circles, 2 variations, H16A, B, and C (Figs. 28, 29, 30, and 31); Leg Raise and Double Leg Rise, H17A and B (Figs. 32 and 33); Double Leg Circles, H18 (Fig. 34); Scissors, H19; Side Leg Raise and Back Leg Raise, H20A and B (Fig. 35); Double Leg Side Raise, H21 (Fig. 36); Side Knee-Chin Kiss and Double Side Knee-Chin Kiss, H22A and B (Figs. 37 and 38); Side Leg Circles and Double Side Leg Circles, H23A and B; and Side Scissors, H24A and B (Fig. 39).

To Reduce the Ankles

Use the same as above plus the special ankle exercises: Ankle Circles, H28; Ankles Aweigh, H29; Ankle Stretch, H30 (Fig. 44); Tendon Stretch, H31 (Fig. 45); and the Charlie Chaplin Walk, Pigeon-Toed Walk, and variation, H32A, B, and C (Figs. 46 and 47).

A special exercise that is particularly good for draining edema from ankles and legs and for helping varicose veins is performed in this way:

Lie on the back on either the floor or a hard bed. Support the head and shoulders with pillows. Bend the knees and grasp the legs just above the ankles.

. . . the most commonly performed cosmetic surgery—the face lift—can be postponed or avoided entirely with a program of good nutrition, general exercise, massage, hydrotherapy, and special facial exercises.—**H.J.R.**

The Cayce Head-and-Neck Exercises

The head-and-neck exercises described and illustrated in Chapter 6, if performed faithfully each day, will stimulate the circulation to the entire face, head, and neck; keep the throat and jaw line firm; and prevent the formation of double or multiple chins.

*—***H.J.R.**

Open the thighs as wide as possible and support arms on open thighs, which will help push them more widely apart; hold them there. Then rotate the ankles, first clockwise, and then counterclockwise. Move the feet up and down, up and down. The wider apart the thighs, the more benefit from the exercise, for the main arteries and veins in the groin are thus opened and circulation increased to the legs.

To Reduce the Fanny (Buttocks)

Do:

The Fanny Walk (H36) and the Fanny Bounce (H37), Chapter 7, p. 136. Also use the percussion massage, similar to that prescribed for hips.

Exercising the Face

The only way to alter the facial features that you were born with is through plastic surgery, and increasing numbers of young girls and boys as well as age-battling men and women are going this route to correct nature's errors. Certainly the growing skill of plastic surgeons is a great blessing where there is serious deformity from burns, accidents, and war-created injuries.

However, the most commonly performed cosmetic surgery—the face lift—can be postponed or avoided entirely with a program of good nutrition, general exercise, massage, hydrotherapy, and special facial exercises. The face, like every other part of the body, is made up of bones, blood vessels, connective tissue, fat, nerves, and voluntary muscles (twenty-six). When the muscles become flabby, the face droops, sags, and ages. Negative thoughts and poor circulation accelerate the appearance of lines, wrinkles, blemishes, and muddy color, while poor elimination will not only produce blackheads, pimples, and dry or oily skin, but is one of the chief causes of major skin diseases.

Marjorie Craig, who for years has guided the beauty and exercise program at Elizabeth Arden's, says in her excellent book, *Face-Saving Exercises,*[2] "A firm face is the symbol of youth, but a firm face need not be the property solely of the young. If muscles of the body can be brought back to tone—and they can be—so can muscles of the face and by the same means: exercise."

Cayce and I go further and say that spirit, serenity, and positive thinking as well as good health can be reflected in your face.

Toning, conditioning, and exercising the face can be done best by "making faces," blowing up balloons, and using the Cayce head-and-neck exercises.

Blowing Up Balloons

This exercise, which I use primarily for asthma, emphysema, and other respiratory problems, is an excellent facial exercise for keeping cheeks firm, eliminating telltale squirrel pouches, and keeping the muscles around the lips elastic.

Making Faces

Try to follow balloon-blowing, which purses the lips, with grinning and smiling, which stretches the muscles in the opposite direction.

The Nonsurgical Face Lift

We have inherited an unexpected beauty bonus from Cayce, which we have found is an excellent nonsurgical face lift.

The following procedure was recommended to a sixty-seven-year-old man for a dropped palate—a not unusual complaint found in the aging. However, Miss Billings used it on her seventy-year-old mother for a palate complaint and found that a fringe benefit was a rejuvenated appearance of her entire face. It certainly seems to correct middle-age sag.

The man, Case 3632-1, had asked, "What is the cause of the cough and what treatment will relieve it?"

Cayce replied, "Tie up a piece of hair in the center of the head. Keep it tied up like a wig. Tie this tighter each day. Every three days, make it a little bit tighter, a little bit tighter; it'll soon stop the cough and raise the palate."

It will also raise your entire face—giving you a face lift.

All the expressions that register emotions can be used to exercise the face. Just perform them very slowly and rest and relax the muscles between movements:

For Forehead: First frown, then look surprised—alternate movements.

For Nose: Wrinkle the nose "like a bunny" or as you do when smelling something unpleasant.

For Eyes: Use the eye exercises in Chapter 7, particularly the Eye Squeeze. Also practice the Eyebrow Lift, raising brows as high as you can.

For Cheeks: Blow up balloons.

Wink one eye and hold hard and then the other. Show contempt or disbelief by twisting mouth to one side while winking the eye on the same side; then do the same on the other side. Laugh out loud: Ha, ha, ha.

Stick your tongue out and down as far as you can—really stretch.

For Mouth: Use the Cayce head-and-neck exercises. Stretch the lips over the teeth and pull out widely in a grin. Stretch hard.

Do as singers do and practice the vowels going up and down the scale singing as loudly as you can (also benefits cheeks).

Oh–Oh–Oh–Oh–Oh

Ah–Ah–Ah–Ah–Ah

Eeh–eeh–eeh–eeh–eeh–

Ooh–ooh–ooh–ooh–ooh

Pout as hard as you can, bringing the lower lip up over top lip.

(Q) Should I continue the mud packs?
(A) These are well occasionally; not too often . . . Once a month, for the very pleasure of it, we would have the mud pack.

(1968-7)

For Chin: To avoid developing a double chin, use the Cayce head–and–neck exercises.

Also check your posture.

Chin-Writing: Place pen or pencil between teeth. Lift the chin. Move the chin in circles and straight lines as though you were using it as an imaginary pen to write the alphabet. Now write words with the chin—your name or "Hello" or some short phrase. Change the words daily for variety. Do it slowly and not too strenuously. These movements will eliminate fat and flabbiness in the neck and chin and make for a firm contour.

Two or more people can make a game out of this. One can ask questions with the voice; the other players answer with chin–writing. Sample question:

What is today's date? Answer with figures.

You can try chin–writing on a sheet of paper tacked on the wall at head level, sitting or standing. Or you may use a thin paintbrush and try to paint with it.

Facial Massage and Mud Pack

Be careful when getting a massage that you do not break down muscles or tissues of the face. Cayce, when asked if patting of the tissue of the face would help "to keep the muscles from sagging," replied, "It does. The patting of the tissue is the better." (811–4)

Consult Chapter 9 on massage for the correct way to massage the face. Cayce was asked:

(Q) How can people avoid aging in appearance?
(A) The *mind!*
(Q) How can sagging facial muscles be avoided? How corrected?
(A) By massage and the use of those creams as indicated, over the chin and throat, around the eyes and such conditions [of sagging]. Occasionally, the use also of the Boncilla or mud packs would be very good. (1947-4)

. . . about twice a month . . . we would have the mud packs; face and neck, and across the shoulders and upper portion about the neck; especially extending over the area of the thyroids—as an astringent and as a stimulation for a better circulation throughout the system. (1968-3)

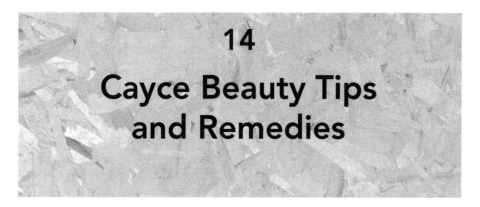

14

Cayce Beauty Tips and Remedies

Beauty Problems

Beauty begins with cleanliness—inner as well as outer. Therefore, I suggest that you initiate your new beauty program with the apple diet cleansing routine as described in Chapter 11 on "Internal Cleansing."

Skin Blemishes

Cayce was asked:

(Q) What can be done locally for impurities on face?
(A) . . . Keep the eliminations open. (452-2)

There might be used bleaches, or cleansing creams, but these would eventually give more trouble than the blackheads are causing in the present. Get to the basic conditions of these, as is now being accomplished through the use of the fumes, the rubs, and now the Violet Ray [hand machine, bulb applicator]. (2072-9)

First, in the blood supply we find indications of the inclination toward poor eliminations through the alimentary canal; and this is inclined to produce toxic forces that cause a poor coordination between the superficial and the deeper circulation.

Hence those disturbances as a rash, or blackheads, or pimples, or large pores—all of these are at times indicated. (2154-2)

If skin eruptions and problems persist after a thorough internal housecleaning, instead of spending money on creams and lotions, see your doctor, have a physical checkup, and have your thyroid checked. Cayce often recommended the ingestion of from 1 to 5 drops of Atomidine for these problems, together with correction of the diet, hydrotherapy, exercise, osteopathy, and

Let there not be too much activity in the middle of the day, or too much [of] the sunshine. The early mornings and the late afternoons are the more preferable times. For the sun during the period between eleven or eleven-thirty and two o'clock carries too great a quantity of the actinic rays that make for destructive forces to the superficial circulation . . . (934-2)

(Q) What can be done to clear up the skin?
(A) Make for the better eliminations. (480-22)

(Q) Is there not a treatment or method that might be used by the entity for the removal of blackheads from the face?
(A) The general building up of the body forces and the establishing first of correct coordination of eliminations. These [blackheads] will gradually be removed.
(2072-9)

If skin eruptions and problems persist after a thorough internal housecleaning, instead of spending money on creams and lotions, see your doctor, have a physical checkup, and have your thyroid checked.—**H.J.R.**

massage. *But under no circumstances should Atomidine ever be taken except under the supervision of a doctor.*

Beauty-Full Diet

Diet occupied the center stage in all of the Cayce skin remedies. In many readings he cautioned against the overconsumption of animal flesh, fats, and sweets. He urged that the diet consist chiefly of vegetables, nuts, and fruits—particularly when one was trying to correct skin problems.

> We would keep those foods that carry full quantities (though not excessive) of calcium and iodine. These will be the more helpful if they are assimilated from foods than by the administration in other manners. For, the affectation or the helpful influence passes then through the entire activity of the assimilating and distributing of energies. By that assimilation through the body.
>
> (619-10)

Face and Body Lotions, Soaps, Etc.

A sixteen-year-old girl asked Cayce, "What can I do to improve skin condition of face and back, and of scalp and hair?" The answer:

> At least once a week, after a good thorough workout of body in exercise—following the bath afterward, massage the back, the face, the body, the limbs with Pure Peanut Oil. Then this will add to the beauty. *And know, if ye would take each day, through thy experience two almonds, ye will never have skin blemishes, ye will never be tempted even in body toward cancer nor toward those things that make blemishes in the body forces themselves.* And *the oil rubs once a week, ye will never have rheumatism nor those concurrent conditions from stalemate in liver and kidney activities.* [Italics added.] (1206-13)

> For making or keeping a good complexion—this for the skin, the hands, arms and body as well—we would prepare a compound to use as a massage (by self) at least once or twice each week.
>
> To six ounces of peanut oil, add:
>
> | | |
> |---|---|
> | Olive Oil | 2 ounces |
> | Rose Water | 2 ounces |
> | Lanolin, dissolved | 1 tablespoonful |
>
> This would be used after a tepid bath in which the body has remained for at least fifteen to twenty minutes, giving the body then [during the bath] a thorough rub with any good soap—to stimulate the body-forces. As we find, Sweetheart or any good Castile soap, or Ivory, may be used for such.
>
> Afterwards, massage this solution, after shaking it well. Of course, this [amount] will be sufficient for many times. Shake well and pour in an open saucer or the like; dipping fingers in same. Begin with the face, neck, shoulders, arms; and then the whole body would be massaged thoroughly with the solution; especially in the limbs—in the areas that would come across the hips, across the body, across the diaphragm.

This will not only keep a stimulating [effect] with the other treatments as indicated [hydrotherapy, massage, and osteopathy] taken occasionally, and give the body a good base for the stimulating of the superficial circulation; *but [the solution] will aid in keeping the body beautiful; that is, as to [being free from] any blemish of any nature.* [Italics added.] (1968-7)

(Q) How may I avoid the skin eruptions?
(A) Keep good eliminations and use such cosmetics as do not become too great astringents. (1206-15)

To one tablespoon of melted cocoa butter add, while it is in the liquid:

Rose Water .... 1 tablespoonful

Compound Tincture of Benzoin..... 1 tablespoonful

Keep this to massage into these tissues. The activity of these ingredients will be to *enliven* and to make for—well, this would be a very, very good skin cleanser for anyone! (1016-1)

(Q) How may I avoid the skin eruptions?
(A) Keep good eliminations and use such cosmetics as do not become too great astringents . . .

In the diet beware of too much of fats of any nature, or sweets, and do keep good eliminations. (1206-15)

(Q) What soap, manner of cleansing, creams and makeup would be least harmful and most helpful in correcting and beautifying the skin?
(A) Pure Castile soap is the better as a cleanser. As a cleansing cream or the like, the Genuine Black and White products are nearer to normal. (2072-6)

As to the face lotion, we find that a cream that is less acid will be the more beneficial. A test of these may be easily made before they are used. Both the red and the blue litmus test are the better way for testing same. And any that is wholly alkaline and non-acid is preferable. (275-37)

(Q) Give a good skin freshener.
(A) To one half pint of Olive Oil add one ounce of Rose Water, a few drops of Glycerine and one ounce of a 10% solution of Alcohol, and shake these well together. This is a skin invigorator. (404-8)

Dry Skin

(Q) Can you suggest any treatment for dryness of hands and skin?
(A) Use any good oil, as Sweet Oil or such, on the hands and over the body— *Peanut oil (sweet oil)* it will change this. The better change should come within from the better assimilation of that eaten, which will be found to be more improved by the exercises of stretching arms above the head or swinging on a pole would be well. This doesn't mean to run out and jump up on a pole every time you eat, but have regular periods. When you have the activities, do have these exercises, for they will stimulate the gastric flow and let that eaten have something to float in; that is, eat some more! (2072-14)

Deodorants
The use of pure soaps is preferable to any attempt to deodorize. Any that allays perspiration certainly clogs the activity of respiratory and perspiratory system. (2072-6)

If You Would Have Beautiful Skin

The greatest enemy to a beautiful complexion is the sun. Cayce cautioned against overexposure to its rays:

To treat sunburn, Cayce advised the following:

Any good lotion would be well for the sunburn; such as soda water, or any application that would act as a balm, in the forms of some character of oils that remove the fire from the affected areas—such as Glyco-Thymoline. (3051-1)

There is no better than plain, pure apple vinegar!
Of course, the use of any of the detergents or oils; the Sun Tan Oil, or Unguentine or any of these applications would be very well. But if proper precautions are taken, there is none much better than the pure apple vinegar. (601-22)

When asked for a remedy for skin breaking out from sun, he gave this reply:

Use Palmolive soap baths, followed with a small amount of Pure White Vaseline rubbed on any rough places. (1709-10)

As for the acute conditions—we would daub or apply spirits of camphor by using tufts of cotton.
Then in an hour or two hours afterward have a tepid bath, and then apply peanut oil. (303-33)

Freckles

(Q) For freckles?
(A) You'd better try to keep your freckles and not try to get rid of them. Genuine Black and White [brand of products] for skin is preferable for such, but these [freckles] are in the pigment of the skin, and unless you wish to upset something else, don't attempt to bleach more [freckles out] than you would have from the regular conditions. These are partially liver conditions but don't be touchy about freckles, they're good for you. (5223-1)

Superfluous Hair

(Q) Would you give me a formula for destroying superfluous hair, but which does not injure the skin in any way?
(A) There's no such animal! This may best be done by diet, *and* the applications to the skin for keeping the pores open *and* the body-actions better. (1947-4)

(Q) Since diet has not caused hair on lips to diminish, is there anything which will prevent this that can be used externally? Will cutting or bleaching increase growth?

(A) Do not shave off, do not attempt to bleach or dye, but use this mixture:

    Cocoa Butter .... 3 drams [1 dram=1/8 oz.]
    Calomel .... 2 grains
    Epsom Salts .... 20 grains

Mix these thoroughly, as with [mortar] and pestle. Massage this ointment gently in the areas where there are the disturbances from superfluous hair, and after leaving on for fifteen to twenty minutes, rub off. This used as an ointment will remove hair without injury to the body. To be sure, mercury is in the calomel, and this is a poison, but with this combination and in this quantity there is not sufficient for a body to absorb enough to become detrimental to the body-forces.

After this is used, as the base for a better skin condition use the Genuine Black and White cream. (2582-4)

For this body, then, we find it would be well to use the Atomic Iodine, or Atomidine [*do not use except under supervision of a doctor*]; one to two drops in half a glass of water before the morning meals and at night just before retiring, in periods of 4 to 5 days [taken for 4 to 5 days]—then leave off for a week, then take again . . .

The diets would consist often of the seafoods; once or twice a week, you see. Only the potato peeling, or the very small potato used with the peeling is preferable to the pulp of same. All those vegetables that make for the carrying of iron and silicon; as squash, cucumbers, radishes, the oyster plant, or such natures, should be a portion of the diet quite often—if there would be kept the proper balance as related to those activities of the glands that make for the growth of the hair. For if these [foods] are kept with the normal activities, we will find these will not only produce the *proper* growth of the hair but will cause its normal or natural color . . . [to stay]. Naturally, though, this is a long-drawn-out method and must be a persistent and consistent thing upon the part of the users of same. (920-2)

Q) How can one permanently remove superfluous hair?
(A) This, as we find, arises from a general condition that is from the activity of the diet—and from this activity of the glands that makes for the growth of same in or upon the body. (920-2)

Rashes

(Q) What causes breaking out on wrists, and should anything specifically be done for that?

(A) This as we have found, as indicated, if the eliminations are set up, should disappear. If this is washed occasionally in this combination it would be well, though the bathing tends to make for greater irritation. But after bathing, use this as a combination—and it's very well for anyone that has a rash or heat or a humor in the blood.

    To 2 oz. of Rosewater, add:

            Glycerine .... 30 minims
                                    (minim is a drop)
            10% solution of Calcium .... ½ ounce

This should be shaken together and rubbed on the hands, wrists, or those portions of the body that are disturbed. (555-8)

After the bath, do dust with the powder that carries Balsam in same. This is healing, but don't tend to dry up too much. (2752-1)

Then dust over this the Stearate of Zinc with the Balsam [a talcum powder containing tolu or Peruvian balsam and zinc stearate], which we find is made or combined by Johnson and Johnson. Or we may obtain this combination in the older concern, Eimer & Amend. (322-5)

Heat Rash (Babies)

This [Stearate of Zinc] will keep down those disturbances from heat. (2781-1)

[And for a two year old] . . . will relieve the itching. (5520-6)

Should there continue to be the irritation of the skin, use some good powder—as Stearate of Zinc powder—with Balsam. Use this for the rash that occurs on parts of the body. (69-6)

Hair and Scalp

Hair Loss, Baldness, and Graying

Hair loss and baldness, which afflict 80 percent of American men, are now quite common occurrences in women. A prominent New York hairdresser has reported that 30 percent of the salon's women clients are bald or going bald. I can vouch for the effectiveness of Cayce's cure for baldness inasmuch as I began growing new hair on my own head at the age of seventy–five.

The treatment I used was one that he recommended in many readings:

(Q) What causes the [hair] falling out . . . and what can be done to prevent it?
(A) This is lack of an activity through the glands that are secreting from the system the elements necessary to make for activity in those portions of the thyroids that affect the circulation to those portions of the system.

The diet affects this principally, though those portions where this is indicated would be stimulated by a massage—which may be had with properties that aid the scalp circulation; such as a small quantity of the crude oil. Rub a small quantity of this into the scalp once or twice a month; this should be sufficient to renew the cells that produce this—if there is the stimulation through the gastric flow in the digestive forces and the stimulation through the general distribution of the circulatory forces of the body.

Each time after the crude oil massage, when the oil is rubbed in, cleanse same with a twenty percent solution of [grain] alcohol [with] water added.
(480-23)

Crude oil is not the kind you get at a gas station. To procure it, consult the supply sources at the back of the book. The reason grain alcohol is preferred to the denatured variety is because "this will not dry–as does that which has been denatured." (275-30)

(Q) What oil should be used on scalp before washing?

(A) As we find (and have given oft), the crude oils are the most satisfactory for stimulating the scalp, to prevent falling hair, to add luster, and to stimulate the growth. Following the oil shampoo there should be the cleansing with alcohol; that is, one to twenty, but this should be preferably of the pure *grain*, for any of the ingredients such as in pyro or those that make for the denaturing produce breaking and burning of the hair. (276-4)

We would also begin taking Atomidine internally as a purifier for the glands and to stimulate better thyroid activity. This may change the heart's regularity for the time but if it is properly administered and the osteopathic corrections are made properly we will find changes wrought in the activities in the epidermis and as associated or related to the hair. (3904-l)

See doctor

Alternate Treatment

For the scalp we would prepare a close-fitting cap—oil cap—to be used once a week or left on over night, when the scalp would be massaged with pure hog lard. Not that which has been mixed with vegetable matter, but the pure pork or hog lard. Massage this in at night. Sleep with it in the hair and scalp. Using the cap as protection. In the morning have a thorough shampoo with Olive Oil shampoo, massaging the scalp afterward with white Vaseline cut with a little alcohol solution—just sufficient to cleanse same; about a drop of grain alcohol to an ounce of water—just enough to change the activity of same. [Or just enough to rinse most of the Vaseline out of the hair.] (3904-1)

Improvement in the diet can also help to stimulate the glandular activity to overcome baldness, and Cayce made such diet recommendations:

Do eat more of seafoods, more carrots, and—while certain times will have to be chosen for such—do eat onions and garlic. (3904-l)

Do use the diets that carry iodine in their natural forms. Use only kelp salt or deep-sea salt. Plenty of seafoods.

Not too much sweets. The egg yolk but not the white of egg should be taken. (4056-1)

In the diet eat the soup from the peelings of Irish potatoes. Add more often the raw vegetables such as lettuce, celery, watercress, radishes, onions, mustard greens and all of those that may be prepared as salads and the like. Carrots will make better conditions in combination with these for the sparkle of the eye and for the general vision. (4086-1)

Internal cleansing was also stressed by Cayce in the cure for baldness:

Have the full evacuation of alimentary canal at least once a day and do at least once a month purify the colon by the use of high enemas. These may be taken by self, provided the colon tube is used . . .

To Increase Hair Growth

(Q) What should body now do to cause hair to grow on front of forehead?

(A) Won't have much brains there and hair, too, see? This may be assisted, though, by using any vapor rub, or that such as Listerine will keep the hair in a healthy, normal condition, see? (257-11)

(Q) What will thicken the hair?

(A) Massage [the scalp] with crude oil—cleansing [it] with a twenty percent solution of grain alcohol—[this] will thicken [the hair] and bring better conditions to the scalp. (4501-1)

Dandruff

(Q) Is there any special treatment recommended for dandruff and can it be entirely cured?

(A) If this will be used, this may entirely cure same: To 4 ounces of same [pure water] add 20 minims of 85% alcohol, with that of the Oil of Pine, 2 minims. This should be rubbed thoroughly into the scalp, so there is the proper reaction from same. Then, with this still damp from same, massage thoroughly into the scalp small quantity of white Vaseline. Then wash the head thoroughly with that of a tar soap. Do this about once each week. It will disappear. (261-2)

Do these, be very careful with the general eliminations.

Keep away from all those things such as hard drinks, carbonated water or the like and we will gain better health and have better superficial circulation.

(4086-1)

(Q) To keep hair from graying or falling out?

(A) Don't worry about the hair, just keep it nice and smooth. Take care of it more often with either Drene hair tonic or Olive Oil Hair Tonic, followed with the shampooing with crude oil and tar soap. These while making irritation at first will maintain the better conditions for the body. (5261-1)

Shampoos and Tonics

(Q) What soap should be used on hair for washing?

(A) Preferably that carrying the tar content as its base, or Packer's Tar, or any that have a tar and glycerine content . . .

(Q) What hair tonic would be good for my scalp?

(A) Preferably the alcohol, that we have indicated, for this is the active principle in any of those tonics that are manufactured. So this in its perfect state, without the addition of any other oils, is well; followed, of course, with a gentle rub with the pure white Vaseline. (276-4)

Scalp and Hair Massage

Do not overlook the importance of exercise and massage in maintaining beautiful, luxuriant hair. The Cayce head–and–neck exercises are excellent for stimulating circulation. And the cat crawl and the torso circle, as described in Chapter 6 and illustrated in Chapter 7 (Figs. 5A and 5B) will stimulate the glands, benefiting hair, skin, and nails.

To massage the scalp, place the fingertips of both hands on scalp. Then move the scalp up and around in circles. Do not move the fingers in a rubbing motion—the purpose is to loosen the scalp from the skull and increase circulation.

Sometimes we find Cayce recommending the scalp massage to be taken this way:

During that period give the scalp a thorough massage with crude oil, using the electrically driven vibrator with the suction applicator. This should be done very thoroughly, not hurriedly, and should require at least thirty to forty minutes for the massage with the crude oil and then the application of white Vaseline and then the electrically driven vibrator using the suction cup applicator. (4056-1)

Cayce instructed the patient to repeat the procedure after five days, during which he was to take each morning, for five days, one drop of Atomidine.

Then, after a two–week rest, another complete series, but "between each two series allow two weeks to elapse. Doing these, we will find that in six to eight months it will begin to stimulate the activities for the growth of hair over the scalp and on body."

Again, the Atomidine, which Cayce recommended in 610 readings because, he said, it "will purify the glandular system so as to resist adverse influences" (1521–2), should not be taken except by a doctor's prescription. There can be grave danger in overstimulating the thyroid gland without professional supervision.

Eyes

To Improve Vision

There are a number of Cayce recommendations to improve the eyesight and to bring out the full beauty of the "windows of the soul."

"[Take plenty of] carrots, green peas and green beans, onions, beets." These were recommended to be taken each day. They "have a direct bearing upon the application of that assimilated for the optic forces." (3552–1)

Do add to the diet about twice as many oranges, lemons and limes as is part of the diet in the present. These also supplement with a great deal of carrots especially as combined with gelatin, if we would aid and strengthen the optic nerves and the tensions between sympathetic and cerebrospinal systems. (5401-1)

(Q) How can I improve my vision?
(A) When we remove the pressures of the toxic forces we will improve the vision. Also the head and neck exercise will be most helpful. Take this regularly, not taking it sometimes and leaving off sometimes, but each morning and each evening take this exercise regularly for six months and we will see a great deal of difference. Sitting erect, bend the head forward three times, to the back three times, to the right side three times, to the left side three times, and then circle the head each way three times. Don't hurry through with it, but take the time to do it. We will get results. (3549-1)

(Q) How may my eyes be strengthened so as to eliminate the necessity of reading glasses?
(A) By the head and neck exercise in the open, as ye walk for twenty to thirty minutes each morning. Now do not undertake it one morning and then say "It rained and I couldn't get out," or "I've got to go somewhere else," and think there aren't those despot conditions that rebel at not having their morning walk! (2533-6)

For Granulated Eyelids

(Q) What should be done for granulated eyelids?
(A) Use a weak solution of boracic acid. About twice each week use those [poultices] of scraped Irish potato, bound of an evening over the eye. (409-22)

Q) What is the best diet for this body?
(A) That which is a well balanced diet. But often use the raw vegetables which are prepared with gelatin. Use these at least three times each week. Those which grow more above the ground than those which grow below the ground. Do include, when these are prepared, carrots with that portion especially close to the top. It [that is, this part of the carrot] may appear the harder and the less desirable but it carries the vital energies, stimulating the optic reactions between kidneys and the optics. (3051-6)

Eye Strain

(Q) What should be done to relieve my eyes?
(A) Bathe these with a weak Glyco-Thymoline solution. Use an eyecup, and two parts of distilled water (preferably) to one part of the Glyco-Thymoline. This irritation is a part of the kidney disturbance that has come from the upsetting in the digestive forces. (3050-2)

We would use Murine as an eyewash about once each week [for this condition]; preferably Saturday evenings or Sunday mornings, so that there is rest from the use of the eyes following same. This is only as a stimulation to the flow of [or from] the mucous membranes about the eyeball itself. (1968-3)

(Q) What is the best procedure for care of teeth?
(A) Have local attention and then take care of the teeth. Use an equal combination of salt and soda for massaging the gums and teeth. Don't use a brush [for massaging]. Use your finger. (3484-1)

Cataracts

(See Chapter 11 on "Internal Cleansing" for directions on preparing the potato pack.)

Sties and Inflammations

Not long ago a woman in Riverside, Illinois, reported to Virginia Beach that hot castor oil packs are effective in treating sties: "I have seen at first hand how hot castor oil packs disburse the inflammation in sties, having tried this treatment from the files, on a limited basis, on my family."

Last summer I had a severely ruptured eye that did not respond to treatments with Glyco-Thymoline and raw potato packs, but it did clear up beautifully with hot castor oil packs.

Others have reported improvement in early stages of cataracts when these were treated with castor oil packs.

Mouth and Teeth to Prevent Tooth Decay

(Q) Give care of teeth so I will have less decaying.
(A) Use as a massage for the gums and teeth an equal combination of common table salt and baking soda; about once a month add one drop only of chlorine to a pint of water and rinse the mouth with this. Do not swallow it, but rinse the mouth and then brush the teeth. This will preserve them, even aid in filling cavities. (2981-2)

*— * If not taking medi for thyroid probs.*

(Q) How to prevent tooth decay [which I've had an awful lot of the past three years]?
(A) Have them attended to, and add to the system occasionally Atomidine as a manner of gaining better control of the activity of the glands which formulate the circulation through teeth and structural portion of the body. One drop 5 days at a time and then skip 2 weeks. Then again do this through a whole year, you'll have your teeth in very good fix if local attention is given to the rest. (5313-4)

★ For normalcy in the salivary glands

(Q) Are teeth forming normally?
(A) These are very good. We would find that a weakened solution of Ipsab for the gums would tend to relieve the pressure and make for normalcy in the salivary glands, as well as strengthening the tissue in the mouth. This should be reduced at least half, and the gums massaged with a tuft of cotton with same. This also adds to the amount of saline, calcium and iodine, for the activity of the glands in mouth and throat. (299-2)

Also, during this period of the formation of the teeth, keep sufficient quantities of iodine in the food values for the body, as well as calcium, and so forth. It will be found that a massage of the gums occasionally with those properties known as Ipsab will be helpful . . . as these processes are carried on through the activity of the thyroid operations in the body. (314-2)

(Q) What can I do to keep my teeth for life?
(A) You won't. For already these have begun to need local attention. If there is kept the proper balance in the vitamins, it will help—but these precautions should begin—well, during the period of gestation is when they should begin, but for a body should begin at least in the first or second year.

The general care of same [teeth] with a good dentifrice, as well as a good massage for the gums will aid. Use the Ipsab at least twice a week for the gums . . . Massage the gums with Ipsab, though, and we will have a better chance for keeping the teeth much longer. (3436-1)

Cayce had some highly original ideas about teeth—for example, he said, "Cycles change for the teeth during the second year of each 7-year cycle. During that year take at least 3 to 4 series of Calcios doses or its equivalent, to supply calcium, and it will aid not only the teeth but all the activities of the thyroid gland." (3051-2)

Calcios is an easily assimilated form of calcium. The same effect, however, should be available through the increased ingestion of calcium-rich foods, particularly vegetables and seeds.

Toothache and Sore Gums

In one of his trances, Cayce was given the formula and the name for a preparation called Ipsab, which is now prepared and available through many retail outlets. (See back of book for sources of supply.) Cayce recommended the use of Ipsab in most problems involving the gums and teeth. The principal ingredient is prickly ash bark, which the Native Americans called "toothache bark" and to which Cayce referred in the same manner.

In one reading, he gave this formula:

To 6 ounces of distilled water, add two ounces of Prickly Ash Bark. Reduce by simmerings (not boiling) to 2 ounces. Strain and add powdered Common Salt until we have a very thin paste. Rinse or rub gums with this once every 2 days until this trouble in the mouth and gums has subsided. (4436-2)

Another version is in liquid form and contains in addition to the above ingredients, calcium chloride, peppermint, and iodine. (See back of book for sources of supply.)

We would use same [Ipsab] not upon cotton, for this body, but upon the finger use it and massage; not only the gums where the teeth are but where they are not! And we will find that the stimulation to the activities of the throat itself, to the salivary glands, to even the tonsil area, will be materially aided by the activity of the combination of the calcium with the iodine in same, as well as the antiseptics that arise from the vegetable forces in same as combined with sodium chloride. (569-23)

Ipsab has been very effective in many cases of canker sore. Another Cayce remedy, which many doctors as well as I have found efficacious, is the application of Atomidine with a cotton swab to the canker, combined with a frequent mouthwash made from Glyco-Thymoline mixed with water.—**H.J.R.**

Bleeding Gums and Canker Sores

Use Ipsab to keep *these [teeth] clear from the tartar* and [*to stop the bleeding from the gums*]. (257-13)

The following is the treatment of early acute cases where infection is present, gums are bleeding, and teeth are loose but not decayed beyond repair:

1.   Massage gums thoroughly for five minutes twice a day with Ipsab. Repeatedly apply a liberal quantity of Ipsab to the tip of the finger and massage the gums vigorously on all surfaces. In extreme cases, take a small tuft of cotton that has been dipped in Ipsab and use a pair of tweezers to rub this saturated cotton between the gum and each tooth that is very loose. This will ensure the contact of Ipsab with the growing organisms. After the massage, rinse out the mouth with an undiluted solution of Glyco–Thymoline, followed by tap water. *Do not swallow any of these solutions.*

2.   Brush the teeth once each day in the evening before retiring with a mixture composed of equal parts of common table salt and sodium bicarbonate. Brush the teeth each morning after breakfast with any good dentifrice.

3.   Eat a large raw vegetable salad each day.

4.   Have corrective dental work done on any carious teeth.

Ipsab has been very effective in many cases of canker sore. Another Cayce remedy, which many doctors as well as I have found efficacious, is the application of Atomidine with a cotton swab to the canker, combined with a frequent mouthwash made from Glyco–Thymoline mixed with water. Also swab the canker with full–strength Glyco–Thymoline. In this connection, here is what Case 257 wrote: "I don't know whether it's the massage with the Ipsab for the gums, or whether it's the frequent and regular use of Glyco–Thymoline as a mouthwash, but I just never have those awful canker sores in my mouth any more like I used to . . . "

Other mouthwashes frequently recommended by Cayce were Listerine and Lavoris.

We have also found castor oil to be very healing to all mucous membranes, including those of the mouth, and some patients have reported good results from its use on canker sores.

Pyorrhea

(Q) What can I do about pyorrhea condition in my teeth?
(A) Use Ipsab regularly each day and rinse mouth out when it is finished with Glyco-Thymoline. (5121-1)

The receding gums and those tendencies towards pyorrhea would be allayed by the consistent use of Ipsab as a massage for the teeth and gums. Also these should be treated, some locally, with the dentist's paraphernalia [and also]—the small wads of cotton saturated with the Ipsab and applied in the areas where the conditions are indicated at the base or edge of the gums. (3696-1)

This will *purify* and make for such a condition as to assist in correcting the trouble where there has been the softening of the teeth themselves—or the enamel on same. (1026-1)

Case 257, whom we quoted earlier, also wrote the following in the same letter: "Thanks to Ipsab, the eighteen teeth I was supposed to lose about five years ago according to two dentists' prognosis in Ohio, all are still with me, each and every one! I still have to keep up the pyorrhea fight, though, but now I only have to use the Ipsab once a week—*some weeks I forget to do it at all!"*

Other Tooth Disorders

(Q) What can I do to prevent the teeth from wearing down?
(A) Use more of an alkaline-reacting diet; as quantities of orange juice with a little lemon in same, as four parts orange juice to one part lemon; grapefruit, raw vegetables, potato peel . . . (365-3)

For local disturbance, use Ipsab as a massage for gums; using this just 3 times a week. Then use any good dentifrice; preferably that of the same combinations of [chemicals as contained in] Ipsab, but without the iodine in same—Ipana. (3051-1)

(Q) What causes the gray film on teeth?
(A) The chemical balance in the system and the throw-off or discharge from breath in the lungs. This [the breath] is a source from which drosses are relieved from the system, and thus passing through the teeth produce [evidences of] same on the teeth. Keeping such cleansed with an equal combination of *soda and salt at least* three to four times a week will cleanse these [teeth] of this disturbance. The use of Ipsab as a wash for mouth and gums will further aid in keeping these conditions cleansed; and use any good dentifrice once or twice a day. [Italics added.] (457-11)

(Q) What should be done about her teeth, the existing condition of enamel? Is it due to her diet, or can some correction be made by dentist?
(A) . . . We would include with the diet, twice a day, those properties that are found in Calcios [or increase calcium-rich foods]. This would be most beneficial. [Take] about half a teaspoonful, level; taken twice each day, *with* the meal. (903-31)

(Q) Does gold in mouth help to cause bitterness?
(A) It does! No teeth should ever be filled with heavy metals, as gold. (325-55)

Where there is indicated that pus sacs are a portion of the roots of the teeth, remove 'em! For they only become a storehouse for poisons. (325-54)

Q) What can I do to keep my fingernails from splitting?
(A) Add the vitamins necessary so that the glandular forces, and especially the thyroid, are improved.
        (2448-1)

Halitosis

Bad breath in most cases comes from improper elimination and/or decaying teeth. Cayce recommended internal cleansing with colonics, packs, a well-balanced diet, and in a number of cases ingesting Glyco-Thymoline in water as an intestinal antiseptic:

(Q) How can I get rid of bad breath?
(A) By making for better conditions in eliminations. Take Glyco-Thymoline as an intestinal antiseptic. Two, three times a day. Put six drops of Glyco-Thymoline in the water. This is a throwing off into the lung, into the body-forces, poisons from this changing in cellular activity, or through the body, of lymph forces that become fecal. (5198-1)

Nails

Proper diet and good eliminations and circulation are essential for the growth and maintenance of good nails. Particular attention must be paid to obtaining adequate amounts of calcium and minerals in the diet. In extreme cases be sure to check your thyroid metabolism with your doctor.

This Cayce remedy for nail care has helped some patients:

(Q) What should be done for breaking of nails?
(A) We would massage the fingers around the cuticle with the Atomidine. This will tend to color for a while, but with the treatments that have been indicated, and the rubs [massage] and the diets—with this used once or twice a week so as to allow that already begun to grow, we should have better condition . . . (3025-1)

For the calcium intake in this case, Cayce recommended Calcios (as previously mentioned, a calcium preparation) and an antacid preparation, Acigest (no longer made) in half a teaspoonful stirred in a glass of raw milk, preferably homogenized. There are other antacids on the market similar in chemical composition.

Take a few doses or drops of Atomidine occasionally; say once a month, just before the [menstrual] period, take one drop of Atomidine in half a glass of water before the morning meal, for three to five days.

Also massage the fingernails with Atomidine. It may stain for a bit at first; but get the system going better and we will find this will be different.
        (2448-1)

(Q) What causes the deep ridges in thumbnail and what treatments . . . ?
(A) These are the activities of the glandular force, and the addition of those foods which carry large quantities of calcium will make bettered conditions . . . Take often chicken neck, chew it. Cook this well, the feet and those portions of the fowl, and we will find it will add calcium to the body. Also eat bones of fish, as in canned fish. Also parsnips and oyster plant; all of these, of

course, in their regular season. Wild game of any kind, but chew the bones of same . . . (5192-1)

(Q) What should be done to correct the nail-biting habit?
(A) This is the effect of nervousness—from the gnawing that has been indicated that has been existent for some time in the system, see? And with these corrections, and with the tendency for the body to watch or be careful with self, this [habit] may be eliminated . . . For, if we take away the cause the habit is more easily changed. *For, we correct habits by forming others! That's everybody!* [Italics added.] (475-1)

Feet and Legs

Callouses, Corns, and Bunions
(Q) What caused growth on foot, and what should be used if it repeats itself?
(A) This was from irritation; and that best for the reduction of same, as we find, would be a massage with baking soda which has been dampened with spirits of camphor. This will be good for anyone having callous places or any attendant growths on feet; for it will remove them entirely! (276-4)

Bathe the limb from the knee down with warm olive oil. Then apply the saturated solution of spirits of camphor, with bicarbonate of soda. Even spread it on, as a very thin layer, see? bandaging this with a *thin* cloth . . . about the limb and foot, see? Let this remain over the evening, or night, see?
(3776-13)

Ingrown and Infected Toenails
These . . . [ingrown toenails] would respond to the dampening of baking soda with spirits of camphor and putting a small quantity of same on cotton, or alone, under the tip of the nail, close to the irritated place. This will remove the condition if used daily or nightly. (1770-4)

 . . . for the conditions of toes and nails, use baking soda moistened with Castor Oil. Put this under the points or edges where ingrown toenails give disturbance. This may make it sore for one time, but rub off with Spirits of Camphor. These may make for roughening but it will rid the body of those tendencies of ingrown toenails. (5104-1)

Once each week we would use the Atomidine as a massage for the soles of the feet, and as a dressing for the toenails . . . this will change the disturbance with ingrowing nails. Lift up the nail and put small parts of cotton saturated with Atomidine under the edge of the toenail. Use this at least once each week. (2988-1)

(Q) [What can be done] for the infected toenails?
(A) These applications suggested will be the more helpful, but as an ointment

(Q) What can I do to cure callous or bunion on my left foot?
(A) As we would find, an application morning and evening [will do it]—not bound on, but massaged thoroughly; and this means not just dabbing on and leaving same, but take three to five minutes of massaging. First, for five to ten days, use common baking soda wet or saturated with spirits of camphor. Then, after this has been used until the soreness is removed, use equal parts of Olive Oil and Tincture of Myrrh, and it'll be like baby's foot! Massage each of those into the portion where there is the disturbance. (574-1)

(Q) What causes excessive dryness or peeling of skin on bottoms of feet?

(A) Poor circulation. Hence the needs for the massage and oil rubs, which should include the limbs—of course—and especially the feet, with adjustments in the muscular forces and bursa of the feet [Peanut Oil and Olive Oil; equal parts]. (1770-5)

here we would use Carbolated Vaseline and then the Cuticura Ointment over same. (5068-1)

Athlete's Foot

A grateful patient wrote, "Just a note to tell you that I have discovered another use for good old ATOMIDINE—it has completely cured my athlete's foot. I remembered you warning about never putting a bandage over a sore after putting on Atomidine, so I made sure the toes were good and dry and well-aired before putting on shoes and stockings. Worked like a miracle."

Also recommended for athlete's foot in a number of Cayce readings is Ray's Ointment, a lotion made up of Nujol, witch hazel, sassafras oil, and pure kerosene. (See back of book for source of supply.)

Pain in Feet and Limbs

[If the feet and limbs give a great deal of trouble] we would apply Mullein Stupes over those areas of the ankle and foot. Put these on hot and then bind about with padding or wadding to keep the heat. Apply these stupes at least twice each day. Preferably use the green or fresh mullein. This would be bruised, put in very hot water and allowed to stand a few minutes, then dipped out and applied between gauze over the affected area. (2227-3)

Fallen Arches

Each evening before retiring, bathe the feet and limbs to the knees in a very mild tannic acid; which may best be made (for such conditions) from coffee grounds. When they are ready to be thrown out, put on a cupful to a gallon and a half of water. Let boil for ten minutes, pour off [the liquid], and allow to cool sufficiently so that the lower limbs may be bathed in it. Massage the limbs and the feet, especially the heels and the arches and toes, all the time they are in the solution, see? The whole quantity being used, of course. Drain the dregs off, or the grounds; and keep the limbs and feet in same for twenty minutes.

After taking them out of the solution, massage them with *this* compound for five to ten minutes; putting the ingredients together in the order named:

Russian White Oil	½ pint
Witch Hazel	2 ounces
Rubbing Alcohol	4 ounces
Oil of Sassafras	3 minims
Tincture of Capsici	2 minims

Massage only the amount the skin will absorb. Shake the solution together, for the tendency will be for the Oil of Sassafras to rise to the top—see? Pour a small quantity in a saucer, and only massage into the feet and to the limbs to the knees, including the knees. And do it yourself! And we'll be rid of all of this trouble, and it'll help the body in many different ways. It'll walk ten miles instead of five! (386-3)

(Q) What is the best thing to do for his fallen arches?

...e condition!
(1735-1)

...e present are
...ody. Thus the
...y great length
...bs and thighs

...o, causes the
...the body.
...on which has
...caused undue

...e lumbar and
...he spine—are
...lencies for the
...so slow in the
...ower limbs.)
...e fresh, green,
...Mullein leaves
...d keep in the
...ounce and a
...een at least every two or three days. Keep
this up, and it will aid in the circulation, in the elimination of the character of
acid in system, and aid in the circulation through the veins—that are disturbing.

When there is the ability to rest, apply the Mullein Stupes to the areas in
knee and along the thigh, and just below the knee where the veins are more
severe. But the Tea taken internally will be more effective.

Do keep up eliminations.

Massage the feet and lower limbs daily in a tannic acid solution, or that
preferably obtained from using old coffee grounds—which carries a mild tannic acid as well as other properties that would be beneficial—that is, the
coffee made from same, see? Boil these and use these, as well as the liquid, to
bathe feet in—of evenings.

Do have the corrections osteopathically made in lumbar-sacral axis, *and*
the coccyx area; and coordinate the rest of the body, for the tiredness and for
the relaxing of the nerves, when these are done. (243-38)

(Also see exercises in Chapter 7 for legs, feet, and ankles; and sitz baths,
Chapter 10.)

(Q) What are those terrible pains from, in toes next [to] small one on each
foot, particularly the left one?
(A) Poor circulation through the lower limbs. The varicose veins, of course,

fail to carry the circulation, thus causing the swelling of limbs and the disturbance of the body. (243-39)

Moles, Warts, and Cysts

(Q) What treatment would remove the mole on my chest, or is this advisable?

(A) The massage with Castor Oil twice each day; not rubbing hard, but *gentle* massage around and over the place. And it will be removed.
(573-1)

(Q) Should moles on the back be removed? If so, by whom and what method?
(A) As we find, these are not to be disturbed to the extent of material or outside influence.

The massaging . . . with just the Castor Oil will prevent growth . . . [Persistence with massaging] will remove same entirely. (678-2)

(Q) What should be done for the small mole or soft growth on left side of back, just below the shoulder blade, that gets irritated at times and is painful?
(A) Use a small quantity of Castor Oil with a little soda mixed in same. This will make it sore for a day or two, then it will disappear.
(Q) Just rub it on?
(A) Just rub it on, two or three days apart, for two or three times. (4033-2)

Mrs. [934] wrote the following:
"The castor oil massage worked beautifully. That great big old brown mole just dried up and fell off. It was in the middle of my right cheek and looked like a bug. It didn't seem to take any time. Just about ten days, I guess."
Mrs. T.L., Sr., wrote this:
"Castor oil is being applied to my husband's mole which is on his face and it shows signs of lightening.
"My mother–in–law also is using the castor oil on her breast mole which she says is now flaking off after two weeks of application."

(Q) The small growth on the first finger of my right hand is still there. Should anything further be done?
(A) This may be massaged with pure Castor Oil and be removed, see?
(Q) How often?
(A) About twice a day; before retiring and when arising. (261-10)

(Q) What causes the warts on the hand and how may they be removed?
(A) This . . . happens to most every individual in those periods of the change that comes about for glandular reaction; and it is the effect of localizing of centers that attempt to *grow*—as they do!

As we find, they may be removed by touching same with a (20%) solution of Hydrochloric Acid. But do not pick at them as the discoloration takes place, and as they begin to deteriorate! Rather let them wear off than pick at them, see? For such would allow too great a chance for infection by the irritating, and cause disturbance; otherwise they will disappear.

In touching them with the Acid it is preferable to use either a glass pestle (that is, a small round piece of glass) or a broom straw. (487-22)

(Q) How can [1179] get rid of her warts?
(A) Apply a paste of baking soda with Castor Oil. Mix together and apply of evenings. Just the proportions so it makes almost a *gum;* not as dough but more a gum, see? A pinch between the fingers with three to four drops in the palm of the hand, and this worked together and then placed on—bound on. It may make for irritation after the second or third application, but leave it off for one evening and then apply the next—and it will be disappearing! (1179-3)

This is the treatment for planter's wart for P.L.H., age six, by her mother, B.S.H., a member of the A.R.E.: "Dr. J.A. White removed the wart with an electric needle; one week later it was back. I applied Castor Oil and Baking Soda–paste twice a day for about two hours for five days. About seven days later I observed my child's foot and the wart was completely gone."

B.L.W., of Chelan, Washington, wrote as follows:

"Two weeks ago I went to a dermatologist with some darkened spots on my face (around a hundred small spots). They are a form of tiny, flat warts which spread. He prescribed an acid mixture and demonstrated on a few places on my face how carefully it was to be put on with a toothpick which had to be dipped into the solution. Four hours later I had one of the worst reactions the doctor had ever seen to this medicine. Large burning blisters. I threw the acid away and am now using cold–pressed castor oil. Am happy to report that the warts are already beginning to come off."

Mrs. L.E.B., of West Palm Beach, Florida, sent this information:

"The book on Edgar Cayce gave spirits of camphor for warts, moles, corns. My poor music teacher had a wart on her face. It was getting so big it pushed her glasses out. I told her about this. She used it and it's gone. She sends her grateful thanks for saving her $50 she did not have."

Plantain Salve for Warts and Moles

As we find, these we would do in the present:

First, we would give the suggestion that there be prepared an ointment from the leaves of young Plantain, at this particular season of the year [July], growing in the vicinity where this body lives [Kentucky]. Yes, it is this herb, that you desire oft to get rid of, in the yard, garden or walk. Do not use the seed, so much, in the ointment. Gather the tender leaves, about the quantity that may be crammed, not too tightly, into a pint [measuring] cup. Then put this into a quart enamel container (with an enamel or glass top) and add one pint of sweet cream, poured off the top of milk.

Cook this until it is rather thick. Do not allow to burn.

(Q) What is the best way to remove warts?
(A) This one on the right knee is gradually leaving. Put equal portions of castor oil and soda on the fingertip, massage this, it'll make it sore but it'll take it away also.
(308-13)

Then use it as an ointment over the areas where these protuberances gather at times—for they do vary. They become as warts or moles that become infected and sore, and run. This Ointment will tend to dry same. (3121-1)

The plantain mentioned above is a weed. The leaves grow flat on the ground, the flower comes up in the spring and summer like a wild dandelion. One common identification mark is the lengthwise ribbing on the leaves. It is also excellent for burns and has been known to heal the abrasions in some skin cancers.

(Q) What caused and may anything be done to eliminate the red spot on my nose?
(A) This is from a broken cell. Do not irritate it too much, or this may turn to a mole or wart—which would be a disfiguration to the body.
We would keep a little camphor, or camphor-ice on same of evenings. (288-51)

(Q) What causes the little place on this eyelid and what will remove it?
(A) Cyst as from breaking of cellular forces. Massage with the pure Castor Oil. (1424-4)

(Q) What causes the lump on the left eyelid?
(A) An accumulation from broken cellular tissue. This as we find will disappear as there are the corrections for the flow of circulation through the whole of these areas . . . [osteopathy]. (1523-5)

Rev. L.L. of Barnardsville, North Carolina (1424-4), sent this message:
"For cysts I'm using castor oil on eyelids and thank God it is working. I'm grateful to Edgar Cayce for this help."

Massage Mixtures for Scars

(Also see p.184.)

(Q) Will continued use of Camphorice gradually eliminate scar on arm [resulting from severe burn two years ago]?
(A) Camphorice, or better—as we find—Camphorated Oil. Or make the [body's] own Camphorated Oil; that is, by taking the regular Camphorated Oil and adding to it, in these proportions:

    Camphorated Oil .... 2 ounces
    Lanolin, dissolved .... ½ teaspoonful
    Peanut Oil ....1 ounce

This combination will quickly remove this tendency of the scar—or scar tissue. (2015-10)

These may be aided in being removed by sufficient time, precaution, and persistence in activity; by the massage over those portions of small quantities at a time of Tincture of Myrrh and Olive Oil, and Camphorated Oil. These would be massaged at different times, to be sure; one one day and the other the second day from same—see? In preparing the Olive Oil and Tincture of Myrrh, heat the Oil and add the Myrrh—equal portions, only preparing such a quantity as would be used at each application. The Camphorated Oil may be obtained in quantity. Only massage such quantities as the cuticle and epidermis will absorb. This will require, to be sure, a long period, but remember the whole surface may be entirely changed if this is done persistently and consistently. In the massaging, do not massage so roughly as to produce irritation. The properties are to be absorbed. Do not merely pat the solution on, but do not use tufts of cotton or other properties to dab it on—dip the fingertips into the solution, and it won't hurt the fingers either—it'll be good for them! And then massage into affected portions . . .

Olive oil—properly prepared (hence pure olive oil should always be used)—is one of the most effective agents for stimulating muscular activity, or mucous membrane activity, that may be applied to a body. Olive oil, then, combined with the Tincture of Myrrh will be very effective; for the Tincture of Myrrh acts with the pores of the skin in such a manner as to strike in, causing the circulation to be carried to affected parts where tissue has been in the nature of folds—or scar tissue, produced from superficial activity from the active forces in the body itself, in making for coagulation in any portion of the system, whether external or internal. And, as indicated in the specific [scar] conditions referred to in relation to this body [this massage] will be most effectual. The Camphorated Oil is merely the same basic force [olive oil] to which has been added properties of camphor in more or less its raw or original state, than the spirits of same. Such activity in the epidermis is not only to produce soothing to affected areas but to stimulate the circulation in such effectual ways and manners as to combine with the other properties in bringing what will be determined, in the course of two to two and a half years, a new skin. (440-3)

Olive oil—properly prepared (hence pure olive oil should always be used)—is one of the most effective agents for stimulating muscular activity, or mucous membrane activity, that may be applied to a body. (440-3)

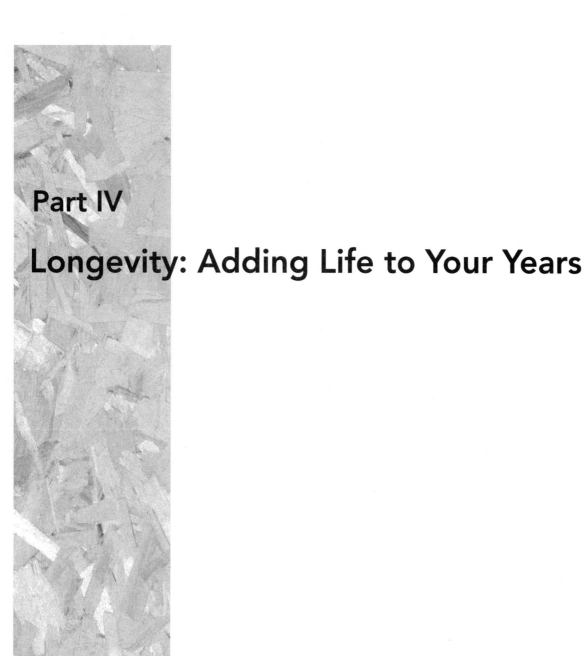

Part IV

Longevity: Adding Life to Your Years

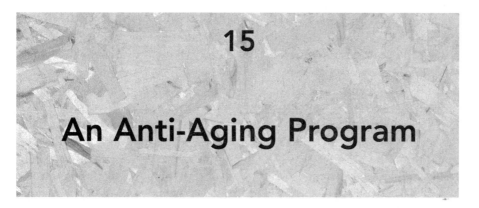

15

An Anti-Aging Program

One of the most exciting mystery stories of our time will not be found anywhere on the TV weekly schedule, crowded as it is with all manner, shapes, and sizes of detectives pursuing villains. Nevertheless, an increasing army of modern sleuths are fanning out all over the world, tracking Public Enemy No. 1 of humankind in remote mountain fastnesses in the Caucasus, in Hunzaland of western Pakistan, in Vilcabamba in Ecuador, and in hundreds of gleaming laboratories all over the world. That enemy is the mysterious and elusive aging factor.

What makes us age? What is the name and identity of this thief that steals the bloom from the prettiest cheek, the color from hair, the blood from the heart, the sound of song from the ears, the memory from the brain, the very air from the lungs, and the grace and flexibility of our bodies and limbs until, like Socrates, we moan, "I cannot eat, I cannot drink; the pleasures of youth and love are fled away; there was a good time once, but now that is gone, and life is no longer life."

In Camelot, no one ever grew old. With the help of Merlin's magic, everybody just "youthened" with the passing years. And that is the dream that our modern Merlins, clad in white coats, armed with their microscopes, measuring devices, and glass retorts, are pursuing—the ephemeral "Fountain of Youth," which brought Ponce de León to Florida and which ever after has remained a haven for those fleeing the nemesis of time. Ponce de León, like other explorers of his time, was a little confused on geography, for the mythical fountain was said to lie somewhere in southern India. Other seekers of eternal youth may have been as far off the mark as he was. For in every age, there have been necromancers who have offered every conceivable remedy to outwit Father Time—the semen of crocodile; testicle and heart of lion or tiger; genitalia of wolf; philosophers' stones; amulets; nauseous secret concoctions sold as elixirs; cakes baked in the shape of genitalia with magic spices; the exotic mixture

305

Li himself attributed his longevity to the herb Fo-ti-Tieng, which he claimed had powerful rejuvenating qualities, along with ginseng root, and he consumed only vegetables grown above the ground and fruit. In addition to his complete vegetarianism, Li was said to have had a calm and serene attitude toward life.

—H.J.R.

gotu kola

✻

called "Orvietan," so popular in the time of Louis XIV; geracomy (sleeping with virgins, as King David, according to the Bible, is reputed to have tried with little success); and even castration, since eunuchs seemed to age more slowly than their more virile brothers.

It was the Chinese who invented alchemy, and one of its goals, in addition to learning how to transmute base metal into gold, was to discover the elixir that would rejuvenate and restore youth. Many Chinese believe that the elixir has already been discovered in Fo-ti-Tieng, a herb (*Hydrocotyle asiatica*) found only in certain jungle districts of the Eastern tropics. Fo-ti-Tieng means "elixir of life" or "long-life elixir." It owes most of its reputation to the fact that a famous Chinese herbalist, Li Chung Yun, lived (it is said) to be 256 years of age, dying in 1933, and he used the herb daily throughout his life. The *New York Times* carried an extensive story about this remarkable man, whose age was apparently confirmed by the Chinese government after thorough investigation by the head of Chang-Tu University. Li had outlived twenty-three wives and was living with the twenty-fourth at the time of his death.

Li himself attributed his longevity to this herb, which he claimed had powerful rejuvenating qualities, along with ginseng root, and he consumed only vegetables grown above the ground and fruit. In addition to his complete vegetarianism, Li was said to have had a calm and serene attitude toward life. Nevertheless, other Chinese venerables have partaken of both the Fo-ti-Tieng and ginseng root and set great store by their rejuvenating properties.

Some Western research has been done on this plant, but perhaps more should be undertaken.

Another herb said to be equally as effective as the Chinese plant is gotu kola, grown principally in India, the islands of the Indian Ocean, and some parts of southern Africa.

The *Ceylon Daily News* of December 22, 1932, ran an article calling gotu kola "The Secret of Perpetual Youth." The article described the plant as "a small herb that creeps along the ground, having fan-shaped leaves of a pale-green color. It is claimed that this vegetable will increase the vitality of seventy and eighty [year olds] to that of forty. The leaves have a marked energizing effect on the cells of the brain and can preserve it indefinitely. The leaves are not a stimulant but a brain food."

The aging and old fare quite well in Oriental cultures and in tribal and peasant societies. In Japan, the elders wore red silk lining in their kimona sleeves upon attaining a certain age as a mark of respect and eminence. In the mountain communities that are now being studied so extensively, the "long-living ones" are cherished, usefully employed, and their wisdom honored in counsel until their stay on this plane is completed.

In marked contrast, age is much feared in modern Western industrial societies. For in addition to the penalties of declining vigor and faculties, and the increase of chronic disease, there are other handicaps and prejudices that seriously tarnish the gold in the "golden age." Early retirement pinches income and shelves talent and ability that should be contributing the richness of maturity, experience, and wisdom to the general welfare of the community as well as to one's own personal life. The aging are banished to playpens set up by real–estate developers to keep the "retirees" occupied with shuffleboard so they will not be underfoot in the households, businesses, and marketplaces of their younger relatives. Expensive illnesses eat away at savings that could be better employed in stimulating useful activity and enterprise. The onset of serious disease is terrifying when the prospect of inhumane nursing homes looms as the solution to the family's inability or unwillingness to cope with chronic and terminal illness. Perhaps the greatest tragedy of all is the onset of senility in a still–functioning body.

Must this be so? Can we escape this common fate?

The answer must be yes, because throughout the ages there are outstanding exceptions—men and women who are miracles of mental, physical, artistic, and creative energy at an age that extends far beyond the biblical "three score and ten."

In the annals of the ageless, much is recorded about the ability of males to produce progeny in their seventh, eighth, and ninth decades, and after the century mark, for while women measure youth by their beauty and looks, men measure youth by virility and sexual vigor. Peter Albrecht had seven children after he remarried in his eighty–fifth year and lived to be 123; Gurgen Douglas, a Swede, had eight children after he remarried in his eighty–fifth year—one of whom was born in Douglas's one hundred and third year. Even in modern times many men father children in their sixth and seventh decades. Dr. Harvey, the famous English physician who studied Thomas Parr and other long–living individuals, reported that the condition of their circulation and genitalia was very good.

In 1956, Javier Pereira, an elderly male from Colombia, South America, was brought to the New York Hospital–Cornell Medical Center for study. Mr. Pereira, a Chibcha Indian of a long–lived tribe, which produces many members living past 100 years of age, remained in the hospital for two weeks while doctors probed, tested, X–rayed, and pondered on his 167 years of age and excellent condition. Doctors Frank Glenn and Arthur J. Okinaka in 1964 published an excellent report on the study of Mr. Pereira.[1] Dr. Glenn observed that the Chibchas, like the residents of Vilcabamba, are mostly farmers living largely on cereals, fruits, and some milk products. They eat little meat and drink large amounts of coffee made from locally grown coffee beans. The patient was also said to have smoked "black tobacco" and chewed "cocoa."

In our own time and in our own society all of us have admired those prodigies of talent and "agelessness," the late Pablo Picasso, Pablo Casals, Bernard Baruch, Harry S. Truman, Igor Stravinsky, Bertrand Russell, Winston Churchill, Konrad Adenauer, and the perennial thirty–nine–year–old Jack Benny; artist Marc Chagall, Charlie Chaplin, Mae West, Gloria Swanson, Golda Meir, Marlene Dietrich, Leopold Stokowski, Jimmy Durante, and Jack Benny's equally youthful pal, George Burns. The list could go on endlessly and I apologize to anyone I have omitted. The example of all of these remarkable individuals is an inspiration that offers hope to everyone. Perhaps of even greater importance is the fact that if some can do it—i.e., beat Father Time—there must be secrets still

Living Proof

Titian produced some of his greatest paintings at the age of ninety-nine; Roscoe Pound wrote five volumes on American jurisprudence after he was eighty-six; Alonzo Stagg mowed his lawn with a hand mower at the age of ninety-eight; Thomas Parr, a Shropshireman of Old England, not only threshed grain at 130 years of age and lived to be 153, but he was accused and tried for committing a sexual offense at the age of 102. Drakenberg, a Dane, buried in the cathedral in Aarhus, Denmark, lived to 146 years of age, and at 130 the much-married evergreen fell in love and made advances to a sixteen-year-old girl; the Italian baron Baravicino de Capellis married when he was eighty-four for the fourth time and had seven children before he died at an age somewhere over 107.

In the annals of the ageless, much is recorded about the ability of males to produce progeny in their seventh, eighth, and ninth decades, and after the century mark, for while women measure youth by their beauty and looks, men measure youth by virility and sexual vigor.—H.J.R.

locked away in nature that can open the magic door to prolonged youth and life for most of humankind.

This hope is what has sent so many doctors, journalists, and film crews to the three enclaves of longevity and youthfulness, where entire populations seem to have found the secret. In Hunzaland, in Vilcabamba, and in the Abkhazia region of Georgia, and in fact elsewhere in Georgia—the mountainous region of Russia—most of the population, instead of the exceptional and rare individual, live to a human's full current potential into the nineties and well past 100, free of heart trouble, cancer, and the other crippling chronic diseases that mar the later years of more than half of the men and women of the United States and other industrialized societies.

In Vilcabamba—an Incan word meaning "sacred valley"—investigators found that 16.4 percent of the population was over sixty years of age (compared with 10 percent in America); and nine of the 819 inhabitants were over 100. The "longevos" and all others are farmers, who work hard and vigorously throughout their lifetime. There is no such word or concept as retirement. Their diet is very low in animal protein and fat, running around 1,200 calories, and is composed chiefly of fruits, vegetables, and grains. But they do make a strong local rum drink from sugar cane, which is grown in the valley, and they drink coffee and chew coca leaves.

The local medicine man cures with home remedies, including tobacco and whiskey—for treatment of a variety of complaints—the coca leaves, and the waters of a mineral spring that is supposed to have great curative properties.

Although there is absolutely no sanitation (one resident admits to not having had a bath in ten years) and infant mortality is very high, the adults do not have the common diseases that inflict their countrymen living in cities. Most of the population is European—not of Indian descent—and the genetic strain of longevity has been well protected by the insulation of the valley.

Hunza, ruled by a hereditary line of leaders known as Mirs, is one of the most inaccessible places on the earth. Unfortunately, many researchers in the past thirty-five years have penetrated its mountain seclusion and consequently the extraordinary perfect health of the Hunzas is beginning to be affected by civilized acquaintance with sugars and other contaminating influences.

A Pakistani nutritionist who has surveyed the diet of fifty-five adult males in Hunza puts the daily diet average at 1,923 calories: 50 grams of protein, 36 grams of fat, and 354 grams of carbohydrate. Meat and dairy products account for only 1 percent of the total.

From other reports we gather that the diet is composed of grains, leafy green vegetables, root vegetables, dried legumes, fresh milk and buttermilk, clarified butter and cheese, fresh and sun-dried apricots and mulberries, and grape wine. Oil extracted from apricot seeds is used in cooking.

Like the Vilcabambans, the Hunzas work hard to wrest a living from the rocky hills and "one sees an unusual number of old people vigorously and agilely climbing up and down the steep slopes of the valley."

Renee Taylor in *Hunza Health Secrets* [2] points out that the remarkable thing about the populace is that it is free from heart attacks, cancer—and war.

The Hunzakuts are genetically pure through their isolation, so that longevity has been transmitted and can be traced in their ancestry.

In Abkhazia, however, the genetic factor is less important, for many people over 100 are not only Georgian but also Russian, Jewish, Armenian, and Turkish. Abkhazia is only one of the three Soviet republics that make up the Georgian region: the others are Georgia and Armenia. In this entire region, a great many more old people are found in the mountainous areas than at sea level.

Dr. G.Z. Pitzkhelaur, head of the Gerontological Center in the Republic of Georgia, has reported that the 1970 census placed the number of centenarians for the entire Caucasus between 4,500 and 5,000. In terms of percentages, in Abkhazia almost 3 percent of the population lives to over 100 years of age.

In the Caucasus considerably more milk products (especially yogurt and cheese) are consumed, since they have an active dairy economy; but the cheese is very low in fat content and the total fat intake is only forty to sixty grams per day. This compares with an average American intake of 157 grams daily.

Considering the other factors that enter into longevity, the Abkhazians have no word at all for "old people." Those who reach and surpass 100 years of age are referred to as "long-living people." Everyone works hard right up to the day of demise. There is little stress in their lives—although like all the other mountain peoples they work very hard—and competition is unknown.

There is an Abkhazian saying that "without rest, you cannot work: without work, the rest may not give you any benefit." In addition to hard, physical labor, daily hikes, swimming, and horseback rides are enjoyed even by the old.

In the very first opening words of this book, I quoted Edgar Cayce's words on life expectancy, which he felt should range in contemporary times from 121 to 150 years of age, and now we find most gerontologists and scientists agreeing with him. Why, then, are we only enjoying a life expectancy of 71.2 years for men (around 76.1 for women), which is higher than it has been but still many years short of our full life potential?

Obviously our lifestyle in the modern Western world falls far short of the youth-perpetuating habits of the mountain people of the Caucasus, Ecuador, and Hunzaland. Nor can we, if we would, all find our own mountain to live on. But we can discipline ourselves to duplicate those elements that make for long years of healthy, disease-free, youthful, vigorous living, and throughout the pages of this book we have been giving you the very secrets and guidelines you need to attain these goals.

When Cayce was asked, "Is it possible for our bodies to be rejuvenated in this incarnation?" he gave this reply:

Possible. For, as the body is an atomic structure, the units of energy around which there are the movements of the atomic forces that—as given—are ever the sentiment or pattern of a universe, as these atoms, as these structural forces are made to conform or to rely upon or to be one with the spiritual import, the spiritual activity, they revivify, they make for constructive forces.

The soul cannot die; for it is of God. *The body may be revivified, rejuvenated.* And it is to that end it may, the body, *transcend* the earth and its influence. (262-85)

There is an Abkhazian saying that "without rest, you cannot work: without work, the rest may not give you any benefit." In addition to hard, physical labor, daily hikes, swimming, and horseback rides are enjoyed even by the old.—H.J.R.

. . . for each cell in the atomic force of the body is as a world of its own and each one—each cell—being in perfect unison, may build to that necessary to reconstruct the forces, of the body in all its needs. (93-1)

Remember the body does gradually renew itself constantly. Do not look upon the conditions which have existed as not being able to be eradicated from the system . . . Hold to that *knowledge* and don't think of it as just theory—that the body *can,* the body *does* renew itself! (1548-3)

Let us pause for a moment now and compare the wisdom of the more primitive way of life and the Cayce concepts with the findings of modern science.

The most popular—at least the most highly publicized—methods of rejuvenation in this century up to now have been based on the work of prominent "youth" doctors, such as Dr. Paul Niehans of Switzerland and Dr. Ana Aslan of Romania. Dr. Niehans, the eminent cell therapist whose famous patients included Konrad Adenauer, Somerset Maugham, and Pope Pius XII, injected his aging patients with the fresh chopped-up embryos of lambs, which are supposed to rejuvenate the organs and cells. Dr. Aslan injects her patients with a procaine mixture.

Both therapists (whose patients swore by the effectiveness of the respective therapies) put them on rigid regimens of no alcohol, no smoking, and no sunbathing (which is very aging, as we pointed out in the chapter on beauty tips).

In addition, Dr. Ana Aslan, when treating patients at her Romanian retreat in Bucharest, retains her patients over a period of time during which they are disciplined and regulated as to diet, exercise, rest, and careful observation. Her T.L.C. (tender, loving care) may explain why Dr. Aslan has gotten better results than other doctors who have tried the procaine treatment on their patients. She also has patients return for "booster" shots—which is what I term "shoulder-tapping"—and it always has a very beneficial effect in sustaining improvement in patients. Dr. Alex Comfort, the eminent British gerontologist, and other scientists have suggested that it is the "care" and attention the patients receive, the added exercise, and the improved diet and rest, rather than the procaine itself that produces the results. We shall have to await the verdict of further research.

Dr. Aslan's product, Gerovital 3, is now being tested with human patients in clinics in a number of centers in the United States in an effort to obtain licensing for use from the FDA. Such respectable researchers in gerontology and pharmacology as Drs. Josef P. Hrachovec and M. David MacFarlane, scientists at the University of Southern California, and others report that the effective element in the procaine may be something that inhibits monoamine oxidase (MAOI). MAOI is an enzyme that seems to be correlated to depression in people over the age of forty-five and may be one of the elusive villains of the aging process itself—a subject we will discuss in greater detail later in this chapter. Dr. Nathan S. Kline, associate professor of psychiatry at Columbia University's College of Physicians and Surgeons and director of the research center at

Rockland State Hospital, Orangeburg, New York, is coordinating the research on Gerovital 3. However, when and if the drug is licensed it will be as an antidepressant, not as a cure for aging.

Although Dr. Niehans recently died at a ripe old age—in his eighties—(without availing himself of the benefits of his lamb–embryo injections, according to his biographers), his work is being carried on at his Swiss La Prairie Clinic, and other youth doctors have adopted his methods. When others did not achieve the same remarkable results that Dr. Niehans reported, he attributed their failure to the fact that they were using dried instead of fresh–killed material or that they were not doing it properly, or some other reason. The famous novelist Somerset Maugham did recover from senility when he took the treatment and followed the discipline of no smoking or drinking; but the third time he was treated, upon relapsing into his bad smoking and drinking habits, he was not helped at all. Therefore, since cell therapy has not been subjected to the rigid clinical testing that Ana Aslan's work is now undergoing, it is difficult to pass judgment on it. We don't know whether it is the lamb embryos or the discipline that helps. One must consider also the charisma of the doctor, which influences the mind and spirit of the patient. And no one who believes in Edgar Cayce's work would underestimate the value and role of those two elements—for body, mind, and spirit are one.

To return to the more prosaic and scientifically based methods of unraveling the mystery of why we age and what causes aging, we find that if current research has not yet found all the answers, at least it has dispelled many misconceptions and turned up some valid clues that can help us cope with the problems of aging until the cure is found.

One of the first misconceptions to be dispelled is that people die of "old age." Dr. Robert H. Dorenmuehle of Duke University's Center for Aging says, "People do not die of old age—only disease."

The late Dr. Edward L. Bortz of Philadelphia's Lakenhau Hospital, former president of the AMA and the American Geriatrics Society, used to say: "There is no known case of death from old age. No pathologist has ever established at the autopsy table that a person dying of old age (natural causes) had body tissues correct and adequate in every way except that they had worn out in the process of aging. People do not die of old age, they die of diseases which occur with the passing of time. All these are recognizable."

Theoretically, as mentioned in Chapter 1, it is possible for humans to live forever. Each day our body manufactures trillions of new cells. The only cells that do not reproduce are those of the muscles and the brain. Tumor and cancer cells have been kept alive in laboratory solutions for many years and may be eternal. Cayce, in some of his readings, said that people in biblical times lived up to 1,000 years.

There should be a warning to *all* bodies as to such conditions; for would the assimilations and the eliminations be kept nearer *normal* in the human family, the days might be extended to whatever period as was so desired; for the system is *builded* by the assimilations of that it takes within, and is able to bring resuscitation so long as the eliminations do not hinder. (311-4)

This is right in line with the latest research on aging, which is studying what happens to the cells when a person grows old. When we are on our deathbed, we are full of cells only twenty-four hours old. There is a growing belief among scientists that what happens to the cells that die may contain the secret of aging and mortality, as Cayce suggested in his emphasis on "elimination."

When young cells are put into a chemical solution, they live and subdivide fifty times—the life span that is programmed into them genetically by the DNA and RNA. When the same cells are put into a deep freeze after twenty subdivisions and then defrosted, they continue to subdivide until they reach their full program of fifty subdivisions. On the other hand, if the cells are taken from an old person, they subdivide from ten to twenty times and then die.

Some geneticists, especially those active in the newly exploding field of molecular biological science, theorize that the life span is programmed into the genes—and that is why long-lived persons come from long-lived parents, grandparents, and ancestors.

Why do fruit flies die in forty days; the mayfly in twenty-four hours; the mouse after three years; the human after seventy years (although one's normal span should be at least 110 or more years); the turtle at 200 years? The genetic code says, "So much—no more. Like a phonograph record, your song is ended—you are through."

Other geneticists say no to this fatalistic view. They believe that, like scratches on our life phonograph record or tape, errors occur in the repeated copying of the genetic message and this interferes with the communication of the correct life-giving messages. Dr. Josef P. Hrachovec subscribes to this latter view and says in his book, *Keeping Young and Living Longer,* [3] "The human body is designed to function efficiently to an age numbering in three figures. But most people are robbed of achieving this potential by the accumulated effects of a variety of stresses. Permitting these stresses to act upon us day after day, month after month, year after year, comprises the disease-inducing, life-shortening errors which sap our strength and shorten our lives . . . Preventive maintenance functions to allow us to achieve the potential life span past 100 years—that is our birthright."

Dr. Williams, the biochemical nutritionist, concedes that heredity is important and "may be a serious stumbling block to continued good health and longevity . . . and [a person] may be barred from longevity, provided he eats and lives very much like his neighbors. If, however, by using unusual expedients he can get a suitable assortment of everything his bodily cells need, he may be able to retain a measure of youth until old age, even though initially he may have been handicapped by heredity." [4]

Dr. Williams is saying here that we can overcome the obstacle or handicap of heredity. His solution is adequate nutrition.

Dr. Clive M. McKay of Cornell University and his co-workers in experiments carried on as far back as 1932 proved that by underfeeding rats one could increase their life span by 33 percent. The example of the "longevos" of

Vilcabamba and the "long–living ones" of Georgia and Hunzaland who live on such a limited–calorie diet would seem to support the theory for humans as well as laboratory rats.

However, Dr. Williams has pointed out that when rats are underfed, they live longer because they mature at a *slower* pace and *later* age. "With human beings, underfeeding with good food might result in a delay of maturity (perhaps it would be necessary to raise the voting age to thirty). The social practicality of increasing life span in human beings by underfeeding seems dubious," he concludes.

Nevertheless, no one disagrees that obesity is a serious threat to longevity and that as one grows older it is wise to cut the intake of calories provided essential nutrients are included. Dr. Nathan Shock of the Gerontology Research Center of the National Institute of Child Health and Human Development puts it this way: "If you could suddenly wave a wand and eliminate all the obesity in the population, you'd be more likely to increase life span than by almost any other means."[5] Keeping your weight down reduces the risk of stroke, hypertension, heart attacks, diabetes, and other killers that are on the increase after the age of sixty.

Dr. Denham Harman of the University of Nebraska is pursuing villains called "free radicals"; these produce in cells a heavy deposit of lipofuscin, also known as age pigment. Dr. Harman told a national conference on aging, sponsored by the Huxley Institute on March 6, 1972, that the deposit is "very characteristic of the senile period." He went on to say that "rather than discuss whether senility and memory loss is a psychiatric or a biochemical problem, for all changes—functional or organic—are basically due to chemical reactions, I should like to consider a possible approach for slowing the rate of degradation in the brain and elsewhere so as to increase our years of healthy, productive life.

"There are two aspects of this problem," he continued. "One is to slow the rate of degradation (deterioration) of the body as a whole; and two, to be sure that the brain deteriorates in step with or behind the remainder of the body, so that the higher functions are essentially intact until death."

Dr. Harman cites, as examples, the burning of gasoline and the development of rancidity in butter to illustrate free radical reactions. In humans, this process produces harmful peroxides when lipids (fats) combine with oxygen.

Dr. Harman warns that polyunsaturated lipids (oils), such as those in safflower and corn oils, would be expected to increase the level of free radical reactions as compared with comparable amounts of lard or olive oil. This was confirmed experimentally by feeding mice and rats diets in which the sole source of lipid was lard, olive oil, corn oil, or safflower oil. *Increasing the degree of unsaturation of dietary fat caused the animals to die significantly faster.*

This bombshell of information directly contradicts all the educational admonitions of medical authorities trying to save us from premature death from heart attacks because of cholesterol–clogged arteries. It seems to leave us on the horns of a most uncomfortable dilemma: either you risk cardiovascular disease and arteriosclerosis from animal (saturated) fats or you court an earlier death because the polyunsaturates combine with oxygen to produce noxious

Dr. Harman cites, as examples, the burning of gasoline and the development of rancidity in butter to illustrate free radical reactions. In humans, this process produces harmful peroxides when lipids (fats) combine with oxygen.

—H.J.R.

. . . we ought to be able to take a couple of millimeters of blood from a person, run tests to see what his hormone levels are, then give him a cocktail of juices to remedy some of the imbalances involved in aging.—**Dr. Caleb E. Finch**

peroxides that will shorten the life of your cells—and yours with it.

However, do not despair. Help is at hand. As Dr. Williams points out in *Nutrition Against Disease:* [6]

"Lipid (fat) peroxidation, the formation of harmful peroxides from the interaction between oxygen and highly unsaturated fats (polyunsaturates) needs to be controlled in the body. Both oxygen and the polyunsaturated lipids are essential to our existence, but if the protection against peroxidation is inadequate, serious damage to various body proteins may result.

"Vitamin E is thought to be the leading agent for the prevention of peroxidation and the free radical production which is associated both with it and with radiation. Vitamin E, along with a relatively large number of other antioxidants—ascorbic acid (vitamin C) ubiquinones, sulfhydryl compounds, and the trace element selenium—do their jobs in a complicated manner. They protect the body against the damaging products formed when oxygen reacts directly with the highly unsaturated fatty substances which are essential parts of our metabolic machinery . . .

"As a practical matter, providing plenty of vitamin E and ascorbic acid—both harmless antioxidants—is indicated as a possible means of preventing premature aging."

Vitamin C, or ascorbic acid, is frequently mentioned in connection with the deterioration and loss of flexibility in the collagen that accounts for the stiffening of joints as we grow older.

"Since ascorbic acid is absolutely essential for the building of healthy collagen," Dr. Williams advises, "it seems probable that an abundant supply of this vitamin would tend to slow down the form of deterioration which accompanies impaired collagen production."

Dr. Caleb E. Finch of the University of Southern California is tracking the hypothalamus, deep inside the brain, as the secret aging agent. Dr. Finch has reported that changes in levels of such nerve hormones as noradrenaline coincide with age. He suspects such changes could affect the nearby pituitary gland, the body's master endocrine regulator, affecting in turn the other endocrine glands throughout the body, including the adrenals, ovaries, and testes. In the future, he suggests, "we ought to be able to take a couple of millimeters of blood from a person, run tests to see what his hormone levels are, then give him a cocktail of juices to remedy some of the imbalances involved in aging."

There is also the interesting work being done by Dr. Roy L. Walford on the theory that as we grow older, the body's immune system becomes deranged and the cells of the organism fight themselves, and in fact, the body kills itself.

Dr. Walford has doubled the life span of certain fish by reducing the temperature of its water habitat by five or six degrees. Other researchers agree that this seems to suggest that lowering human body temperature by only a degree or two could add an extra twenty-five to thirty years of life. Just how to do this—by drugs, hibernation, or some other method—still remains to be researched.

Other scientists believe that the cells after a definite number of divisions lose their generative power and kill the whole organism. As the cells deteriorate and lose their quality, waste matter collects in the cell with every division. As this waste collects, it interferes with the chemical process, and the cells begin to make tiny mistakes during the dividing process. The body then develops defense mechanisms against these wastes which, as the body ages, Dr. Walford claims, causes the cells of the organism to fight themselves and in fact kill the body.

When biochemists find a way to eliminate this waste matter from the cell before it damages the chemical process, there will be no reason for the cells to stop dividing forever and thus sustaining eternal life. (Thus far only cancer cells seem capable of eternal life in culture.)

Remember Cayce's reiterated admonition to cleanse the body—to *eliminate* in order to *regenerate.*

Let us see how current Cayce was with contemporary cellular research, when, many, many years ago, he said this:

> If a cell is left in the system that should be eliminated, or if it is of that condition of inactivity, then all the cells gathered about it cannot heal that cell. It *must* produce sufficient of the lymph or leukocyte . . . [to] move it out of the system, to let the new supply take its place! . . .
>
> Just as a comparison . . . a rotten apple left in a barrel may make all of these rotten; yet no matter how many sound ones are put about it, the rotten one will never be made sound. (243-7)

While none of us may even want eternal life on this planet, it is encouraging to know that so many scientists are now hard at work to solve the mystery of aging. Indeed, the outlook is very optimistic for extending youthfulness into our middle and later years.

Dr. Bernard L. Strehler, professor of biology and director of biological research and training at the Gerontology Center of the University of Southern California, asks (referring to the process of aging), "Will we someday learn how to turn the switches back on?"

His answer is extremely optimistic. "The way things are going in medical science nowadays, I would not be at all surprised if by the turn of the twenty-first century we have learned how."

A number of exciting leads were reported at the conference on "The Crisis in Health Care for the Aging," previously referred to.

Dr. Richard C. Adelman, Ph.D., of the Fels Research Institute and Department of Biochemistry of Temple University School of Medicine in Philadelphia reported that there is increasing evidence that the immune system "probably exerts a critical influence on growth and that breakdown in biological communication may be responsible not only for cancer and many other diseases but also for aging."

It thus becomes increasingly clear that the breakthrough in research on aging will probably also solve the mystery of cancer, and vice versa, since the two are closely linked.

Dr. Eleanor A. Jacobs, Ph.D., clinical assistant professor, Department of Psychiatry, School of Medicine of the State University of New York at Buffalo, and clinical psychologist at the VA Hospital in Buffalo, reported considerable success in reversing senility and memory loss by feeding oxygen to people under "increased barometric pressure," in special chambers designed for this purpose. Dr. Edwin Boyle, Jr., research director of the Miami Heart Institute, reported similar success from "immersing [the patient] in pure oxygen at 3 atmospheres of pressure—about the same as 30 pounds of pressure in an automobile tire and the equivalent of diving about 60 feet in scuba gear." Dr. Boyle concedes that not all patients so treated respond well, but many "were smarter."

Because the hyperbaric chambers are so expensive and available to only a privileged few, studies are underway on the possibilities of trace-metal metabolism, the biogenic amines, the sulfur-containing amino acids, and the antioxidant vitamins, especially ascorbic acid and vitamin E, which may achieve the same result and become more easily available and distributed.

Other experiments that show promise of being useful in solving the mystery of aging or treating its symptoms and reversing its course are being conducted with DMSO, a membrane penetrant that passes through every tissue of the body except the fingernail and tooth. "DMSO reduces pain by impeding conduction in some of the smaller nerve fibers," according to Dr. Stanley W. Jacob, associate professor of surgery at the University of Oregon Medical School, who reported on it. It is alleged that it has "anti-inflammatory properties, dissolves scar tissue, improves blood supply and scientists have demonstrated that a patient can actually be fed by dissolving protein, fat, and carbohydrate in DMSO and applying this mixture to the skin."

It is reported elsewhere that DMSO is a powerful sexual stimulant for the male and that a few drops on the skin can cause even an impotent male to respond with an erection. (This report is unverified and since the compound is not available in this country and has not been licensed by the FDA we have no reliable clinical data on it. It may be an exaggeration, since impotence is compounded of many psychological as well as physiological factors.)

Dr. Alex Comfort, director of the Gerontology Research Group of University College in London, a world-recognized gerontologist, who is better known to American TV audiences and book buyers as the author of *The Joy of Sex*,[7] summarized the entire subject at the conference with such precision and so succinctly that I would like to quote him:

"The average person, asked if he'd like to live to 150 would answer, 'Hell, no,' because he knows what he'd be like at 150. We are not trying to prolong life without regard to the quality of what we're prolonging. What we're trying to do is prolong adult vigor so that aging happens later.

"Towards this goal, there are a number of fundamental lines of attack. They are all going on now, and they all require more funding to make them go on faster.

"The first is regulative enzymology, the study of why metabolic processes change with age.

"The second is the study of error theory, based on the assumption that there may be failures in the accuracy of bodily copying processes causing faulty development in later years (through the DNA and RNA).

"Third is immunology. Why do immune mechanisms go wrong with age? Do the cops become less effective, or the robbers more numerous, or both? At the moment it seems to be both. In our study of this area there is real chance of an important advance.

"The fourth is the nature of the dietetic effect. Since 1930 we have known we could make mice and rats live 40 percent longer by manipulating the caloric content of the diet (downwards).

"The last line of attack is the antioxidant effect. Dr. Harman has the idea that if the effects of radiation resemble those of aging, antiradiation drugs might slow down natural aging—in particular those drugs which prevent oxidative attack. We do just that in preserving rubber or butter by adding substances called antioxidants which slow down the perishing process.

"So there's a bevy of ongoing experiments which in three to five years should give us a better idea of the underlying process of aging or at least what it is not."

While the scientists are deciding why you are aging, it may be important to you to keep as healthy and youthful as possible now with the knowledge and tools at hand. I sincerely believe that everything we have learned from Cayce, tested clinically throughout the years, and reported in the pages of this book, can help you do just that.

All agree on the importance of nutrition in maintaining good health and youthful vigor. In addition to the sound guidelines set forth in Chapter 5 on diet and nutrition, Cayce had a few more useful ideas that are worth heeding on nutrition and aging:

The ordinary conclusions of the activity of Gold, when assimilated, is incorrect—for these feed directly to the tissue of the brain *itself,* and given properly—silver and gold may almost lengthen life to its double, of its present endurance. (120-5)

Good sources of gold are shellfish, carrots, and oyster plant (salsify), highly regarded by Cayce for all of its mineral properties.

Also there may be obtained from the turtle egg those influences for longevity that may be created in certain cellular forces in the body. (659-1)

In *Nutrition Against Disease*, Dr. Williams says that "while no one seriously entertains the idea of a philosopher's stone which will prolong life indefinitely the evidence at hand indicates that well–rounded nutrition, including generous amounts of vitamin C and vitamin E, can contribute materially to extending the healthy life span of those who are already middle aged. The greatest hope for increasing life spans can be offered if nutrition—from the time of prenatal development to old age—is continuously of the highest quality."[8]

The average person, asked if he'd like to live to 150 would answer, "Hell, no," because he knows what he'd be like at 150. We are not trying to prolong life without regard to the quality of what we're prolonging. What we're trying to do is prolong adult vigor so that aging happens later.
—**Dr. Alex Comfort**

While the scientists are deciding why you are aging, it may be important to you to keep as healthy and youthful as possible now with the knowledge and tools at hand. I sincerely believe that everything we have learned from Cayce, tested clinically throughout the years, and reported in the pages of this book, can help you do just that.—**H.J.R.**

... while no one seriously enter-tains the idea of a philosopher's stone which will prolong life in-definitely, the evidence at hand indicates that well-rounded nutri-tion, including generous amounts of vitamin C and vitamin E, can contribute materially to extending the healthy life span of those who are already middle aged. The greatest hope for increasing life spans can be offered if nutrition— from the time of prenatal devel-opment to old age—is continuously of the highest quality. —Roger J. Williams in *Nutrition Against Disease***

A Favorite Cayce Saying
*After breakfast, work a while.
After lunch, rest a while.
After dinner walk a mile.*
(3624-1)

Cayce was much preoccupied with the glandular system and attrib-uted great importance to the pi-tuitary when Gray's Anatomy *was describing it as something of no use after the first years of growth. Cayce also attributed much importance to the Peyer's patches—a series of aggregated lymph nodules in the lining of the small intestine.* —H.J.R.

Dr. Ronald Walker of Surrey University's Department of Biochemistry, com-menting on the work of Dr. Comfort and other researchers who are experi-menting with feeding antioxidants in substantial amounts to laboratory animals, warns, "We do not yet know how antioxidants affect such things as loss of bodily functions. We have to be cautious because of potential side effects . . . I would recommend that people search out many of the natural foods that contain large amounts of them. The best diet would come from a vegetable source rather than a meat source."

This advice is certainly consonant with Cayce's repeated advice to get your nutrients from natural foods rather than pills, except in severe cases of illness.

Exercise

Dr. Hrachovec, in *Keeping Young and Living Longer*,[9] says that "exercise is the closest thing to an anti-aging pill now available." Dr. Herbert A. DeVries, who also works at the Gerontology Research Center at U.S.C., has done experiments proving that the changes in function of various organs in the human body that we associate with age are very similar to the changes that can be pro-duced in very young men simply by keeping them inactive.

In Chapters 6 and 7, I devoted considerable attention and space to the exer-cise principle, as well as instruction in specific ones. They can keep you youth-ful, fit, healthy, and vigorous throughout the years. I would like to remind "youtheners" of the special value to you of the Cayce cat, pelvic circle, and head-and-neck exercises that are all good stimulants for the glands. Also take note of the bicycle-riding to control and avoid incontinence. Cayce included exercise as part of essential therapy in almost 1,400 readings, and I can say from my own personal experience that exercise has kept me fit so that now in my eightieth year I can still outwork most of my younger students, standing on my feet all day and giving manipulation to patients.

Cayce and I have always been strong advocates of the benefits for men of colonics, sitz baths, and breach-beating as a protection from and treatment for prostatitis. I have used these therapies with repeated success on older patients and they are also equally effective preventive measures. Cayce believed that a man who took a colonic every month would never have this trouble common to aging males. Instructions for colonics (or enemas) are to be found in Chapter 11, and also instructions for sitz baths. Breach-beating, which is percussion massage on the buttocks, is described in Chapter 8, on massage and manipu-lation.

Cayce was much preoccupied with the glandular system and attributed great importance to the pituitary when Gray's *Anatomy* was describing it as some-thing of no use after the first years of growth. Cayce also attributed much importance to the Peyer's patches—a series of aggregated lymph nodules in the lining of the small intestine.

Dr. William McGarey relates in one of the medical research bulletins that Allan Goldstein, director of the Biochemistry Division of the University of Texas Medical Branch at Galveston, reported that thymosin levels in the blood decrease dramatically with age—"significantly between twenty-five to forty-five years of age." Thymosin is a hormone produced by the thymus gland, and Goldstein found that injecting this hormone into mice increased their immunity and resistance to disease. The thymus gland is the master of the immune system and it has been known for years that cells from the thymus migrate to other portions of the body (such as to the Peyer's patches) and become centers of lymphatic activity.

Peyer's patches are best marked in the young, become indistinct in middle age, and sometimes disappear altogether in advanced life. The Cayce readings suggest that these patches tend to become fewer in number as the body grows weaker and that the regular use of castor oil packs over the abdomen tends to rejuvenate these glands and thus serve as a major factor in the rejuvenation of the entire body.

> When there is over-exercise physically, or especially the mental forces as of worry or anxiety, to be sure it calls on the necessity of these emunctory activities—or those patches that are called by a man's name [Peyer's patches]. These are then lessened in their number and thus make a quickening or an anxiety, causing the flow of blood in the heart . . . to dilate. (294-212)

> Now in the physical forces of the body (as seen and understood, in the nervous systems of the body) there are those glands that secrete fluids which in the circulation sustain and maintain the reaction fluid in the nerve channels themselves. (271-5)

Dr. McGarey goes on to explain that "merging all these bits of information together, one might say that lack of tensions, or not being able to handle them properly might be directly related to the number of Peyer's patches present in one's body, which in turn could well have a strong influence on how one lives. Castor oil packs, one might postulate, could well have an influence on the length of one's life."

The human being is more than a body, and a program for adding years to one's life and life to one's years must consider many other factors. Most of my former patients and clients who lived or who are living into their eighties and nineties have been active and working at their business or professions. David Dubinsky, in his eighties, was able to beat off a youthful mugger; Bob Hope, in his seventies, looks as good as he did when he worked out at Reilly's, and in an interview he confessed he has had to wage the "battle of the bulge" against overweight all of his life. Hard work and exercise, temperate eating, and challenge keep him going.

Gloria Swanson is noted for her crusades for better, natural, and purer food. Her mental attitude, expressed in an interview with Mrs. Brod some years ago for the *Philadelphia Bulletin*, is a good Rx for youthfulness for all. "Never grow old—grow up," she told Mrs. Brod. Former Vice-President Nelson Rockefeller attributes his youthful vigorous good health and stamina to heredity (his father lived to eighty-six and his grandfather to ninety-eight). He has never

The Cayce-Reilly Blueprint for Longevity

1. Health maintenance.
2. Balance of mental and physical activities.
3. Emotional discipline.
4. Striving for ego expression through challenge.
5. Motivation for useful living.
6. Giving and receiving love and friendship.
7. Intelligent adaptation, such as adjusting to one's financial condition.

Gloria Swanson is noted for her crusades for better, natural, and purer food. Her mental attitude, expressed in an interview with Mrs. Brod some years ago for the Philadelphia Bulletin, *is a good Rx for youthfulness for all. "Never grow old—grow up," she told Mrs. Brod—***H.J.R.**

smoked, drinks only aperitif wine, never has weighed more than fifteen pounds more at his highest point from his lowest point during an exhausting political campaign, tries to hike, horseback ride, and play golf in the open, and finally he attributes a great deal to his personal osteopath, Dr. Kenneth Riland.

"I see Dr. Kenneth Riland about twice a week," Mr. Rockefeller wrote me. "This is the best possible preventive medicine and keeps one relaxed, which is very important in face of the pressures and responsibilities of public life.

"I am also convinced that health and vitality depend as much on one's state of mind as on the state of body. I am intensely interested in what I do. I thrive on solving problems. Philosophically, I am an incorrigible optimist and finally, my whole outlook is conditioned by a positive religious faith that was instilled in me by devout and loving parents from childhood."

Rockefeller concluded, "Good health is basically sensible living and purposeful living—which are, in my judgment, the best medicines ever compounded."

I think enough has been said in all the foregoing pages to guide you on proper health maintenance and balance of physical and mental activity. In addition to exercise, I would like to add the importance of having a sense of humor. Abraham Lincoln once said, "With the fearful strain that is on me night and day, if I didn't laugh, I should die." Mahatma Gandhi said, "If I had no sense of humor I would long ago have committed suicide."

One also must maintain a proper perspective on the troubles large and small that plague us all our lives. As people get older, they should have more wisdom and better judgment. The trouble is that most of them become toxic and, as a result, become irritable rapidly. One must watch that irritation. "No" has a much more detrimental effect on an older person than it has on a younger one. One way to offset this is to have a good philosophy of living—just project yourself a hundred years from now and you won't have anything to worry about. The Irish have an expression I like: "A hundred years to back it—you can't tell which were the bones that wore the ragged jacket."

The Chinese also have a wise saying: "The power that people have to hurt me, I give them." It is a good maxim to remember when things start piling up on you.

So much for emotional discipline and balance. Now we come to the concept of "challenge" and motivation for useful living.

Dr. Roy M. Hamlin, a research psychologist at the Danville, Illinois, Veterans Administration Hospital, completed a study that shows that people live for as long as they feel needed. "If the older individual has a need for the years beyond seventy, he will retain competence and live longer," Dr. Hamlin reports.

Justice William O. Douglas, in an article titled "Towards Greater Vitality," says, "Vitality thrives on challenge, provided there is hope."[10]

One does not have to climb mountains as Justice Douglas does, for challenge can be found anywhere. In our own small community, we have Pat Curran, a man who retired from the Mobil Oil Company after forty years and came to live here. First he winterized his summer cottage and when that challenge was completed, he became active with the Golden Age Club of Milton,

New Jersey. In a short time he galvanized all of its members into volunteering for every conceivable kind of civic, church, and charitable activity. He has organized trips and recreation that keeps those golden-agers hopping physically and mentally.

"We took a bus ride to the Amish country," Mr. Curran told Mrs. Brod, "and that made a twelve-hour day that would be taxing for someone in their thirties. Our people are in their late sixties, seventies, and eighties. The average seventy or eighty year old sits in a rocking chair, dozing off, growing older every minute. Not this group. It is the zest for life, the desire for life, and the drive that count. We have sick people, too, but they get out with the others and forget their aches and pains. When one of our ladies fell getting on a bus and cut her leg, the accident showed us that we had to learn something about first aid and carry a first-aid kit with us—so we all took the course.

"One of the things I try to do with these people is to instill a lot of confidence and self-respect and dignity into their lives," Mr. Curran went on. "As a general rule the older you get the more you are shunted aside."

There is a full-scale revolt against this shunting aside by society brewing in the country today. Groups like the AARP (the American Association of Retired Persons) and the Grey Panthers are mobilizing to change the compulsory retirement laws and bring about other reforms that will enable healthy, vital people to continue to function in the mainstream of society.

Dr. Wendell M. Swenson of Mayo Clinic and the Mayo Foundation comments on the confusion that exists today within the science of psychology concerning the gerontic abilities of humans. "It was not long ago that psychology courses taught that man's intellectual capacity achieved a peak at about the age eighteen to twenty years and that, after this, his mental powers tended to decline or deteriorate first in small degree, but later rather considerably and rapidly. But recent studies, particularly those serial evaluations of intellectual capacity during advancing age carried out at the University of California, have shown that this view is not particularly true. The data are significant in that studies of a large number of persons from college age until the age of fifty to fifty-five years, with the same tests, demonstrated virtually no changes in intellectual capacity."[11]

There is no reason why people should retire at fifty-five or sixty years of age if they are healthy and wish to continue in active employment.

However, until that day of change comes, it is important "not to retire," but to change activities—even if they are nonpaid, voluntary ones.

Finally, follow the advice of Cayce, who in answer to the question, "How can I best prepare for old age?" replied thusly:

By preparing for the present. Let age only ripen thee. For one is ever just as young as the heart and the purpose. Keep sweet. Keep friendly. Keep loving, if ye would keep young. (3420-1)

Grow old along with me!
The best is yet to be
The last of life for which the
first was made
Our times are in his hand.
—Robert Browning

DR. HAROLD J. REILLY was founder–director of the Reilly Health Institute in Rockefeller Center. For many years he worked personally with Edgar Cayce, applying treatments recommended in Cayce's psychic readings. More than 3,000 physicians have referred patients to him or his institute for treatment.

RUTH HAGY BROD is a syndicated columnist, foreign correspondent, and author of a number of books, including *Ena Twigg: Medium*.

Notes

Chapter 1

[1]Max Bircher–Benner, M.D., *The Prevention of Incurable Disease* (Greenwood, S.C.: Attic Press, 1969), p. x.
[2]*Ibid.*

Chapter 3

[1]Hans Selye, M.D., "How to Avoid Harmful Stress," *Today's Health* (July 1970).
[2]Roger J. Williams, *Nutrition Against Disease* (New York: Bantam Books, 1973), p. 32.
[3]Bircher–Benner, *The Prevention of Incurable Disease*, p. 23.
[4]*Ibid.*, p. 25.
[5]See Ted Burke, "Recipes for Rejuvenation," *Harper's Bazaar* (March 1973), p. 154.
[6]Atomidine (atomic iodine) is a molecular iodine mentioned in earlier chapters. See the source of supply at the back of this book.
[7]*Medical Research Bulletin*, vol. II, no. 9 (May 1972).

Chapter 5

[1]Jess Stearn, *Edgar Cayce–The Sleeping Prophet*, p. 103.
[2]Roger J. Williams, *Nutrition Against Disease* (New York: Pitman, 1971), p. 49.
[3]*Ibid.*, p. 123.
[4]*Ibid.*, p. 45.
[5]Patapar paper is a vegetable–based parchment used for cooking, which should be available at cooking supply stores. Also see the source of supply at the back of this book.
[6]Cathryn Elwood, *Feel Like a Million* (New York: Pocket Books, 1965). [NOTE: This book is out of print, but sprouts can be researched on the Internet, in books, or at local health food stores.]
[7]*Ibid.*, p. 289.
[8]Anne Read and Carol Ilstrup, *A Diet/Recipe Guide* (Virginia Beach, Va.: A.R.E. Press, 1967).

Chapter 6

[1]Dr. Roger J. Williams, *Nutrition Against Disease*, p. 101.
[2]Dr. Kraus was the physician–in–charge of the Therapeutic Exercise Institute of Rehabilitation and Physical Medicine at New York University–Bellevue Medical Center, and former chief of the Clinic, Physical Therapy, Columbia Presbyterian Hospital.
[3]Carlson Wade, *Magic Minerals: A Key to Better Health* (West Nyack, N.Y.: Parker Publishing Co., 1967), p. 183.
[4]William FitzGibbon, "Striding: The Most Natural Exercise of All," *Reader's Digest* (January 1972), p. 152.

Chapter 7

[1]Ronald M. Deutsch, "A Key to Feminine Response in Marriage," *Reader's Digest*

(October 1968), p. 114.
[2]*Ibid.*, p. 115.

Chapter 9

[1]Douglas Graham, *A Treatise on Massage* (St. Louis, Mo.: J.H Chambers & Co., 1890), p. 40.

Chapter 10

[1]Frederick M. Rossiter, *Water for Health and Healing* (Riverside, Calif.: H.C. White Publications, 1972), p. 34.

Chapter 11

[1]McGarey, *Edgar Cayce and the Palma Christi*, vol. 2, no. 7. (Also see *The Oil That Heals*, by Dr. McGarey.)
[2]*Ibid.*, no. 10.

Chapter 12

[1]Grace Lichtenstein, "A Nation of Fat Heads," *Esquire* (August 1973), p. 94.
[2]Neil Solomon and Sally Sheppard, *The Truth About Weight Control: How to Lose Excess Pounds Permanently* (New York: Stein & Day, 1972).
[3]Corinne H. Robinson, *Normal and Therapeutic Nutrition*, 14th ed. (New York: Macmillan Publishing Company, 1972), p. 421.
[4]Jean Mayer, "Correlation Between Metabolism and Feeding Behavior and Multiple Etiology of Obesity." *Bulletin of the New York Academy of Medicine* 33 (November 1957), p. 744.
[5]Robinson, *op. cit.*, p. 420.
[6]Williams, *Nutrition Against Disease*, pp. 100–102.
[7]Jean Mayer, "So You Think You Are Exercising Enough," *Family Health* (July 1973), pp. 34–35.
[8]E.M. Abrahamson and A.W. Pezet, *Body, Mind, and Sugar* (New York: Pyramid Books, 1951).

Chapter 13

[1]Maurice Zolotow, *Marilyn Monroe: A Biography* (New York: Harcourt, Brace & Co., 1960).
[2]Marjorie Craig, *Miss Craig's Face-Saving Exercises* (New York: Random Rouse, 1970).

Chapter 15

[1]Frank Glenn and Arthur Okinaka, "Surgical Problems and Pulmonary Function in the Geriatric Patient. Including Observation on a Man Purported to Be 167 Years Old," *Journal of the American Geriatic Society*, vol. xii, no. 7 (July 1964), p. 632.
[2]Renee Taylor, *Hunza Health Secrets* (New York: Award Books, 1969), p. ix.
[3]Josef P. Hrachovec, *Keeping Young and Living Longer* (Los Angeles: Sherbourne Press, 1972), p. 4.
[4]Williams, *Nutrition Against Disease*, pp. 140–141.

[5]Reported in *Newsweek*, April 16, 1973.

[6]Williams, *op. cit.*, pp. 141–142.

[7]Alex Comfort, *The Joy of Sex* (New York: Crown, 1972).

[8]Williams, *op. cit.*, p. 144.

[9]Hrachovec, *op. cit.*, p. 129.

[10]William O. Douglas, "Towards Greater Vitality," *Modern Maturity* (May 1973), p. 54.

[11]Wendell M. Swenson, "The Many Faces of Aging," *Geriatrics* (October 1962), p. 661.

Bibliography

Abrahamson, E.M., and Pezet, A.W. *Body, Mind, and Sugar.* New York: Pyramid Books, 1951.

Atkins, Robert C. *Dr. Atkins' Diet Revolution: The High Calorie Way to Stay Thin Forever.* New York: David Mckay Co., 1972.

Baker, M.E. Penny. *Meditation: A Step Beyond with Edgar Cayce.* Garden City, N.Y.: Doubleday, 1973.

Bircher–Benner, Max, M.D. *The Prevention of Incurable Disease.* Greenwood, S.C.: Attic Press, 1969.

Bolton, Brett. *An Edgar Cayce Encyclopedia of Foods for Health and Healing.* Virginia Beach, Va.: A.R.E. Press, 1998.

Burke, Ted. "Recipes for Rejuvenation," *Harper's Bazaar* (March 1973).

Carter, Mary Ellen. *My Years with Edgar Cayce: The Personal Story of Gladys Davis Turner.* New York: Harper & Row, 1972.

Comfort, Alex. *The Joy of Sex.* New York: Crown, 1972.

Craig, Marjorie. *Miss Craig's Face-Saving Exercises.* New York: Random Rouse, 1970.

Davis, Gladys Turner. *An Edgar Cayce Home Medicine Guide.* Virginia Beach, Va.: A.R.E. Press, 1983.

Deutsch, Donald M. "A Key to Feminine Response in Marriage," *Reader's Digest* (October 1968).

Douglas, William O. "Towards Greater Vitality," *Modern Maturity* (May 1973).

Editors of A.R.E. Press. *Edgar Cayce's Diet and Recipe Guide.* Virginia Beach, Va.: A.R.E. Press, 1991.

Elwood, Cathryn. *Feel Like a Million.* New York: Pocket Books, 1965.

FitzGibbon, William. "Striding: The Most Natural Exercise of All," *Reader's Digest* (January 1972).

Gabbay, Simone. *Nourishing the Body Temple: Edgar Cayce's Approach to Nutrition.* Virginia Beach, Va.: A.R.E. Press, 1999.

_____. *Visionary Medicine.* Virginia Beach, Va.: A.R.E. Press, 2003.

Gammon, Margaret. *The Normal Diet.* Virginia Beach, Va.: A.R.E. Press, 1957.

Glenn, Frank, and Okinaka, Arthur. "Surgical Problems and Pulmonary Function in the Geriatric Patient. Including Observation on a Man Purported to Be 167 Years Old," *Journal of the American Geriatric Society,* Vol. xii, No. 7 (July 1964).

Graham, Douglas. *A Treatise on Massage.* St. Louis, Mo.: J.H Chambers & Co., 1890.

Hrachovec, Josef P. *Keeping Young and Living Longer.* Los Angeles: Sherbourne Press, 1972

Jarvis, D.C., M.D. *Folk Medicine.* New York: Crest, Fawcett World, 1969.

Kahn, David, and Oursler, Will. *My Life with Edgar Cayce.* Garden City, N.Y.: Doubleday & Co., 1970.

Karp, Reba Ann. *Edgar Cayce Encyclopedia of Healing*. New York: Warner Books, 1999.

Kirkpatrick, Sydney. *Edgar Cayce: An American Prophet*. New York: Riverhead Books, 2001.

Lichtenstein, Grace. "A Nation of Fat Heads," *Esquire* (August 1973).

Mayer, Jean. "Correlation Between Metabolism and Feeding Behavior and Multiple Etiology of Obesity." *Bulletin of the New York Academy of Medicine* 33 (November 1957).

_____. "So You Think You Are Exercising Enough," *Family Health* (July 1973).

McGarey, William A., M.D. *Edgar Cayce and the Palma Christi*. Virginia Beach, Va.: A.R.E. Press, 1990.

_____. *Edgar Cayce on Healing Foods for Body, Mind, and Soul*. (rev. ed.) Virginia Beach, Va.: A.R.E. Press, 2002.

_____. *The Oil That Heals: A Physician's Successes with Castor Oil Treatments*. Virginia Beach, Va.: A.R.E. Press, 1999.

_____. *Physician's Reference Notebook*. Virginia Beach, Va.: A.R.E. Press, 1991.

_____*The Edgar Cayce Remedies*. New York: Bantam Books, 1983.

Read, Anne, and Ilstrup, Carol. *A Diet/Recipe Guide*. Virginia Beach, Va.: Edgar Cayce Foundation and A.R.E. Press, 1967.

Read, Anne; Ilstrup, Carol; and Gammon, Margaret. *Edgar Cayce on Diet and Health*. Edited by Hugh Lynn Cayce. New York: Warner Books, 1969.

Reilly, Harold J. *Easy Does It*. New York: Thomas Nelson & Sons, 1957.

_____. *The Secret of Better Health*. New York: Carlyle House, 1941.

Robinson, Corinne H. *Normal and Therapeutic Nutrition*. 14th edition. New York: Macmillan Publishing Company, 1972.

Rossiter, Frederick M. *Water for Health and Healing*. Riverside, Calif.: H.C. White Publications, 1972.

Rowe, James N. *Five Years to Freedom*. Boston: Little Brown & Co., 1971.

Schindler, John A. *How to Live 365 Days a Year*. New York: Prentice Hall, 1954.

Selye, Hans, M.D. "How to Avoid Harmful Stress," *Today's Health* (July 1970).

_____. *The Stress of Life*. New York: McGraw Hill, 1956.

Smith, A. Robert. *Hugh Lynn Cayce: About My Father's Business*. Norfolk, Va.: The Donning Company, 1988.

_____. *The Lost Memoirs of Edgar Cayce: My Life as a Seer*. New York: St. Martin's Press, 1999.

Solomon, Neil, and Sheppard, Sally. *The Truth About Weight Control: How to Lose Excess Pounds Permanently*. New York: Stein & Day, 1972.

Stearn, Jess. *Adventures into the Psychic*. New York: Coward, McCann & Geoghegan, 1969.

_____. *Edgar Cayce—The Sleeping Prophet*. Virginia Beach, Va.: A.R.E. Press, 1997.

_____. *A Prophet in His Own Country*. New York: Bantam, 1989.

Stillman, Irwin, and Baker, Sam. *The Doctor's Quick Weight Loss Diet*. Englewood Cliffs, N.J.: Prentice–Hall, 1967.

Sugrue, Thomas. *Stranger in the Earth*. New York: Holt, Rinehart & Winston, 1948.

_____. *Starling of the White House*. New York: Simon and Schuster, 1942.

_____. *There Is a River*. Virginia Beach, Va.: A.R.E. Press, 1997.

_____. *Watch for the Morning*. New York: Harper and Brothers, 1950.

Swenson, Wendell M., "The Many Faces of Aging," *Geriatrics* (October 1962).

Taylor, Renee. *Hunza Health Secrets*. New York: Award Books, 1969.

Van Auken, John. *Edgar Cayce on Rejuvenation of the Body*. Virginia Beach, Va.: A.R.E. Press, 1999.

Wade, Carlson. *Magic Minerals: A Key to Better Health*. West Nyack, N.Y: Parker Publishing Co., 1967.

Williams, Roger J. *Biochemical Individuality: The Basis for the Genetotrophic Concept*. Austin: University of Texas Press, 1969.

_____. *Nutrition Against Disease*. New York: Pitman Publishing Company, 1971.

_____. *You Are Extraordinary*. New York: Pyramid, 1971.

Zolotow, Maurice. *Marilyn Monroe: A Biography*. New York: Harcourt, Brace & Co., 1960.

Index

Carter, Mary Ellen, 16
Case work, 39–57
Castor oil massage, 181–182
Castor oil packs, 18, 29, 39, 222, 226–231
    directions for, 237–238
    eye problems and, 231, 290
Cat crawl, 106–107
Cataract, 102
Cayce, Edgar
    biographical sketch, xvii–xviii
    case work with, 39
    philosophy of healing, 23–37
    Reilly on working with, 9–22
Cayce, Gertrude (Mrs. Edgar), 10, 16, 18, 19
Cayce, Hugh Lynn (son), 16, 17, 18–20, 34, 44
Celery, 71, 76
Cells, 311, 312, 314
    fat, 252, 253
Cerebral palsy, 162
Charcot–Marie–Tooth disease, 152
Chibcha Indians, 307
Chin-writing, 280
Choate, Robert, 65
Cholesterol, 68, 255
Cholecystitis, 227
Christakis, Dr. George, 65
Cigarettes. See Smoking
Circulation, 30–31, 140, 141
Citrus fruit juices, 66, 76
Cleansing, internal, 217–244, 281
Coffee, 75, 81, 100, 261, 263
Coffee grounds, use in foot bath, 214
Cold-water packs, 215
Colds, 23, 74
    common, cure for, 241
    prevention of, 241
Colonics, 29, 39, 102, 202, 217, 218
    See also Internal Cleansing
Comfort, Dr. Alex, 310, 316
Complexion guide, 281–286
Constipation. See Elimination
Constipation, massage mixture for, 184
Cooking methods, 82–83
Corn, 71
Corns, 295, 299
Coronary-artery disease, 32
Cough remedies, 243–244
Coulter, Dr. George N., 56
Craig, Marjorie, 278
Curran, Pat, 320–321
Cysts, 298–299

D

Dandruff, 288
Davis, Gladys. See Turner, Gladys Davis
De Laney, Mrs. William, 16
Deodorants, 284
Dermatitis, baths and, 214
DeVries, Blanche, 110
DeVries, Dr. Herbert A., 318
Diabetes, 2, 68, 78, 248, 250
Diet, 26–27, 247–266
    apple, 18, 62, 217, 221, 259, 261
        directions for, 235–236
    banana, 62

basic, 88–92
Cayce principles of, 61–94
grape, 62, 222, 231–232, 260, 263
importance of, 269
skin problems and, 282
Dietary reference intakes (RDIs) (chart), 93–94
Dieter's food choices, 262
DMS0, 316
Dorenmuehle, Dr. Robert H., 311
Douglas, William O., 320
Drinking water, 204
Drugs, reducing and, 248–249
Dry skin
    on feet, 296
    treatment for, 283
Dubinsky, David, 205–220, 319
Duerker machines, 223

E

Elimination, 27–30, 311–312
Emotions, effect of on health, 23–26, 27
Emphysema 102, 250
"Empty-calorie" foods, 65–66
Enemas, 223, 225–226, 236–237
Exercise
    appestat mechanisms and, 255
    assimilation of food and, 27
    general instructions concerning, 115
    importance of, 95–111, 318
    overcoming reluctance to, 111
    posture and, 140–150
    preparation for, 113–115
    preparation for sports through, 138–139
    rolling, 106–107
Exercises, specific, 103–150
    abdominal, 126–129, 132, 276
    ankle, 133–134, 154, 277–278
    arm, 121, 124, 276
    back, 133, 275
        lower, 146–147
        upper, 124
    breathing, 105–106
    bust, 121, 273–274
    buttocks, 136, 278
    developmental, 271–278
    eye, 107, 120–121
    face, 278–280
    foot, 109, 133–136, 275
    head-and-neck, 102, 106, 107–108, 278
    head-to-toe, 120–121
    hemorrhoid, 45, 102, 108
    hip, 130, 136, 276
    horizontal, 105, 108, 126
    isometric, 103
    leg, 130–133
    shoulder, 121, 124
    spine, 275
    spot reducing and, 271–278
    thigh, 277
    towel, 114, 115
    vertical, 105, 115, 121
    yoga, 110
Exercising machines, 249
Expectorants, 243–244
Eyelids, granulated, treatment for, 289

A.R.E. Press

The A.R.E. Press publishes books, videos, and audiotapes meant to improve the quality of our readers' lives—personally, professionally, and spiritually. We hope our products support your endeavors to realize your career potential, to enhance your relationships, to improve your health, and to encourage you to make the changes necessary to live a loving, joyful, and fulfilling life.

For more information or to receive a free catalog, call:

1–800–723–1112

Or write:

A.R.E. Press
215 67th Street
Virginia Beach, VA 23451–2061

Baar Products

A.R.E.'s Official Worldwide Exclusive Supplier of Edgar Cayce Health Care Products

Baar Products, Inc., is the official worldwide exclusive supplier of Edgar Cayce health care products. Baar offers a collection of natural products and remedies drawn from the work of Edgar Cayce, considered by many to be the father of modern holistic medicine.

For a complete listing of Cayce-related products, call:

1–800–269–2502

Or write:

Baar Products, Inc.
P.O. Box 60
Downingtown, PA 19335 U.S.A.

Customer Service and International: 610–873–4591
Fax: 610–873–7945
Web Site: www.baar.com   E-mail: cayce@baar.com

DISCOVER HOW THE EDGAR CAYCE MATERIAL CAN HELP YOU!

The Association for Research and Enlightenment, Inc. (A.R.E.®), was founded in 1931 by Edgar Cayce. Its international headquarters are in Virginia Beach, Virginia, where thousands of visitors come year-round. Many more are helped and inspired by A.R.E.'s local activities in their own hometowns or by contact via mail (and now the Internet!) with A.R.E. headquarters.

People from all walks of life, all around the world, have discovered meaningful and life-transforming insights in the A.R.E. programs and materials, which focus on such areas as personal spirituality, holistic health, dreams, family life, finding your best vocation, reincarnation, ESP, meditation, and soul growth in small-group settings. Call us today at our toll-free number:

1–800–333–4499

or

Explore our electronic visitors center on the
Internet: **http://www.edgarcayce.org.**

We'll be happy to tell you more about how the work of the A.R.E. can help you!

A.R.E.
215 67th Street
Virginia Beach, VA 23451-2061